Series Editors:
David R. Beukelman
Joe Reichle

Practically Speaking

Also in the Augmentative and
Alternative Communication Series:

Supporting Communication for Adults with Acute and Chronic Aphasia
edited by Nina Simmons-Mackie, Ph.D., BC-ANCDS,
Julia M. King, Ph.D.,
and David R. Beukelman, Ph.D.

Transition Strategies for Adolescents and Young Adults Who Use AAC
edited by David B. McNaughton, Ph.D,
and David R. Beukelman, Ph.D.

Autism Spectrum Disorders and AAC
edited by Pat Mirenda, Ph.D.,
and Teresa Iacono, Ph.D.

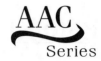

Practically Speaking

Language, Literacy, and Academic Development for Students with AAC Needs

edited by

Gloria Soto, Ph.D.
San Francisco State University
San Francisco

and

Carole Zangari, Ph.D., CCC-SLP
Nova Southeastern University
Ft. Lauderdale, Florida

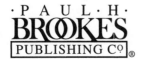

Baltimore • London • Sydney

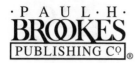

Paul H. Brookes Publishing Co.
Post Office Box 10624
Baltimore, Maryland 21285-0624
USA
www.brookespublishing.com

"Paul H. Brookes Publishing Co." is a registered trademark of
Paul H. Brookes Publishing Co., Inc.

Typeset by Spearhead Global, Inc., Bear, Delaware.
Manufactured in the United States of America by
Sheridan Books, Inc., Chelsea, Michigan.

The individuals described in this book are composites or real people whose situations are masked and are
based on the authors' experiences. In most instances, names and identifying details have been changed to
protect confidentiality. Real names and identifying details are used with permission.

Library of Congress Cataloging-in-Publication Data

Practically speaking: language: literacy, and academic development for students with AAC needs/edited by
  Gloria Soto and Carole Zangari.—1st ed.
      p.   cm.—(Augmentative and alternative communication series)
  Includes bibliographical references and index.
  ISBN-13: 978-1-55766-951-3 (pbk.)
  ISBN-10: 1-55766-951-1 (pbk.)
  1. Children with disabilities—Education—Textbooks. 2. Language arts—Remedial teaching—Textbooks.
  3. Communicative disorders in children—Treatment—Textbooks. I. Soto, Gloria. II. Zangari, Carole.
  III. Title. IV. Series.

LC4028.P73 2009
371.9'0446—dc22   2008049533

British Library Cataloguing in Publication data are available from the British Library.

2025   2024   2023   2022   2021

10   9   8   7   6   5

Contents

III   Supports

Series Preface

The purpose of the Augmentative and Alternative Communication Series is to address advances in the field as they relate to issues experienced across the life span. Each volume is research-based and practical, providing up-to-date and ground-breaking information on recent social, medical, and technical developments. Each chapter is designed to be a detailed account of a specific issue. To help ensure a diverse examination of augmentative and alternative communication (AAC) issues, an editorial advisory board assists in selecting topics, volume editors, and authors. Prominent scholars, representing a range of perspectives, serve on the editorial board so that the most poignant advances in the study of AAC are sure to be explored.

In the broadest sense, the concept of AAC is quite old. Gestural communication and other types of body language have been widely addressed in the literature about communication for hundreds of years. Only recently, though, has the field of AAC emerged as an academic discipline that incorporates graphic, auditory, and gestural modes of communicating. The series concentrates on achieving specific goals. Each volume details the empirical methods used to design AAC systems for both descriptive groups and for individuals. By tracking the advances in methods, current research, practice, and theory, we will also develop a broad and evolutionary definition of this new discipline.

Many reasons for establishing this series exist, but foremost has been the number and diversity of the people who are affected by AAC issues. AAC consumers and their families, speech-language pathologists, occupational therapists, physical therapists, early childhood educators, general and special educators, school psychologists, neurologists, and professionals in rehabilitative medicine and engineering all benefit from research and advancements in the field. Likewise AAC needs are not delineated by specific age parameters; people of all ages who have developmental and acquired disabilities rely on AAC. Appropriate interventions for individuals across a wide range of disabilities and levels of severity must be considered.

Fundamentally, the field of AAC is problem driven. We, the members of the editorial advisory board, and all professionals in the field are dedicated to solving problems in order to improve the lives of people with disabilities. The inability to communicate effectively is devastating. As we chronicle the advances in the field of AAC, we hope to systematically dismantle the barriers that prevent effective communication for all individuals.

Series Editors

Editorial Advisory Board

Volume Preface

The purpose of this book is to provide information to professionals and preprofessional students who serve children with significant communication challenges in school settings. It is the result of many years of combined teaching, research, and delivery of augmentative and alternative communication (AAC) services to students with a variety of abilities, characteristics, and interests. The topics covered in the book reflect our own need for a resource book that includes the necessary information for current and future members of teams serving students with AAC needs in school settings. In some ways, it grew out of frustration at the many obstacles that students with AAC needs and their educational teams face on a daily basis. We believe that a great many of these barriers can be minimized with clear, accurate information about how to facilitate language, academic, and social growth in children who require AAC.

The book focuses on achievement in core language and literacy competencies required for academic and social contexts. It addresses the challenges faced by practitioners, targeting both AAC competence and curricular content. It includes guidelines, strategies, and tools necessary to address student needs, demands of the curriculum, the nature of social contexts, and required technology supports within a complex school environment. Readers will be able to do the following:

1. Use the general education curriculum as a context for goal setting

2. Understand and address the language and communication demands of the curriculum

3. Develop and implement a plan for ongoing, comprehensive language assessment that supports the curriculum

4. Identify benchmarks for alternative assessment and utilize them to develop goals and intervention programs

5. Develop appropriate language, communication, and literacy goals

6. Develop a plan for the management of AAC technology

7. Facilitate teams that function to support student achievement

8. Use strategies for supporting students' ability to develop and maintain meaningful social relationships

9. Modify classroom activities to ensure student participation and achievement

10. Formulate strategies for measuring progress and assigning grades

11. Build a supportive classroom community

The material in the book is written for current and future professionals, primarily educators and speech-language pathologists, challenged with supporting students who require AAC and maximizing their achievement relative to the academic curriculum and social demands of school settings. We anticipate that individuals seeking advanced-level information on assistive technology and the education of students with disabilities will also find value in it as well.

The book was authored by clinicians, teachers, and researchers, many of whom work in the "trenches" providing communication supports in educational settings for children with AAC needs. Their information is both relevant and timely for those working in the dynamic atmosphere of educational settings who wish to better serve students with significant communication difficulties. As

Eric Hoffer observed, "In times of change learners inherit the earth; while the learned find themselves beautifully equipped to deal with a world that no longer exists" (as quoted in Jordan & Follman, 1993).

This book is organized into three sections: assessment, instruction and intervention, and supports. In the first section, Ahlgrim-Delzell (Chapter 1) sets the foundation by exploring some of the key issues that guide educational assessment for students with AAC needs, including legislative mandates and other practice realities. The assessment section continues with the chapter by Downing (Chapter 2), who provides essential information about how the skills of beginning communicators should be assessed. The chapter that follows, by Proctor and Zangari (Chapter 3), looks at assessing specific receptive and expressive language skills in students who use AAC. Foley, Koppenhaver, and Williams collaborated on two separate chapters on literacy assessment, looking at the principles and practices relating to the evaluation of reading (Chapter 4) and writing skills (Chapter 5).

The chapters in Section II, Instruction and Intervention, review key concepts, issues, and strategies for instruction and intervention with students who use AAC. Soto (Chapter 6) takes on the task of relating current thinking on academic adaptations to the specific case of students who use AAC. Kent-Walsh and Binger (Chapter 7) deal with intervention for students who use AAC and are at the early stages of communicative and language development. Zangari and Van Tatenhove (Chapter 8) focus on maximizing the language learning and proficiency of students with more advanced language skills. Erickson and Clendon (Chapter 9) articulate issues and strategies for students at the earlier stages of literacy skill development. More conventional reading and writing skills, and their relationship to the curriculum, are addressed by Light and McNaughton (Chapter 10). An elegant chapter by Hunt, Doering, Maier, and Mintz (Chapter 11) provides important information for communication partners seeking to facilitate social interaction and friendships in students who require AAC. The complex issues involved in integrating AAC with other assistive technology and with the curriculum are tackled by Gillette (Chapter 12).

Section III of this book covers topics important to the support of students who use AAC and their educational teams. Robinson and Solomon-Rice (Chapter 13) describe issues and strategies for effective teamwork and collaboration. Wilkinson and Hennig (Chapter 14) look specifically at aided communication in students who use AAC and address issues of cognition, memory, and attention.

This book was conceptualized and written with certain underlying assumptions. Students with AAC needs are educated in a wide variety of educational situations. Their experiences differ within and across grade levels, educational models, and curricula. In many places throughout the book, we struggled with balancing the "real" and the ideal, recognizing that the principles and practices described here are not uniformly valued or implemented across school districts. Among the most important assumptions reflected in this book is that professionals must be committed to providing access to the general curriculum for all students, regardless of their needs and abilities. The challenge of how to make that happen in a meaningful way is one which, we predict, will be a source discussion for many years to come. We greatly appreciate the opportunity to contribute to that important conversation.

REFERENCE

Jordan, W.R., & Follman, J.M. (Eds.). (1993). Using technology to improve teaching and learning. *Hot Topics: Usable Research* (p. 1). Palatka, FL: NEFEC/SERVE, Regional Vision for Education. (ERIC Document Reproduction Service No. ED355930)

About the Editors

Gloria Soto, Ph.D., Professor, Department of Special Education and Communication Disorders, San Francisco State University, Burk Hall, 1600 Holloway Avenue, San Francisco, CA 94132

Dr. Soto is a full professor in the Department of Special Education and Communication Disorders at San Francisco State University. She has extensive experience serving students with AAC needs in school settings. Her research areas focus on interventions to support the academic, language, and social development of students with AAC needs in general education classrooms and other school settings.

Carole Zangari, Ph.D., CCC-SLP, Director, Tyler Institute, Nova Southeastern University, 3301 College Avenue, Ft. Lauderdale, FL 33314

Dr. Zangari is a professor of speech, language, and communication disorders in the Fischler School of Education and Human Services at Nova Southeastern University, where she directs the Tyler Institute. Dr. Zangari teaches a variety of AAC classes to master's and doctoral students and to practicing professionals in the postmaster's AAC specialization. In addition to AAC, Dr. Zangari has interests in the area of online teaching and support to families and teams serving children with significant communication difficulties.

Contributors

Lynn Ahlgrim-Delzell, Ph.D.
Assistant Professor
Department of Educational Leadership
University of North Carolina at Charlotte
9201 University City Boulevard
Charlotte, NC 29223

Cathy Binger, Ph.D., CCC-SLP
Assistant Professor
Speech and Hearing Sciences
University of New Mexico
1700 Lomas NE
MSC01 1195
Albuquerque, NM 87131

Sally A. Clendon, Ph.D.
Senior Lecturer
Speech Language Therapy Programme
School of Education at Albany
Massey University College of Education
Post Office Box 102 904
North Shore Mail Centre
Auckland, New Zealand

Kathy Doering, M.A.
Instructor
Department of Special Education
San Francisco State University
1600 Holloway Avenue
San Francisco, CA 94132

June E. Downing, Ph.D.
Professor Emeritus of Special Education
California State University, Northridge
3661 North Round Rock Drive
Tucson, AZ 85750

Karen A. Erickson, Ph.D.
Associate Professor and Director
Center for Literacy and Disability Studies
University of North Carolina at Chapel Hill
CB# 7335 TR#46 Mason Farm Road
Chapel Hill, NC 27599

Beth E. Foley, Ph.D., CCC-SLP
Department Head
Communicative Disorders and Deaf
  Education
Utah State University
1000 Old Main Hill
Logan, UT 84322

Yvonne Gillette, Ph.D.
Professor
School of Speech-Language Pathology and
  Audiology
The University of Akron
Akron, OH 44325

Shannon C. Hennig, M.S.
Speech-Language Clinician
TalkLink Wellington
Post Office Box 24 070
Wellington 6142
New Zealand

Pam Hunt, Ph.D.
Professor
Department of Special Education
San Francisco State University
1600 Holloway Avenue
San Francisco, CA 94132

**Jennifer Kent-Walsh, Ph.D., CCC-SLP,
  S-LP(C)**
Assistant Professor and FAAST Center
  Director
Department of Communication Sciences &
  Disorders
University of Central Florida
4000 Central Florida Boulevard
HPA II, Room 101X
Orlando, FL 32816

David A. Koppenhaver, Ph.D.
Associate Professor
Language, Reading, and Exceptionalities
    Department
Reich College of Education
Appalachian State University
124 Edwin Duncan Hall
Boone, NC 28608

Janice C. Light, Ph.D.
Distinguished Professor
Department of Communication Sciences and
    Disorders
The Pennsylvania State University
308 Ford Building
University Park, PA 16802

Julie Maier, M.A.
Instructor
Department of Special Education
San Francisco State University
1600 Holloway Avenue
San Francisco, CA 94132

David McNaughton, Ph.D.
Associate Professor
Graduate Program in Special Education
The Pennsylvania State University
227 CEDAR Building
University Park, PA 16802

Emily Mintz, M.A.
Doctoral Candidate
University of California, Berkeley/
    San Francisco State University
1600 Holloway Avenue
San Francisco, CA 94132

Lisa A. Proctor, Ph.D.
Professor
Communication Sciences and Disorders
Missouri State University
901 South National Avenue
Springfield, MO 65897

Nancy B. Robinson, Ph.D., CCC-SLP
Associate Professor
Department of Special Education and
    Communicative Disorders
San Francisco State University
1600 Holloway Avenue
San Francisco, CA 94132

Patti L. Solomon-Rice, M.A., CCC-SLP
Joint Doctoral Program in Special Education
University of California, Berkeley/
    San Francisco State University
1600 Holloway Avenue
San Francisco, CA 94132

Gail Van Tatenhove, M.S.
Speech-Language Clinician
Private Practice
8322 Tangelo Tree Drive
Orlando, FL 32836

Krista M. Wilkinson, Ph.D.
Professor
Communication Sciences & Disorders
404 Ford Building
The Pennsylvania State University
University Park, PA 16802
(previously Associate Professor,
    Communication Sciences & Disorders,
    Emerson College)

Amy R. Williams, M.A.
Adjunct Faculty
Language, Reading, and Exceptionalities
    Department
Appalachian State University
730 Rivers Street
Boone, NC 28608

Acknowledgments

This book would not have been possible without the collaboration of our contributing authors. For your dedication and commitment to the book, we offer our eternal gratitude. David R. Beukelman's encouragement, guidance, mentoring, and inspiration played an essential role throughout the process. It has been a true pleasure learning from you. We are grateful for the support of the editorial staff at Brookes Publishing Co., especially Astrid Zuckerman, for their vision and patience.

Particular gratitude is due to the many students, professionals, and families with whom we have worked and learned from over the years. You are too many to mention, but you are not forgotten. We are mindful of the words of John Colton Dana when he said "Who dares to teach must never cease to learn" and are so very appreciative of the opportunities to learn from and with you.

To our husbands and children, who have provided us with the encouragement and support throughout this professional endeavor, nothing we do would have meaning without you in our lives.

I

Assessment

1

Educational Assessment Issues

Lynn Ahlgrim-Delzell

_____ Sammi is a first-grade student with a severe intellectual disability. She has cerebral palsy and uses a wheelchair. Her instruction includes functional skills of eating, communicating basic wants and needs, toileting, and following a daily routine. Sammi is nonverbal and is being taught to use pictures to communicate; however, she relies mostly on gestures.

Lyndsey is a fifth-grade student with autism and a moderate intellectual disability. She is nonverbal, can identify about 50 pictures and a few common words, and has a repertoire of about five signs, such as EAT and DRINK. Her instruction includes below grade-level academic skills, such as identifying numbers and letters, and functional skills. She is included in general education physical education, art, media, and music classes.

Camden is a seventh-grade student with autism. He is nonverbal and uses an AAC device, which has an extensive word vocabulary, to communicate. He can navigate through thousands of words and symbols on his AAC device to communicate throughout the day independently. As best as his teachers can tell, he performs slightly below grade level. His general education teachers struggle to provide him with the opportunity to participate in class activities and demonstrate his knowledge because of the AAC device.

Zack is a 10th-grade student who was diagnosed with a mild intellectual disability. He is working toward an alternate diploma offered by his school district, is learning job-related skills such as completing job applications, and is exploring different types of employment. His speech is difficult to understand, so he often uses pictures, word cards, and gestures to supplement his verbal communication. _____

EDUCATIONAL ACCOUNTABILITY

Educational accountability for students who use augmentative and alternative communication (AAC) devices requires some unique considerations. This chapter provides background and suggestions for educators who work with such students. Examples illustrate how these suggestions might look for a diverse group of students.

Legal Tenets of Educational Accountability

Since the late 1980s there has been a period of great educational reform for all students in the United States.[1] Initial reform created higher standards to improve outcomes of students in general education curricula. Recent reform has specifically included all students, with and without disabilities. The

[1]Although this chapter on educational assessment issues is grounded by legal mandates in the United States, the ideas presented can be applied to any educational system that supports students who require the assistance of AAC systems. The _International Classification of Functioning, Disability, and Health_ (ICF) published by the World Health Organization (2001) defined the relationship of factors that contribute to a disability. Two of these factors, environment and participation, are applicable to this discussion of educational issues. The _environment_ component includes the use of products and technology such as AAC systems. The _participation_ component includes having access to resources and being engaged in life experiences. The discussions and ideas presented in this chapter regarding participation in accountability systems, assessment issues including validity of accommodated tests, linking instruction and assessment, Universal Design for Learning, test preparation, grading, and organization relate to the internal issues and are applicable to students who require AAC support wherever they may reside.

reform movement was spawned by a report from the National Commission on Education (1983). This report publicized the poor performance of America's students as a threat to our ability to compete in the global society. It also led to a national agenda to create rigorous educational goals and to measure progress of youth against these goals—the Goals 2000: Educate America Act of 1994 (PL 103-227). This legislation defined national education standards and encouraged states to create their own standards based on the national ones. Professional organizations such as the National Council of Teachers of Mathematics (NCTM; 2000), National Council of Teachers of English (NCTE) and International Reading Association (IRA) (1996), and National Research Council (NRC; 1996) generated standards for the teaching of mathematics, English, and science. Subsequently, states have generated standards based on the standards outlined by Goals 2000 and the professional organizations.

The initial legislation on educating students with disabilities was the Education for All Handicapped Children Act of 1975 (PL 94-142), which was reauthorized in 1997 under the Individuals with Disabilities Education Act Amendments (IDEA 1997; PL 105-17) and again in 2004 as the Individuals with Disabilities Education Improvement Act (IDEA 2004; PL 108-446). The 1975 legislation created requirements such as free appropriate public education (FAPE), least restrictive environment (LRE), and the individualized education program (IEP). The 1997 legislation first mentioned access to the general curriculum and inclusion of students with disabilities in large-scale state and district assessments with the use of alternate assessments. It mandated that IEPs address participation and progress of students in the general curriculum. States were required to utilize alternate assessments to include students with disabilities in their accountability systems beginning July 1, 2000.

Provision of communication supports for students fall under two federal laws—IDEA 2004 and Section 504 of the Rehabilitation Act of 1973 (PL 93-112). IDEA provides special education for students with specific disabilities. Assistive technology (AT) devices and services can be provided to students with these disabilities under IDEA. An AT device is defined in IDEA as "any item, piece of equipment, or product system, whether acquired commercially off the shelf, modified, or customized, that is used to increase, maintain, or improve functional capabilities of a child with a disability" (§ 602[1][A]). Considering AT for communication purposes is part of the development of the IEP. IDEA specifically mentions that the IEP team should consider whether a child requires AT devices and/or services when developing the IEP. The need for such devices and/or services falls under the section of the IEP designated for consideration of special factors. Section 504 provides a much broader definition of disability than IDEA. Therefore, students who do not qualify for special education services under IDEA may be able to receive accommodations and modifications under Section 504 of the Rehabilitation Act of 1973. This act provides accommodations and modifications to avoid discrimination based on the presence of a disability. For all disabilities eligible for services under IDEA, there must be a significant effect on educational performance. A student with a speech-language limitation may be eligible for special education services under IDEA if the impairment significantly affects his or her educational performance. If the speech-language impairment is augmented with a communication device that allows the student to perform at or near grade level, then the student would not be eligible for special education under IDEA but could receive accommodations and/or modifications under Section 504.

Access to the general curriculum and inclusion of students with disabilities in accountability policies was further strengthened by the No Child Left Behind (NCLB) Act of 2001 (PL 107-110), which was a reauthorization of the Elementary and Secondary Education Act of 1965 (PL 89-10). This act required states to establish rigorous academic content standards and academic achievement standards; develop and implement assessments to monitor progress toward these standards; and hold schools, school systems, and states accountable for the progress toward these standards for all students. In the 2007–2008 school year, states were required to assess students in reading/language arts and mathematics in 3rd through 8th grades and at least once in 10th through 12th grades. Science assessments were conducted at least once in 1st through 5th grades, once in 6th through 9th grades, and once in 10th through 12th grades (U.S. Department of Education, 2005). States develop their own assessments based on their established academic content standards. This accountability system is called *adequate yearly progress* (AYP). AYP measures the yearly academic progress of all students and examines the progress of specific subgroups of students based on 1) disability, 2) gender, 3) ethnicity, 4) economical disadvantage, and 5) English proficiency. States are required to include a minimum of 95% of their student population in their state accountability score reporting. Subsequent regulations to help states implement NCLB have allowed states to develop alternate achievement standards for students with the most significant intellectual disabilities (defined as 1% of the general population). These alternate achievement standards must be aligned to the state general academic content standards and promote access to those standards (Title 1, 2003). Additional guidance stipulates that this connection of alternate achievement standards to the state general academic content standards must be grade-level content or prerequisite skills to gain access to the grade-level content (U.S. Department of Education, 2005).

Why Should We Include Students with Disabilities in Accountability Practices?

Students such as Sammi, Lyndsey, Camden, and Zack would have been excluded from state and district testing prior to the implementation of IDEA 2004 and NCLB (Elliot, Erickson, Thurlow, & Shriner, 2000). In many states, policies discourage the participation of students with disabilities in statewide testing (Thurlow, Ysseldyke, & Silverstein, 1995). If students were included in the testing, they often were not included in the reported results (Krentz, Thurlow, & Callender, 2000). Excluding these students from accountability systems that held students, teachers, and schools to high expectations also excluded them from the rigorous curriculum. Being a part of the accountability system and measuring their achievement provides an avenue for receipt of appropriate resources in order to foster their success, not just meet their needs.

Because students such as Sammi, Lyndsey, Camden, and Zack have not had the opportunity to learn academic skills, their potential in learning these skills is yet to be known. These students had been required to master functional life skills prior to considering academic instruction. When academic instruction did occur, it was often terminated when progress was deemed too slow. These are not requirements for typically developing students. Typically developing students who experienced toileting accidents or could not tie their shoes were not excluded from learning to read in first grade. Remediation of academic skills of students in general education classes continues throughout their academic career as long as they need it. Even if students with disabilities cannot master all of the academic skills in each grade level, the acquisition of prioritized academic skills can be beneficial and open additional opportunities because these skills have functional applications.

Consequences for Students with Disabilities Participating in Accountability Systems

High-stakes testing is another way to hold schools, school districts, and states accountable for student performance. It places significant consequences on testing results. For example, a school may replace administrators if it is classified as low performing because it does not meet its assigned performance goals. Teachers at high-performing schools may be given monetary bonuses. Students who do not pass the state-mandated high school exit examination may be denied a traditional diploma. Although NCLB holds states and school systems accountable, state policy dictates consequences for individual students. Thurlow and Johnson defined *high-stakes testing* for students with disabilities:

> Tests should be considered as high-stakes for students with disabilities when the results are used to make critical decisions about the individual's access to educational opportunity, grade-level retention or promotion, graduation from high school, or receipt of a standard diploma versus an alternative diploma (e.g., special education diploma, certificate of completion). (2000, p. 307)

The intended consequences behind high-stakes testing in general are to promote higher standards; to hold schools, teachers, and students to those standards; and to improve educational services for all students. The implications for students with disabilities are not well known. Hypothesized intended positive consequences for including students with disabilities in accountability systems and high-stakes testing include higher expectations and improved instructional effort, instruction, and student outcomes (Thurlow & Johnson, 2000; Ysseldyke et al., 2004). Thurlow (2003) added that obtaining a more accurate picture of education and identifying interventions and other variables that affect student learning could also be a benefit of including students with disabilities in high-stakes accountability systems. By using student scores as an "index of system performance," information could be used to modify curriculum, instruction, and teacher skills to improve future student performance. Inclusion of students with disabilities into existing accountability systems was seen as one way to address long-standing concern over the quality of special education services (Hanushek, Kain, & Rivkin, 1999; Moody, Vaughn, Hughes, & Fischer, 2000; Schulte, Osborne, & Erchul, 1998; Will, 1986). Such emphasis on identifying instructional interventions and other variables to improve future performance has the potential to affect students who use AAC devices as the field becomes more knowledgeable about the various devices and how they affect a student's ability to participate and respond to instruction aligned to the general curriculum.

There are also numerous hypothesized unintended negative consequences for students with disabilities in high-stakes accountability systems. Some of the proposed negative consequences include the following (e.g., Cizek, 2001; Disability Rights Advocates, 2001; Firestone & Mayrowetz, 2000; Stone & Lane, 2003):

1. Narrowing the curriculum to those subjects that are included on the tests
2. Decreasing critical thinking skills as students concentrate on the basics and participate in multiple-choice tests
3. Increasing dropout rates
4. Restricting opportunities for standard diplomas and loss of educational and career opportunities
5. Increasing grade retention
6. Increasing test anxiety
7. Decreasing expectations if students perform poorly on the tests
8. Increasing the stigma of failure and thereby reducing self-esteem

All of these consequences may be an issue for students who use AAC strategies to participate in accountability testing, particularly if the AAC device is not an allowable accommodation for taking the assessment (see Chapter 12). If a student's AAC device is not an allowable accommodation, Table 1.1 provides examples of a variety of allowable accommodations that may be acceptable substitutes. Sometimes individual school principals or districts are unfamiliar with the needs of students with disabilities and set rules or policies that negatively affect these students. For example, a school district that implements a pacing guide for all students in general curriculum classes may intend to produce better performance on state tests by making sure the entire intended curriculum is covered in all of the classes. The side effect of this act may result in poorer performance of students such as Camden who struggle to keep up by forcing the teachers to go at a faster pace with less time for the students who are low performers to grasp material before moving on the next topic. Additional discussion of this problem is addressed later in this chapter.

Unfortunately, there is very little empirical evidence examining the occurrence of any of these possible positive and negative consequences. Although it is certainly possible that any of these consequences, positive or negative, could occur for any individual student, there is no evidence to support their occurrence in any systematic fashion for students with disabilities as a whole. The lack of evidence does not mean that these consequences do not occur. Rather, this lack of evidence is due to the fact there are not any experimental studies to document the occurrence of consequences.

Table 1.1.   Examples of presentation, setting, response, and time/scheduling accommodations

Presentation	Explanation of or repeating directions, large print, magnification devices, sign language, braille, tactile graphics (i.e., raised from page), read-aloud by another person, audiotape/CD, books on tape, audio amplification, videotapes, computerized screen reader, visual cues, notes/outlines, voiced materials (e.g., clocks or calculators with auditory components), computerized adaptive tests, enhanced lighting, highlighting key words, placeholder system
Setting	Reduction of distractions, use of adaptive furniture/equipment, locations to increase physical access to special equipment or to allow use of augmentative and alternative communication (AAC) device without disturbing others, individual/small-group administration
Response	Oral, scribe, word processor, speech to text, brailler, notetakers, tape recorder, recording written responses other than opscan bubbles, monitoring alignment of written responses (recording on correct line, filling in intended bubble), eye-gaze boards, pointing to enlarged options from test booklet, calculators, spelling/grammar checking devices, visual or graphic organizers, programmed AAC device, computerized adaptive tests
Scheduling/time	Extended time, testing breaks, shorter sessions over multiple days, individual schedule of peak performance, ordering of activities, computerized adaptive tests

Source: Thompson, Morse, Sharpe, & Hall (2005).

Ysseldyke et al. (2004) conducted an exhaustive search on empirical evidence of the consequences of high-stakes testing. They found nine empirical studies that tended to be surveys, focus groups, or trends in individual states. There is a great need for additional empirical evidence before we can state if any of the positive or negative consequences have affected students with disabilities.

How Students with Disabilities Participate in State Accountability Tests

The IEP teams for Sammi, Lyndsey, Camden, and Zack determine how these students will participate in their state accountability tests. Regulatory guidance from implementation of NCLB (Title 1, 2003, 2007; U.S. Department of Education, 2005) allows states to develop up to five options for assessing students for AYP. These options include

1. Grade-level assessment based on grade-level achievement standards

2. Grade-level assessment with accommodations

3. Alternate assessment based on grade-level expectations

4. Alternate assessment based on modified grade-level achievement standards

5. Alternate assessment based on alternate achievement standards

Not all states provide all options.

Most students will take the state grade-level assessment based on grade-level achievement standards. Each state provides content standards and grade-level (or clusters of grade levels) expectations for student achievement. For example, in Colorado these standards are called Model Content Standards (Colorado Department of Education, 2008). Each standard is broken down into grade cluster benchmarks for K–4, 5–8, and 9–12. State accountability assessments measure student progress toward accomplishing these expectations. Discussion of each of the other assessment options follows.

Grade-Level Assessment with Accommodations   Some students require accommodations in order to participate in a state's accountability test. *Accommodation* is defined as "practices and procedures in the areas of presentation, response, setting, and time/scheduling that provide equitable access during instruction and assessments" (Thompson, Morse, Sharpe, & Hall, 2005, p. 14). Accommodations allow students to gain access to grade-level learning expectations without changing the content of the expectation by compensating for the effect the disability may have on the student's ability to demonstrate knowledge. Modifications are changes in the learning expectations such as reducing the amount of material the student is expected to learn, reducing the number of items on a test, or shortening homework assignments. Previous discussions regarding adaptations and instructional support for students incorporate both accommodations and modifications. It is important to know the difference between accommodations and modifications in the accountability context because the use of test modifications in a state accountability test may have future consequences for the student. Providing modifications and reducing the learning expectations for a student may affect future diploma options for high school graduation. It may determine whether a student receives a standard high school diploma, nontraditional type of diploma or certificate, or no diploma at all.

It is important for all educators, even elementary teachers, to know the consequences for providing modifications. Reducing the learning expectations of students in elementary school will be cumulative. Not expecting students to master third-grade material will significantly reduce the possibility of mastering grade material in middle school or high school. Providing a student who is taking the grade-level assessment with an AAC device or a braille version of the assessment could be considered an accommodation as long as the assessment itself is not modified in any way. Changing the number of multiple-choice response options from four on the regular grade-level assessment to three options on the AAC device is considered a modification.

There are many different types of accommodations. Thompson, Morse, et al. (2005) provided four categories of accommodations: presentation, setting, response, and time/scheduling (see Table 1.1). Presentation accommodations allow for various changes in how standard print instructional material is presented to the student. Changes in setting allow for increased access to necessary specialized equipment located someplace other than the typical instructional/assessment location. Students who use AAC devices will most often need response accommodations. Time/scheduling accommodations would be common for students with distractibility, physical disabilities, and health issues.

From the assessment options provided by the state, the IEP team determines which one is most appropriate for the student. The state is also required to provide the IEP team with the information necessary to assist the team in deciding which assessment is most appropriate for individual students. Usually this is in the form of eligibility criteria that students need to meet in order to take the specific assessments offered by the state. This means that IEP team members, including family members, need to be familiar with their state grade-level academic content standards, allowable accommodations for the state assessment, and available alternate/modified assessments. Each state has developed academic content standards for individual grade levels or grade-level clusters. Special education teachers and others who may provide services to students in special education classes such as speech-language pathologists (SLPs) and occupational and physical therapists need to gain access to the academic standards for the grade levels of students they serve. Most, if not all, states post these standards on their state education agency web sites.

The IEP team determines the accommodations or modifications that a student will need to participate in the state accountability test, but the state determines whether to use these scores in accountability decisions (Heumann & Warlick, 2001; Thompson, Johnstone, Thurlow, & Altman, 2005). Most states provide lists of allowable accommodations on state accountability tests that are documented in some fashion on the assessment. If a student needs to use a nonallowable accommodation, then the test may be assigned a score of zero, given no score, or automatically assigned to the lowest level of proficiency. This may, in turn, affect grade promotion or diploma options for students who use nonallowable accommodations. Using nonallowable accommodations should be highly discouraged.

Consider Sammi, Lyndsey, Camden, and Zack. As an early communicator, Sammi will most likely be a candidate for modifications of first-grade content standards. Accommodations to provide first-grade material in an alternate format are likely to not be the best route for her. Lyndsey is an early language communicator with an expressive repertoire of approximately 50 symbols. Although she clearly has some academic skills, they are not at the fifth-grade level. Therefore, she, too, is a candidate for modifications. Zack is an advanced linguistic communicator using supplements when conversing with people who do not understand him. He is working on an alternative diploma and is a candidate for modifications. Camden is a more advanced reader and writer functioning near grade level. His AAC device is considered an accommodation because it allows him access to the material by demonstrating his knowledge in an alternate response format. The use of the AAC device does not change the learning expectation. Camden's teachers need to continue to reprogram the device to include new vocabulary from each of the content areas or to teach him other strategies to convey these words (e.g., spelling with word prediction).

For Camden, the question becomes: Does Camden require this accommodation on the state test? If he can read the questions and fill in the bubbles of the response booklets used by his state, then perhaps he may not need any accommodation. If he needs an accommodation, can this accommodation be used on his state accountability assessment? The IEP team will need to familiarize themselves with the accommodations their state allows. If the AAC device cannot be used to take the state accountability assessment (most likely it cannot), then the team should consider what options are available to him. Some questions the team should ask when making this decision include:

1. *Which of the allowable accommodations most resemble the skills the student already has or already uses?*—Significantly changing how a student responds or how information is presented may affect test performance simply because the student is not familiar with the new system. Give the student plenty of opportunities to learn and practice the new accommodation before the test.

2. *Is there an allowable accommodation that can be used during instruction and assessment in the classroom on a consistent basis?*—Selecting an accommodation that is allowable on the state accountability assessment eliminates the need to teach a new system.

3. *Can this accommodation be used at home? At work? In social situations?*—By selecting an accommodation that can be used in a variety of situations, the student receives multiple opportunities to integrate this system into daily life. It also allows others to become familiar with the accommodation and increases the likelihood that it will be used.

4. *Which of the appropriate accommodations is more cost effective?*—Sophisticated communication equipment can be expensive. Can the student use the equipment without fear of damage? Computerized adaptive testing is a very flexible system that can accommodate a variety of presentation, response, and timing needs. Unfortunately, fewer states are offering this accommodation due to budgetary concerns and lack of technology in schools that is needed to support this accommodation (Thompson, Johnstone, et al., 2005).

5. *Which of the appropriate accommodations is user friendly?*—Some accommodations, especially communication equipment, may not be user friendly. A system that can be programmed, maintained, and used with little technological knowledge will most likely be used by more people.

Restricting the use of accommodations, whether in frequency of students who use them or in limiting the types of accommodations allowed on state accountability assessments, is based in controversy surrounding technical adequacy of the assessments. Testing standards developed by national research and testing organizations such as the American Educational Research Association (AERA) and American Psychological Association (APA) suggest that test developers (in this case, states) are responsible for establishing the technical adequacy of an assessment (AERA, APA, & National Council on Measurement in Education, 1999). *Technical adequacy* refers to test properties of reliability and validity. *Reliability* is the extent to which a test reports an individual's score accurately and consistently. *Validity* is a process that estimates the extent to which the test provides an appropriate score interpretation.

One important process in maintaining technical adequacy is standardized procedures in administering the assessment. When accommodations are provided, they may violate the standardized administration of the assessment, and the scores may not be valid and reliable, given particular accommodations. The current thinking about accommodations is that an appropriate accommodation should eliminate the effect of the disability on the individual's performance on the test. A valid accommodation will improve the performance of a student with a specific disability but will not improve the score when provided to a student without the disability. This is called the *interaction hypothesis* (Sireci, Scarpati, & Li, 2005). Take the student who is provided with a read-aloud accommodation in which an individual reads the passage aloud for the student. On a reading assessment in which the student is to read a passage and answer questions, the provision of a read-aloud invalidates the score because the goal of the assessment is reading comprehension, not listening comprehension. On a mathematics assessment, the provision of a read-aloud accommodation may not invalidate the test score because the goal of the assessment is not reading. In this same sense, providing students with AAC devices for testing accommodations may invalidate the test results simply because it changes the manner in which responses to test items are given.

Research on the provision of accommodations is confusing. A synthesis of accommodations research by Johnstone, Altman, Thurlow, and Thompson (2006) and Sireci, Scarpati, and Li (2005) provided inconsistent conclusions regarding specific accommodations. Specific accommodations were found to have a positive effect in some studies and a nonpositive effect in other studies. Evidence for appropriate use of extended time and read-aloud for mathematics accommodations appears to be emerging. Given this state of confusion, states are challenged by how to include scores of students with accommodations while maintaining the validity of those test scores.

Alternate Assessment Based on Grade-Level Expectations

Students who are working toward grade-level achievement standards but are unable to participate in the grade-level assessment, even with accommodations, can take an alternate assessment based on grade-level expectations. These assessments address the same content and student expectations as the grade-level test, just in a different format. For example, Oregon provides a portfolio collection of evidence called a *Juried Assessment* (Oregon Department of Education, 2007) and North Carolina uses a checklist called the *North Carolina Checklist of Academic Standards* (North Carolina Department of Public Instruction, 2007). These assessments are appropriate for students who are working on grade level with accommodations and modifications in the classroom in order to demonstrate their performance when they cannot gain access to the typical pencil-and-paper assessment and the accommodations/modifications they use are not offered on the grade-level assessment. For example, this would be a viable option for a student who uses a word processing program that voices text for demonstrating learning in the classroom if it is not an option for the grade-level assessment.

Alternate Assessment Based on Modified Grade-Level Achievement Standards

For students for whom the grade-level assessment is too difficult and the alternate assessment based on alternate achievement standards would be too easy, another option is an assessment based on modified grade-level standards (Title 1, 2007). This assessment is aligned with the academic content standards but has less rigorous expectations for demonstrating mastery of the grade-level content. These students would be achieving close to grade-level content but not quite meeting the achievement standards set by the state. This would not include out-of-level assessments in which a fifth-grade student would be working on third-grade standards—this is no longer allowed. Examples of an alternate assessment based on modified grade-level standards include *North Carolina's Extend 2* (North Carolina Department of Public Instruction, 2007) and the *Virginia Substitute Evaluation Program* (Virginia Department of Education, 2007). Zack is working below grade level and would not be able to independently read the grade-level assessment. He uses pictures and word cards to communicate. He could possibly participate in this type of assessment by replacing difficult test items with easier ones, eliminating the number of multiple choice options, and allowing him to use his picture and word cards to answer the questions. Up to 2% of a state or district's proficient AYP scores can include alternate assessments based on modified grade-level standards (U.S. Department of Education, 2005).

Alternate Assessment Based on Alternate Achievement Standards   Students with the most significant disabilities can take alternate assessments based on alternate achievement standards. Up to 1% of a state or district's proficient AYP scores can include alternate assessments based on alternate achievement standards. Although still aligned to a state's academic content standards, these standards are based on a less complex and narrower range of content with a different set of expectations (U.S. Department of Education, 2005). These assessments typically fall into one of three categories: 1) portfolio or body of evidence, 2) rating scale or checklist, or 3) performance based (Thompson, Johnstone, et al., 2005). Portfolio is the most common in which a collection of work over time is used to demonstrate student growth. A checklist or rating scale simply requires teachers to record skills performed by the student. Performance-based assessments directly measure specific skills as the students perform them. Both Sammi and Lyndsey are likely candidates for an alternate assessment based on alternate achievement standards because they are performing well below grade level. A student eligible for this type of assessment will most likely have an intellectual disability in addition to being an AAC user.

Browder, Wakeman, Flowers, Rickelman, and Pugalee (2007) provided four criteria for creating alignment between instruction and an alternate assessment:

1. Focus on grade academic content.
2. Connect to student's assigned grade level.
3. Alter the depth or breadth of the achievement level.
4. Distinguish different achievement levels across grade levels.

They reminded the field that focusing on academic content can still include functional activities and materials. When connecting to grade-level content, instruction should align with the state academic content standards for that grade level. Application to grade-level content can consist of prerequisite skills such as those selected for Lyndsey. The depth and breadth of the achievement level refers to the complexity of the response required by the student. The expectations of the student when demonstrating knowledge will differ from grade-level expectations. A student participating in an alternate assessment using alternate achievement standards may be asked to demonstrate knowledge of the big idea but not the smaller details of a concept (depth). The skills selected for this student will not necessarily include all of the subdomains of a given academic content area but only incorporate the major subdomains of that content standard (breadth). For example, state academic content standards for mathematics in fifth grade may include aspects of numbers and operations, algebra, measurement, geometry, and probability. It is necessary to include some of these areas in the alternate assessment with reference to a fifth-grade activity, but not all. Some states mandate a specific number of skills for each area that must be included in the alternate assessment. Refer to your state guidelines to determine the number of subdomains you will need.

Although a student may work the same skill across grade levels, there should also be some distinction in increasing expectations of achievement across the grade levels. For example, Lyndsey, a fifth grader, would be gaining access to the same literature being read in fifth grade with modifications to the vocabulary—adding pictures and objects to supplement the text (criteria 1 and 2). Given a goal to understand text that is read, in fifth grade she may be working on identifying traits associated with the main character (e.g., physical description, emotions, actions) by selecting her answer from three picture/word cards. Last year, she was working on identifying the main character, setting, and theme of the story (criteria 3 and 4), selecting her answer from four picture/word cards.

Standards-Based Individualized Education Programs   Some states require that the alternate assessment skills linked to the state academic content standards be included in the IEP, creating a standards-based IEP document. A standards-based IEP is an IEP that includes individualized goals that are aligned to the state's academic content standards for the assigned grade level of the student (Courtade-Little & Browder, 2005). Some states provide examples of extensions of the state content standards for the IEPs from which the team can select to form the alternate assessment content. For example, Texas provides teachers with a curriculum framework specifically for their alternate assessment at each tested grade level that lists multiple examples of aligned skills for each academic content standard (Texas Education Agency, 2008). Other states leave selection of a skill that aligns to the grade-level content standard to individual teachers.

An IEP can help promote the link between the assessment, state content standards, and instruction (Courtade-Little & Browder, 2005; Nolet & Mclaughlin, 2000). This link is important to make sure whatever is tested on the assessment is also what is taught in the classroom. In the past, the IEP was the curriculum for students receiving special education. Now, with the changes in IDEA, the IEP creates access to the general curriculum. Figure 1.1 illustrates the connection between state academic content standards, the IEP, instruction, and assessment. The IEP documents individual needs for academic instruction as well as functional life skills. There may be individual needs that assist the student to gain access to the academic skills that should be considered as priority skills. Once the skills have been selected by the IEP team, instruction begins. Notice the two arrows between instruction and assessment. Progress as measured by periodic formative assessment is used to refine the instruction throughout the academic year or IEP cycle. Summative assessment at the end of the academic year or IEP cycle is used to refine the IEP.

Communication skills should be considered a priority IEP skill as they create access for all the academic areas. Therefore, the team should consider how the student will use a particular mode of communication for each academic area (mathematics, language arts, and science). Consider not only how the mode will be used, but also the words and symbols that may be necessary to use the communication mode. A system that is accessible and responsive in all settings is more likely to be used. Recall that this system is not only for instruction but is also used for the assessment.

Universal Design for Learning   The concept of UDL can help manage the diverse individual needs and minimize potential barriers to assessments. Three essential qualities for UDL include multiple means of representation, expression, and engagement (CAST, 1998; see Chapter 6 for a more extensive discussion on UDL). Multiple means of representation provides flexible

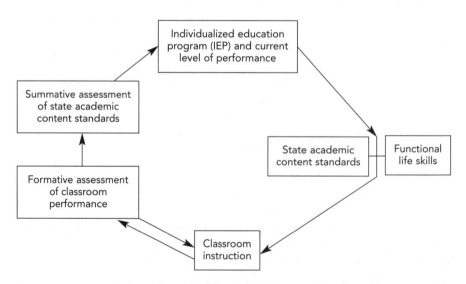

Figure 1.1.   The connection between state academic content standards, individualized education program, instruction, and assessment.

alternatives to reduce barriers to gaining access to instruction. Sammi and Lyndsey would require access to objects, pictures, and gestures. Zack would require text of limited vocabulary. Multiple means of expression provides flexible alternatives to reduce barriers of demonstrating what has been learned. Camden will need to use his AAC device programmed with the vocabulary for the content areas. Multiple means of engagement provides flexible alternatives to reduce barriers to interact with the curriculum. Lyndsey, Sammi, and Zack will need strong connections of new material to familiar material. Planning multiple ways for linking representation, engagement, and expression in instruction and assessment in thoughtful planning can help manage access to learning and assessment of diverse needs of individuals.

CLASSROOM ASSESSMENT ISSUES

Classroom assessment can provide teachers with valuable information about individual student performance and acquisition of skills. Although the state testing is used for inclusion in AYP calculations required by NCLB, classroom assessment can monitor skill acquisition and determine if the individual is on target to master skills by the state testing date and IEP target date.

Teachers can collect three main types of assessment data: portfolios, performance data, and self-evaluation (Airasian, 2005; Anderson, 2003). Recall that portfolios are a collection of student work throughout the year. These can be tests, homework assignments, or any other products generated by the student. The portfolio may also include videotapes, audio tapes, or notes from parents or other teachers. Performance assessments require the student to perform the skill with some accuracy measure of the performance. Self-evaluation asks individuals to reflect on their work in terms of quality, effort, accuracy, goal setting, and use of learning strategies. Self-evaluation can range from an in-depth narrative or a questionnaire format with Likert scales from very good to very poor, to simple use of two picture symbols such as a happy face and a sad face.

Formative and Summative Assessment

Assessment serves a primary function of using data to make decisions. The process may be either formative or summative (Worthen & Sanders, 1997). In formative assessment, data are collected throughout instruction and used to make decisions to improve instruction. Summative assessment data is collected at the end of the instruction period (quarter, semester, or year) to provide a judgment to the merit of the instruction. This judgment is typically the assignment of a final grade for the course. State tests used for AYP calculations and grades assigned at the end of a semester or year-long course are forms of summative assessment. Using a formative assessment is more valuable for teachers because it can be used to gauge student progress and determine strengths and weaknesses in student performance.

Homework and Classroom Assessment   Homework and class assignments, which are two forms of formative assessments, are part of the daily routine of general education classrooms. They assist students in practicing new skills and are valuable only to the extent that learning is enhanced. Homework can raise school achievement when it is carefully planned for skill level, attention, and motivation of the students (Cooper & Nye, 1994), especially in high school students (Cooper, 1989). Research has shown that the completion of homework that is graded and commented on by teachers significantly improves student achievement by as much as 30 percentile points on achievement tests (Marzano, Pickering, & Pollock, 2001). Assignments that are misunderstood or too difficult will actually be counterproductive. Confusing or difficult assignments will probably not be completed and over time may cause the student to fall even further behind. Research recommends that early elementary students spend from 10 to 30 minutes per day on homework and older elementary students spend from 30 to 90 minutes per day on homework (Bond & Smith, 1966; Partin, 2005; Pennsylvania Department of Education, 1973; Strang, 1973). Middle school students should spend from 50 to 120 minutes per day on homework. A typical high school student should spend from 1 to 3 hours per day on homework.

There is no reason to support lack of homework for students in special education classes. Expecting the same amount of time on homework and class assignments, however, is an individual decision that should be made by the IEP team. In cases in which students have been deemed most appropriate for modified or alternate achievement standards, it has already been decided by the team that typical expectations do not apply. It is important that any testing accommodations afforded in the IEP be practiced daily in the classroom in independent work and nightly homework. Some things to consider in regard to homework are

- Budget time so that students spend more time on the important skills. Teachers need to prioritize homework based on individual needs of the students. Teachers also need to communicate with each other to develop a homework schedule assigning courses to particular days of the week.

- Intersperse fun activities with difficult ones. Keeping students motivated is key to getting them to complete homework. If assignments and homework are consistently difficult or not fun, then students will tend not to complete them.

- If students are using AAC, then it may take them longer to complete assignments because they are also managing the communication system. Keep in mind the response mode of the student and how that may extend time spent on assignments.

- Planning ahead is essential to any teacher of a student with AAC needs. The appropriate pictures and/or words need to be readily available to facilitate completion of these assignments.

- It is okay to shorten assignments or provide alternate forms of completing assignments based on individual needs of the student.

- Communicate with parents in regard to expectations, how much time students spend completing assignments at home, and how to improve parental oversight. Some students will need assistance in completing assignments, and availability of this assistance will influence completion of homework assignments. If possible, provide assignments that a student can complete independently or try to limit the amount of involvement of others needed to complete the assignment.

- Encouragement and rewards for completion of assignments will help improve successful completion of future assignments.

- Provide a homework organizer to record assignments and directions and store completed assignments. Provide space for parent comments. Include how students can get help with homework assignments such as telephone numbers, web site addresses, or tutors.

- Create homework teams pairing academically strong students with students needing support.

Organizational Skills

The development of organizational skills can assist students in managing assignments and facilitating learning. Providing organizers will facilitate the learning of many differing types of students. Students can be taught to organize their time (Gall, Gall, Jacobsen, & Bullock, 1990), their environment (Doelling, Bryde, & Parette, 1997), and their assignments (Devine, 1987). Time management involves individual and class schedules posted on desks and walls or in individual planners. Individual schedules should be readily accessible to the student in a format with which he or she is familiar (e.g., pictures, objects, words). Keeping a daily or weekly routine will facilitate students in keeping to their schedule. Monthly planners can be used to record assignments, due dates, and long-range activities. The items in a monthly planner can be added to daily/weekly schedules as needed. Reviewing schedules and giving advanced notice about schedule changes can prevent confusion by preparing students for changes in their daily schedule. Organizing the environment can also provide important cues to student achievement. Some students work better under certain conditions such as lighting or sound level, but they also need structure to their personal work environment to ensure access to the supports they need such as necessary work materials, adaptive equipment, and schedule systems.

A task analysis for completion of assignments can be specific to a large or long-range project or general for completion of daily class or homework assignments. A task analysis breaks up an assignment into smaller steps with an estimated completion time (Mastropieri & Scruggs, 2007). Some students are able to create their own task analysis for assignments, whereas other students may need one developed by a teacher. The following is an example of a generic task analysis for completing a class assignment that Zack might use.

1. Put name on paper.

2. Read instructions carefully.

3. Set timer for 15 minutes.

4. Raise hand to ask a question.

5. Work quietly until timer rings.

6. Put materials away.

7. Put assignment in teacher's desk.

The typed list of steps can be replaced with graphic symbols, pictures, or object reminders.

A specific task analysis for a longer assignment can be placed in a planner that lists all the steps needed to complete the assignment. For example, a task analysis for a book report to be completed at home might be organized for Lyndsey as follows.

• *Monday 7-2*—Select book from school library.

• *Tuesday 7-3*—Read book with Mom; identify picture of main character.

• *Wednesday 7-4*—Read book with Mom; identify picture representing the theme of book.

• *Thursday 7-5*—Read book with Mom; identify picture of main character and theme.

• *Friday 7-6*—Read book with Mom; identify picture of setting of the book.

• *Saturday 7-7*—Read book with Mom; identify picture of setting, main character, and theme.

• *Sunday 7-8*—Same as Saturday.

• *Monday 7-9*—Complete book report by filling in incomplete sentences with the pictures of main character, setting, and theme.

• *Tuesday 7-10*—Turn in book report.

In this example, the teacher prepares a list of questions with answer cards using words and picture symbols and instructions for Lyndsey's mom. On Friday, the teacher sends home a paragraph summary of the book with blanks that Lyndsey must fill in with the answer cards.

Visual organizers such as a Venn diagram or concept map create a conceptual framework within which to organize information. They can be used to map information from a single work or connect information from multiple works. Figure 1.2 illustrates the use of a concept map of a book titled *Jafta* that Sammi's teacher read to the class. They completed the map together after reading the book.

Using Assessment to Shape Instruction

Progress monitoring, the use of frequent data to make educational decisions, is another form of formative assessment. Two types of progress monitoring, curriculum-based measurement (CBM) and classroom assessment, can be valuable tools for teachers. Teachers can use the information from CBM to gauge progress of students against grade-level standards and the information from classroom assessment to gauge progress of students on IEP goals. Effective teachers regularly use assessments of student progress to make teaching decisions. Research has demonstrated that ongoing data collection

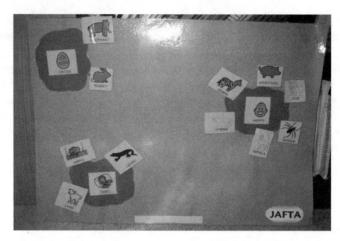

Figure 1.2.   Illustration of a concept map for *Jafta*. (Photo courtesy of Bree Jimenez.)

to assess student progress and use of these data to evaluate effective instruction can improve student outcomes, teacher decision making, and student awareness (e.g., Belfiore & Browder, 1992; Calhoun & Fuchs, 2003; Deno, 2003; Good, Simmons, & Kame'enui, 2001; Snell & Loyd, 1991). Teachers tend not to use progress monitoring (Stiggins, 2001), despite the evidence that it is successful in improving student outcomes.

CBM focuses on grade-level content and is designed to be frequent, quick, and easy probes of student achievement in a variety of content areas. There are a number of commercially available instruments, such as the Dynamic Indicators of Basic Early Literacy Skills (DIBELS; Good & Kaminski, 2002) and AIMSweb (Edformation, 2007), that are based on a generic curriculum and not a specific reading or math curriculum. Advantages of CBM include the ability to conduct error analyses and graphing of student progress. Pictorial representations provide teachers and parents with an easy format to describe student progress and can be motivating to students. Some also provide recommendations based on student performance and estimate the level of risk of future difficulty. More information can be found at the web site of the National Center for Progress Monitoring (http://www.studentprogress.org) regarding specific CBM tools and their use. One disadvantage of these tools may be the need for frequent and easy access to a computer. One issue for students who use AAC is that these commercial measures require standardized administration of the tests. Many of these require verbal responses by students. Deviation from the standardized procedures prevents peer comparison so recommendations and level of risk estimates may not be accurate. This does not mean that the tests cannot be used, but altering administration of the test should be noted in any discussion of test results.

Classroom assessment is another valuable tool that teachers can use to measure student progress. A system for creating measurable skills, collecting data, and evaluating the data (i.e., data-based decisions) is described by Browder (2001) and Snell and Brown (2006). Data can be frequency counts, such as number of correct responses or steps in a task analysis completed independently; percent of correct responses; or time-based rates of duration or latency. In this system, teachers begin by collecting baseline data on student performance prior to instruction. During instruction, data is collected frequently and plotted on a graph with the dates of instruction along the *x* axis (bottom of the graph) and the frequency/time along the *y* axis (left side of the graph). Connecting the plots of student responses is called the *line of progress*. This plot is then compared with an Aim line. An Aim line is drawn from the onset of instruction (where the *x* and *y* axis intersect) to the date the skill is to be mastered. This could be the date listed on the IEP or the date of the alternate assessment. This comparison leads to a decision rule process identifying progress as adequate, slow, variable, or none.

Each type of progress is paired with a specific intervention strategy to improve student performance. This system does not require the use of a computer because graphing can be done on a piece of graph paper. For more detailed information on aligning instruction with data patterns refer to Browder (2001) and Snell and Brown (2006).

Classroom assessment can be individualized toward any student regardless of communication or other needs and any goal as long as the goal is measurable. This makes this technique especially useful to teachers of students with AAC needs. The testing format is the same as the instruction format. In some cases, such as with a list of vocabulary words, assessment data can be taken during instruction. Other skills, such as comprehension of vocabulary words, would need to be assessed in the context with which the words will be used, such as a science lesson or trip into the community.

Depth of Knowledge for Developing Assignments and Assessments

Teachers need to consider the depth of knowledge required by the task when creating assignments and formative and summative assessments for students with disabilities. Different types of assignments and question formats require different types of thinking by the student in order to complete the activity. A common system of describing the depth of knowledge is Bloom's (1954) taxonomy. Additional research is needed to validate how these descriptors can be applied to students with disabilities. Some work in this area is being conducted by the National Alternate Assessment Center (http://www.naacpartners.org). A description of the six levels of depth of knowledge as modified by the National Alternate Assessment Center at the University of North Carolina at Charlotte (Flowers, Karvonen, Browder, & Wakeman, in press) and application to a science activity on magnetism appears in Table 1.2. One study found that alternate assessments tend to contain items at the lower levels of depth of knowledge, but creative application of learning and assessment can generate items that reflect higher levels of learning as well (Flowers, Browder, & Ahlgrim-Delzell, 2006). A series of

Table 1.2.   Application of Bloom's taxonomy to an assessment of magnetism

Level of depth of knowledge	Description	Application
Attention	Touch, look, vocalize, respond, attend	Eyes directed toward magnet, student reached out to touch it
Memorize/recall	List, describe facts, identify, state, define, label, recognize, record, match, recall, relate	Student touched picture of magnet on AAC device when given four picture/word options
Performance	Perform, demonstrate, follow, count, locate, read	Student used a magnet to pick up metallic objects placed on the work table
Comprehension	Explain, conclude, group/categorize, restate, review, translate, describe concepts, paraphrase, infer, summarize, illustrate	Student sorted pictures/words of metallic objects that could be attracted to a magnet from pictures/words of objects clearly not metal using an ACC device
Application	Compute, organize, collect, apply, classify, construct, solve, use, order, develop, generate, interact with text, implement	When given a variety of objects and asked to place a piece of paper on a magnetized dry erase board, student selected the correct tool to hang the paper
Analysis/synthesis/ evaluation	Pattern, analyze, compare, contrast, compose, predict, extend, plan, judge, evaluate, interpret, cause/effect, investigate, examine, distinguish, differentiate, generate	When given a magnet and a variety of metallic objects, student distinguished types of metals that are magnetic (e.g., iron) versus metals that are not magnetic (e.g., aluminum foil) creating two picture/word lists using an ACC device

From Flowers, C., Karvonen, M., Browder, D., & Wakeman, S. (in press). Links for academic learning (LAL): A methodology for investigating alignment of alternate assessments based on alternate achievement standards. *Educational Measurement: Issues and Practice;* adapted by permission.

pilot alignment studies of states' alternate assessments to their content standards confirms this initial finding (Flowers, Browder, Wakeman, & Karvonen, 2006a, 2006b, 2006c).

Grading Student Performance

Grades are an integral part of schooling, judging and communicating the quality of student performance. Grades are typically assigned to individual assignments (formative) and course performance on report cards (summative). They can be assigned by letters (e.g., *A, B, C*), numerals (e.g., 90%), or categories (excellent, good, fair, poor, or pass/fail). Typically, grading takes one of three forms—norm-referenced criteria, performance-based criteria, or percentage-based criteria (Airasian, 2005). *Norm-referenced grading* compares performance of a student with the performance of other students. Many commercially available tests use this method, but teachers who develop grading curves are also using this method. Grading curves place a specified percentage of students in each of the grading categories. Grading based on the normal curve may assign the top 2% of students an *A*, 14% a *B*, 68% a *C*, 14% a *D*, and 2% an *F*. The problem with this method is that it is possible for students to score low on an assignment or course but get an *A* as long as they scored in the top 2% of the class. It can also force some students who score high on an assignment or course into lower grades if they happen to be in a class of high performers in which everyone performed well if they scored in the bottom 14%.

Performance-based grading sets standards of performance that students must obtain to receive a certain grade. When created as a grading rubric and explained to students at the beginning of an assignment or course, this can provide useful information to the student, teacher, and parent. Figure 1.3 shows a grading rubric for a book report used by Lyndsey's teacher that accommodates various student needs.

Notice that this rubric includes many presentation styles without mentioning verbal skills. This presentation could be prepared and delivered via computer software or AAC. The rubric can be individualized by varying the depth of the information being conveyed by the presenter. A similar rubric could be devised for a summative assessment for a grade assignment at the end of a course. An example of a summative rubric is provided in Figure 1.4. Effort and behavior have been left out of this rubric. Acquiring new skills requires some effort and frequent appropriate display of behavior. Extreme lack of effort or inappropriate behavior should be conveyed to the parent and student, perhaps in a separate report, but should not be a part of the course grade reflecting achievement (Anderson, 2003). Lyndsey, a student with autism, has a behavior plan developed with the assistance

A	Student consistently faces and looks toward audience; presentation includes correct identification of title and author, elements of main character, setting, and theme (5/5); presentation organized in order.
B	Student usually faces and looks toward audience; presentation includes correct identification of title and author, elements of main character, setting, and theme (5/5); presentation is less organized with some repetition or is out of order.
C	Student sometimes faces and looks toward audience, looks at floor, or fidgets; presentation includes correct identification of title and author, elements of main character, setting, and theme (4/5); presentation is poorly organized with a lot of repetition or jumping between book elements.
D	Student rarely faces and looks toward audience, looks at floor, or fidgets; presentation includes some correct identification of title and author, elements of character, setting, and theme (less than 4/5); presentation is poorly organized with a lot of repetition or jumping between book elements.

Figure 1.3.   Grading rubric for a book report presentation.

A	Student made substantial progress on all of his or her individualized education program (IEP) skills, consistently completed in-class assignments accurately, and consistently completed homework assignments accurately.
B	Student made good progress on most of his or her IEP skills, mostly completed in-class assignments accurately, and mostly completed homework assignments accurately.
C	Student made some progress on most of his or her IEP skills, completed some in-class assignments accurately, and completed some homework assignments accurately.
D	Student made some progress on some of his or her IEP skills, completed some in-class assignments accurately, and completed some homework assignments accurately.

Figure 1.4.   Summative grading rubric at the end of a course.

of the school psychologist for decreasing her repetitive hand flapping and body rocking behavior. The teacher sends home a progress report summarizing the occurrences of these behaviors separate from Lyndsey's grade reports.

A third common form of grading uses *percentage-based criteria*. Cutoff scores are used based on a percentage of items answered correctly. For example, 90%–100% is an *A*, 80%–89% is a *B*, and so forth. This system may be used in conjunction with percent of mastery of IEP goals based on the criterion of the goal. For example, if the IEP goal states, "Zack will correctly use 10 out of 12 new science vocabulary words during a science experiment," then the criterion is 10. If Zack correctly used 9 of the 10 (90%) by the date in his IEP, then he could be assigned a grade of *A*.

Whatever method is selected, grades should be meaningful so that everyone knows what they mean, explicit in how the teacher arrived at the grade, and fair about how grades are distributed across students (Anderson, 2003). McMillan's (1997) guidelines also included reliance on the most current information, a sufficient number of formative assessments prior to assigning a course grade, and use of informed professional judgment. Occasionally, teachers will need to rely on their professional judgment, in addition to the numerical computation of a grade, in borderline cases.

Preparing Students for Tests

Recall that there should be a link between the expectations of the IEP and academic content standards, the instruction, and the assessments. A strong link between these expectations and instruction help students be well prepared for the assessment. Although there is some negative commentary regarding teaching to the test, there is a difference between teaching to the test and teaching the test (Anderson, 2003). Given that state academic content standards are based on standards developed by national content area organizations such as the NCTE, NCTM, or NRC, the content of these assessments likely reflects the important skills and knowledge identified by these organizations. Good teaching practice ensures that students are competent in their knowledge of the areas identified by these organizations and covered by the assessment. Teaching the test by covering only the items on the test in the fashion in which they are tested, however, is not appropriate. This leads to a tendency to memorize specific answers rather than to understand and generalize the material. Some students do, though, need some specific instruction in order to perform well on tests. In addition to linking instruction to the assessment, there are some things teachers can do to better prepare their students, including reviewing material, familiarizing students with the assessment format, sharing information about the test, and scheduling the test for optimum performance (Anderson, 2003).

Occasionally, review the material before the assessment to help students remember the content that teachers should have covered early in the course. Refreshing students' memory of specific content and main ideas and connecting previously learned information to new information can enhance performance by allowing students to practice skills and clear up any misunderstandings. The key is for the learning to become a part of long-term learning and not short-term memory. For students with disabilities, a review of previously mastered material may need to occur frequently on first learning the material and can taper off as time goes by and the student demonstrates maintenance of the skill. Regardless of which type of assessment a student will take, this refresher will serve as an advantage to the student.

In the ideal situation, the format by which the student will take the assessment is the same format in which it has been instructed and practiced. This may not be true for students with disabilities who will be taking the typical state assessment, though, as these are commonly pencil and paper tests in opscan (fill in the bubble) or narrative form. Familiarity with the assessment format is important so that student performance is not adversely affected by unfamiliarity with the format. Assessing a student in a format with which he or she is not familiar will most likely lead to test results that are not commensurate with his or her optimum performance. If it is necessary for a student to be assessed in a format that is not typically used during instruction or student practice of skills, then the teacher can provide specific time for the student to practice the new format.

For a student such as Camden who may be able to take the typical state grade-level assessment in an opscan format, his teacher can have the class practice taking these tests in formative classroom assessments throughout the year. Opscan formats require some skill in filling in the intended bubble. Although directions for filling in bubbles are presented prior to an assessment, practice may be needed to completely fill in the bubble, erase and change an answer, or eliminate stray marks that may affect recognition of the intended answer by the scoring machine. If a bubble sheet separate from the question booklet is required for recording answers, then practice lining up answers for the intended question because it is easy to lose one's place. The teacher can also develop and provide practice for a system of periodic checking to ensure questions and answers line up correctly. This can help ensure that performance is not affected by incorrect placement of answers.

Sharing information about the assessment can also help prevent unfamiliarity of the test from affecting student performance. Information such as how long the test will take, how many questions, types of questions, what day or days the testing will occur, and what outside tools (e.g., calculator, communication device) are allowed can help a student better prepare for the assessment. This will require the IEP team to be familiar with the particular assessment the student will be taking and the procedures for the assessment. Providing such information applies to both formative teacher-made assessments as well as summative state assessments.

If possible, scheduling the assessment at a particular time of day may contribute to optimal student performance. Many students with significant disabilities may perform better in the morning and easily tire in the afternoons. Students with attentional difficulties may need multiple testing sessions. A student with health issues such as seizures may need flexible assessment sessions to accommodate for seizure activity. It may be easier to individualize a testing schedule for younger students in elementary school where the student is with the same teacher all day rather than for blocks of specific time in the middle and high school years. But if the scheduling is likely to affect student performance, then the teaching team should document such accommodation in the student's IEP.

Another scheduling implication involves disrupting a student's daily routine. Many students in special education utilize an individualized schedule. Lack of advanced warning of the disruption may negatively affect a student's performance. Providing an advanced warning of the disrupted schedule can be accomplished by reviewing the revised schedule with the student, providing a universal symbol for a change in the schedule, or developing a specific symbol to reflect assessment times. Using Social Stories (Gray & Garand, 1993) is another technique that may be applied to the testing situation. Social Stories are individualized short stories with specific elements that have been used to improve the behavior of students with autism spectrum disorders in a variety of situations (e.g., Barry & Burlew, 2004; Kuoch & Mirenda, 2003; Moore, 2004; Scattone, Wilczynski,

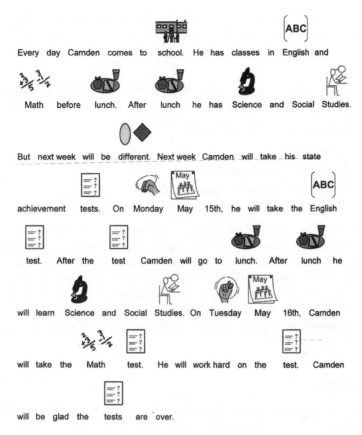

Figure 1.5. Example of a Social Story for Camden using Writing with Symbols (Mayer-Johnson, 2000). The Picture Communication Symbols © 1981–2008 by Mayer-Johnson LLC. All Rights Reserved Worldwide. Used with permission.

Edwards, & Rabian, 2002). Using the Social Story format and guidelines (Gray, 2004), a story can be written describing the assessment situation and expectations of the student and can be read with the student to familiarize him or her with the testing situation and change in daily routine. These stories can be written and adapted as necessary to the individual testing situation, need of the student, and reading ability (see Figure 1.5). For example, teachers can substitute picture symbols or clip art for words or add objects to supplement understanding of the text. An example of a Social Story for Camden follows:

"Every day Camden comes to school. He has classes in English and math before lunch. After lunch, he has science and social studies. But next week will be different. Next week, Camden will take his state achievement tests. The tests show Camden, his teacher, and his mother how hard he has worked this year to learn new things. On Monday, May 15, he will come to his English class with his classmates and Mrs. Branch to take the English test. He will read all the questions carefully and mark his answer in the bubble. When Camden has a question, he will raise his hand and ask the teacher. When the teacher says, 'Time is up,' Camden will put his pencil down and smile. He will work hard. After the test, Camden will go to lunch. After lunch, he will go to science and social studies. On Monday night, he will go to bed early to get a good night's sleep.

"On Tuesday morning, May 16, Camden will come to his math class with his classmates and Mr. Duke to take the math test. He will read all questions carefully and mark his answer in the bubble. When Camden has a question, he will raise his hand and ask the teacher. He can use his calculator to work on the math problems. When his teacher says, 'Time is up,' he will put his pencil down and smile. Camden will work hard. After the test, Camden will go to lunch. After lunch, he will go to science and social studies. Camden will be glad the tests are over. He worked hard all year!"

Some comprehension questions for Camden after reading the Social Story include the following:

1. What day is the English test?
2. Where will you go to take the English test?
3. What day is the math test?
4. Where will you go to take the math test?
5. What can you use to work out the math problems?
6. What should you do if you have a question?

In summary, a teacher can best prepare a student for an assessment by advocating for the most appropriate form of assessment (typical, accommodated, alternate, or modified) and embedding the format and knowledge required into daily instruction and formative assessment strategies. The IEP team should be familiar with the student's needs, state assessment options and allowable accommodations, and consequences of selecting a nonallowable accommodation. Prepare students for novel assessment formats by practicing using the format, providing information about the assessment, and individualizing the schedule of the assessment, all of which can promote optimal student performance.

CONCLUSION

The requirement for participation in statewide tests is mandated in NCLB and IDEA 2004. It requires that all students have access to the general curriculum and participate in state assessments. Subsequent federal guidelines provide for five different types of assessments that states can offer to allow for maximum participation by all students. The implications for students with disabilities are potentially far reaching. The decision regarding what type of test is most appropriate for a student is made by the IEP team. Team members must be knowledgeable in the specific testing and accommodations offered by their state as well as the implications for each type of assessment. Some state assessments will eliminate students from the possibility of diplomas or substitute alternative diplomas. Some test alternatives require the IEP team to select the skills to be included in the assessment. Team members need to be familiar with their state grade-level content standards in order to create the link between the individual needs of the student, the IEP document, and state content standards.

Formative assessment can provide teachers with valuable information regarding student progress. Creating a link between the instruction, formative classroom assessments, and state summative assessments can also facilitate student performance. Formative classroom assessment can be individualized to each IEP goal using a data-based decision model or a CBM purchased commercially. Information from the classroom assessments can be used to modify instruction as needed to improve student performance. Preparing students for state assessments using schedules, implementing Social Stories, providing information about the test, and practicing the testing format can also serve to facilitate student performance.

There is still much we do not know regarding the implications of including students with disabilities in statewide assessments. There has been much negative press about the effects of accountability testing on all students, but there is no research evidenced to support these claims. The increase in expectations of students who had been summarily excluded from the assessment and accountability process is likely to be a long-term benefit. Many of these students are being provided with opportunities never afforded to them before.

REFERENCES

Airasian, P.W. (2005). *Classroom assessment concepts and applications* (5th ed.). New York: McGraw Hill.

American Educational Research Association (AERA), American Psychological Association (APA), & National Council on Measurement in Education (NCME). (1999). *The standards for educational and psychological testing.* Washington, DC: Authors.

Anderson, L.W. (2003). *Classroom assessment: Enhancing the quality of teacher decision-making.* Mahwah, NJ: Lawrence Erlbaum Associates.

Barry, L.M., & Burlew, S.B. (2004). Using Social Stories to teach choice and play skills to children with autism. *Focus on Autism and Other Developmental Disabilities, 19,* 45–51.

Belfiore, P., & Browder, D.M. (1992). Effects of self-monitoring on teacher data-based decisions and on the progress of adults with mental retardation. *Education and Training in Mental Retardation, 27,* 60–67.

Bloom, B.S. (1954). *Taxonomy of educational objectives: The classification of educational goals, handbook 1: Cognitive domain.* New York: McKay.

Bond, G.W., & Smith, G.J. (1966). Homework in the elementary school. *National Elementary School Principal, 45,* 46–50.

Browder, D.M. (2001). *Curriculum and assessment for students with moderate and severe disabilities.* New York: Guilford Press.

Browder, D.M., Wakeman, S.Y., Flowers, C., Rickelman, R., & Pugalee, D. (2007). Creating access to the general curriculum with links to grade-level content for students with significant disabilities: An explanation of the concept. *Journal of Special Education, 41,* 2–16.

Calhoun, M.B., & Fuchs, L.S. (2003). The effects of peer-assisted learning strategies and curriculum-based measurement on the mathematics performance of secondary students with disabilities. *Remedial and Special Education, 24,* 235–245.

CAST. (1998). *Three essential qualities of universal design for learning.* Retrieved February 27, 2003, from http://www.cec.sped.org/osep/appendix.html

Cizek, G.J. (2001). More unintended consequences of high-stakes testing. *Educational Measurement: Issues and Practice, 20,* 19–27.

Colorado Department of Education, Office of Standards and Assessment. (2008, June 6). *Colorado K–12 academic standards.* Available at http://www.cde.state.co.us/cdeassess/documents/OSA/k12_standards.html

Cooper, H. (1989). Synthesis of research on homework. *Educational Leadership, 47,* 85–91.

Cooper, H., & Nye, B. (1994). Homework for students with learning disabilities: The implications of research for policy and practice. *Journal of Learning Disabilities, 27,* 465–536.

Courtade-Little, G., & Browder, D.M. (2005). *Aligning IEPs to academic content standards for students with moderate and severe disabilities.* Verona, WI: Attainment Company.

Deno, S.L. (2003). Developments in curriculum-based measurement. *Journal of Special Education, 37,* 184–192.

Devine, T.G. (1987). *Teaching study skills: A guide for teachers* (2nd ed.). Boston: Allyn & Bacon.

Disability Rights Advocates. (2001). *Do no harm: High stakes testing and students with learning disabilities.* Retrieved June 23, 2007, from http://www.dralegal.org/publications/do_no_harm.php

Doelling, J., Bryde, S., & Parette, H.P. (1997). What are multidisciplinary and ecobehavioral approaches? And how can they make a difference for students with traumatic brain injuries? *TEACHING Exceptional Children, 30,* 56–60.

Edformation. (2007). *AIMSweb.* Retrieved July 7, 2007, from http://www.aimsweb.com/index.php.

Education for All Handicapped Children Act of 1975, PL 94-142, 20 U.S.C. §§ 1400 *et seq.*

Elementary and Secondary Education Act of 1965, PL 89-10, 20 U.S.C. §§ 241 *et seq.*

Elliot, J.L., Erickson, R.N., Thurlow, M.L., & Shriner, J.G. (2000). State-level accountability for the performance of students with disabilities: Five years of change? *Journal of Special Education, 34,* 39–47.

Firestone, W.A., & Mayrowetz, D. (2000). Rethinking "high stakes": Lessons from the United States and England and Wales. *Teachers College Record, 102,* 724–749.

Flowers, C., Browder, D.M., & Ahlgrim-Delzell, L. (2006). An analysis of three states' alignment between language arts and math standards and alternate assessment. *Exceptional Children, 72,* 201–216.

Flowers, C., Browder, D., Wakeman, S., & Karvonen, M. (2006a). *Alternate assessment alignment pilot study: Report to State A Department of Education.* Retrieved July 7, 2007, from http://education.uncc.edu/access/GCAManuscripts.htm

Flowers, C., Browder, D., Wakeman, S., & Karvonen, M. (2006b). *Alternate assessment alignment study: Report to State B Department of Education.* Retrieved July 7, 2007, from http://education.uncc.edu/access/GCAManuscripts.htm

Flowers, C., Browder, D., Wakeman, S., & Karvonen, M. (2006c). *Portfolio alternate assessment alignment study: Report to State A Department of Education.* Retrieved July 7, 2007, from http://education.uncc.edu/access/GCAManuscripts.htm

Flowers, C., Karvonen, M., Browder, D., & Wakeman, S. (in press). Links for academic learning (LAL): A methodology for investigating alignment of alternate assessments based on alternate achievement standards. *Educational Measurement: Issues and Practice.*

Gall, M.D., Gall, J.P., Jacobsen, D.R., & Bullock, T.L. (1990). *Tools for learning: A guide for teaching study skills.* Alexandria, VA: Association for Supervision and Curriculum Development.

Goals 2000: Educate America Act of 1994, PL 103-227, 20 U.S.C. §§ 5801 *et seq.*

Good, R.H., & Kaminski, R.A. (Eds.). (2002). *Dynamic Indicators of Basic Early Literacy Skills* (6th ed.). Eugene, OR: Institute for the Development of Educational Achievement.

Good, R.H., Simmons, D.C., & Kame'enui, E.J. (2001). The importance of decision-making utility of a continuum of fluency-based indicators of foundational reading skills for third-grade high-stakes outcomes. *Scientific Studies of Reading, 5,* 257–288.

Gray, C.A. (2004). Social Stories 101: The new defining criteria and guidelines. *Jenison Autism Journal: Creative Ideas in Practice, 15,* 2–21.

Gray, C.A., & Garand, J.D. (1993). Social Stories: Improving responses of students with autism with accurate social information. *Focus on Autistic Behavior, 8,* 1–10.

Hanushek, E.A., Kain, J.F., & Rivkin, S.G. (1999). *Do higher salaries buy better teachers?* Paper presented at the Annual Meeting of the American Economic Association, New York. (ERIC Document Reproduction Service No. ED437710)

Heumann, J.E., & Warlick, K.R. (2001). *Guidance on including students with disabilities in assessment programs.* (Memorandum OSEP 01-06). Washington, DC: U.S. Department of Education, Office of Special Education Programs. (ERIC Document Reproduction Service No. ED450540)

Individuals with Disabilities Education Act Amendments (IDEA) of 1997, PL 105-17, 20 U.S.C. §§ 1400 *et seq.*

Individuals with Disabilities Education Improvement Act (IDEA) of 2004, PL 108-446, 20 U.S.C. §§ 1400 *et seq.*

Johnstone, C.J., Altman, J., Thurlow, M.L., & Thompson, S.J. (2006). *A summary of research on the effects of test accommodations: 2002 through 2004* (Technical Report 45). Minneapolis: University of Minnesota, National Center on Educational Outcomes.

Krentz, J., Thurlow, M.L., & Callender, S. (2000). *Accountability systems and counting students with disabilities* (Technical Report 29). Minneapolis: University of Minnesota, National Center on Educational Outcomes.

Kuoch, H., & Mirenda, P. (2003). Social Story interventions for young children with autism spectrum disorders. *Focus on Autism and Other Developmental Disabilities, 18,* 219–227.

Marzano, R.J., Pickering, D.J., & Pollock, J.E. (2001). *Classroom instruction that works: Research-based strategies for increasing student achievement.* Alexandria, VA: Association for Supervision and Curriculum Development.

Mastropieri, M.A., & Scruggs, T.E. (2007). *The inclusive classroom strategies for effective instruction.* Upper Saddle River, NJ: Merrill/Prentice Hall.

Mayer-Johnson. (2000). *Writing with Symbols.* Solana Beach, CA: Author.

McMillan, J.H. (1997). *Classroom assessment.* Boston: Allyn & Bacon.

Moody, S.W., Vaughn, S., Hughes, M.T., & Fischer, M. (2000). Reading instruction in the resource room: Set up for failure. *Exceptional Children, 66,* 305–316.

Moore, P.S. (2004). The use of Social Stories in a psychology service for children with learning disabilities: A case study of a sleep problem. *British Journal of Learning Disabilities, 32,* 133–138.

National Commission on Education. (1983). *A nation at risk: The imperative for educational reform.* Washington, DC: Author. Retrieved March 5, 2007, from http://www.ed.gov/pubs/NatAtRisk/index.html

National Council of Teachers of English & International Reading Association. (1996). *Standards of the English language arts.* Urbana, IL: Author.

National Council of Teachers of Mathematics (NCTM). (2000). *Principles and standards for school mathematics.* Reston, VA: Author.

National Research Council. (1996). *National science education standards.* Washington, DC: National Academies Press.

No Child Left Behind Act of 2001, PL 107-110, 115 Stat. 1425, 20 U.S.C. §§ 6301 *et seq.*

Nolet, V., & Mclaughlin, M.J. (2000). *Accessing the general curriculum including students with disabilities in standards-based reform.* Thousand Oaks, CA: Corwin Press.

North Carolina Department of Public Instruction. (2007). *North Carolina testing program.* Retrieved July 23, 2007, from http://www.ncpublicschools.org/docs/accountability/policyoperations/nctpassessmentoptions.pdf

Oregon Department of Education. (2007). *Assessment and testing topics.* Retrieved July 23, 2007, from http://www.ode.state.or.us/teachlearn/testing/admin/juried/asmtjuriedmanual200607.pdf

Partin, R.L. (2005). *Classroom teachers survival guide* (2nd ed.). San Francisco: Jossey-Bass.

Pennsylvania Department of Education. (1973). *Study on homework: Homework policies in the public schools of Pennsylvania and selected states in the nation.* Harrisburg, PA: Author.

Rehabilitation Act of 1973, PL 93-112, 29 U.S.C. §§ 701 *et seq.*

Scattone, D., Wilczynski, S.M., Edwards, R., & Rabian, B. (2002). Decreasing disruptive behavior of children with autism using Social Stories. *Journal of Autism and Developmental Disorders, 12,* 535–543.

Schulte, A.C., Osborne, S.S., & Erchul, W.P. (1998). Effective special education: A United States dilemma. *School Psychology Review, 27,* 66–77.

Sireci, S.G., Scarpati, S.E., & Li, S. (2005). Test accommodations for students with disabilities: An analysis of the interaction hypothesis. *Review of Educational Research, 75,* 457–490.

Snell, M., & Brown, F. (Eds.). (2006). *Instruction of students with severe disabilities* (6th ed.). Upper Saddle River, NJ: Merrill/Prentice Hall.

Snell, M.E., & Loyd, B.H. (1991). A study of the effects of trend, variability, frequency, and form of data on teachers' judgments about progress and their decisions about program change. *Research in Developmental Disabilities, 12,* 41–62.

Stiggins, R.J. (2001). The unfulfilled promise of classroom assessment. *Educational Measurement: Issues and Practice, 20,* 5–15.

Stone, C.A., & Lane, S. (2003). Consequences of a state accountability program: Examining relationships between school performance gains and teachers, student, and school variables. *Applied Measurement in Education, 16,* 1–26.

Strang, R. (1973). *Homework: What research says to teachers.* Washington, DC: National Educational Association.

Texas Education Agency, Student Assessment Division. (2008, April 30). *Texas Assessment of Knowledge and Skills–Alternate (TAKS-Alt) Resources.* Available at http://www.tea.state.tx.us/student.assessment/resources/taksalt/index.html

Thompson, S.J., Johnstone, C.J., Thurlow, M.L., & Altman, J.R. (2005). *2005 state special education outcomes: Steps forward in a decade of change.* Minneapolis: University of Minnesota, National Center on Educational Outcomes.

Thompson, S.J., Morse, A.B., Sharpe, M., & Hall, S. (2005). *Accommodations manual: How to select, administer, and evaluate use of accommodations for instruction and assessment of students with disabilities.* Washington, DC: Council of Chief State School Officers.

Thurlow, M. (2003). Biting the bullet: Including special-needs students in accountability systems. In S.H. Fuhrman & R.F. Elmore (Eds.), *Redesigning accountability systems for education* (pp. 115–137). New York: Teachers College Press.

Thurlow, M.L., & Johnson, D.R. (2000). High-stakes testing of students with disabilities. *Journal of Teacher Education, 51,* 305–314.

Thurlow, M.L., Ysseldyke, J.E., & Silverstein, B. (1995). Testing accommodations for students with disabilities. *Remedial and Special Education, 16,* 260–270.

Title 1: Improving the academic achievement of the disadvantaged: Individuals with Disabilities Education Act Final Rule, 68 Fed. Reg. 236 (December 9, 2003).

Title 1: Improving the academic achievement of the disadvantaged: Individuals with Disabilities Education Act Final Rule, 72 Fed. Reg. 67 (April 9, 2007).

U.S. Department of Education. (2005). *Alternate achievement standards for students with the most significant cognitive disabilities: Non-regulatory guidance.* Washington, DC: Author. Retrieved March 3, 2007, from http://www.ed.gov/policy/elsec/guid/altguidance.doc

Virginia Department of Education. (2007). *Procedures for participation of students with disabilities in Virginia's accountability system.* Retrieved June 23, 2007, from http://www.doe.virginia.gov/VDOE/Assessment/Participation_Guidelines_for_SWD.pdf

Will, M. (1986). Educating children with learning problems: A shared responsibility. *Exceptional Children, 52,* 411–415.

World Health Organization. (2001). *The International Classification of Functioning, Disability, and Health (ICF).* Retrieved July 23, 2007, from http://www.who.int/classifications/icf/site/intros/ICF-Eng-Intro.pdf

Worthen, B.R., & Sanders, J.S. (1997). *Program evaluation: Alternative approaches and practical guidelines* (2nd ed.). New York: Longman.

Ysseldyke, J., Nelson, J.R., Christenson, S., Johnson, D.R., Dennison, A., Triezenberg, H., et al. (2004). What we know and need to know about consequences of high-stakes testing for students with disabilities. *Exceptional Children, 71,* 75–94.

2

Assessment of
Early Communication Skills

June E. Downing

Students who do not use speech fluently often struggle to convey their thoughts and wishes (Downing, 2005; Sigafoos, Arthur-Kelly, & Butterfield, 2006; Snell, Chen, & Hoover, 2006). Their difficulties can result from a number of related or uniquely different causes. They may not have learned a symbolic means of communication and, therefore, expressing any kind of abstract ideas becomes especially challenging. They may have significant physical disabilities that make it difficult to demonstrate what they know. They may not have been provided with the necessary augmentative and alternative communication (AAC) supports to give them another means of communication. They may have serious health concerns that have preoccupied the focus of care providers. In general, they may have been raised in an environment where communication has not been supported or encouraged for a variety of reasons. Despite the lack of strong communication skills, however, these students have much to say and need to be supported to express themselves.

When students do not use speech, they will communicate via alternative means, whether aided (device use) or unaided (gesture, manual signs). Students who use AAC convey their thoughts and wishes through a variety of means including, but not limited to, body movements, facial expressions, conventional gestures, vocalizations, pictures, objects, and devices that can range from low to high technology. For many students with emergent communication skills, clearly expressing what they wish to say to others, especially when unfamiliar, can be extremely difficult and frustrating. The necessary first steps to support their communication efforts are understanding how they are communicating, what they are trying to say, to whom they are communicating, and under what conditions. Therefore, assessment of students' communication skills is a critical step in the intervention process.

This chapter presents recommended practice in assessing students of all ages who are beginning communicators and may use AAC in a limited manner. The rationale for using authentic assessment for these individuals is explained as well as a description of strategies used to obtain important assessment information. Examples of assessments of different students from preschool through high school within typical educational environments are used to clarify recommended practices.

IMPORTANCE OF ASSESSING BEGINNING COMMUNICATION SKILLS

Identifying strengths and determining critical first steps in intervention can be challenging given the often unique and at times subtle communication strategies of students who are just beginning to express themselves. A careful analysis of present communication skills, however, is necessary to ensure that strategies used to increase these skills are most effective.

Being able to effectively communicate with others has an effect on all areas of life. In fact, effective communication could be considered a hallmark of a quality life (Lund & Light, 2006; Threats & Worrall, 2004). Most obviously, communication allows a person to control his or her environment (social and physical) at least to some extent. Communicating allows individuals to obtain basic needs (e.g., food, drink, warmth) as well as desires (e.g., toys, free time, certain people, special outings). Communication is fundamental for allowing an individual to convey decisions and choices that have an effect on his or her life to others and thus forms the foundation for learning self-determination skills. When communication skills are limited and/or not clear to others, as is the case with many students who need AAC, the frustration can often lead to the emergence of undesired behaviors, such as self-injurious behavior and aggression against things and others (Sigafoos et al., 2006; Wacker, Berg, & Harding, 2002). Over time, if individuals feel helpless in their ability to have an effect on others and meet their basic needs, then such behaviors can become more frequent and interfere with positive social interactions. Such a correlation between communication and challenging behavior has been clearly documented in the research (Hetzroni & Roth, 2003; Sigafoos, O'Reilly, Drasgow, & Reichle, 2002; Wacker et al., 2002). When students cannot easily make their needs and thoughts known quickly and efficiently to others, frustration is inevitable. These students may resort to whatever means available to them (e.g., screaming, kicking, hitting, destroying property) to convey this frustration as well as attempt to say what they need to say. Giving these students more effective and conventional means of communication could obviously reduce frustration and improve their quality of life.

Finally, communication skills enhance the social environment by helping individuals understand and respond to others. Light, Arnold, and Clark (2003) wrote that a major purpose of communication is to obtain social closeness with others. Such social closeness and the development of friendships is a recognized quality-of-life indicator for all individuals. Although strong communication is not a prerequisite to forming friendships, it can certainly enhance them.

Communication plays a critical role in supporting the learning of all students. It allows students to receive information and acquire knowledge. Students obtain new information and correct misconceptions by communicating with others who are more knowledgeable. Experiences are discussed and become the foundation for early literacy experiences. Low educational expectations have been noted for students with special education needs, especially for those with more complex challenges (Roach, 2006; Spooner & Browder, 2006; Wehmeyer & Agran, 2006). The No Child Left Behind (NCLB) Act of 2001 (PL 107-110) and the Individuals with Disabilities Education Improvement Act (IDEA) of 2004 (PL 108-446) have given a greater focus on accountability and on maintaining high expectations for all students to learn (see Chapters 1 and 6).

PURPOSE OF ASSESSMENT

The most practical use for educational and communicative assessment is to determine how best to support students' learning. Assessment not only identifies deficit areas and compares developmental levels of same-age children or adults without disabilities but also identifies demands and expectations of students' frequented environments and assesses students' performance within these critical environments. Such a process is highly individualized as it focuses on students as unique participants in various activities. Students do not need to attain a series of developmentally sequenced skills prior to receiving quality intervention support—a *candidacy model* (Cress & Marvin, 2003; Snell, 2002). Instead, assessment and intervention should be closely linked and dynamic, changing as students learn new skills and are involved in different activities. Assessment must consider present needs as well as communication needs of the future.

TYPES OF ASSESSMENTS

Various types of assessment tools and processes exist for determining communication strengths and limitations of students who are beginning to communicate. Although some assessment tools evaluate student skills in isolation of a meaningful context, a preferred practice is to evaluate the students in meaningful contexts as the most optimal environment for determining strengths (Siegel & Allinder, 2005). For instance, although students may not respond to a command to perform a skill (measuring receptive communication), the fact that the command occurred outside of a meaningful activity, routine, or environment could easily be confusing. For example, in a testing situation, students, when asked to comply with the request to wave good-bye, may just sit there and not respond. They may see no purpose in performing the act. When the same students, however, are asked to wave good-bye to their teachers as they leave school, they may do just that. Those assessing students are more apt to determine their best communication abilities when the students can rely on environmental cues and expectations and are in comfortable and familiar environments. Motivation also plays a key role in performance; therefore, capturing students' communication skills when the students are highly motivated to engage in communicative exchanges should produce the best results.

CAUTIONS REGARDING THE USE OF STANDARDIZED AND NORM-REFERENCED ASSESSMENT TOOLS

A standardized and norm-referenced assessment tool holds to the premise that all students will display similar skills at similar ages and in a specific developmental order (Siegel & Allinder, 2005). Although such tools may give a general understanding of students' skills along a developmental continuum, they may fall well short of documenting true communicative skills and potential. Students may fail to display desired skills because they do not understand the reason to do so, see no reason to comply, or find the physical effort of responding too challenging. They may not demonstrate their best skills just to please an assessor, especially if the assessor is someone unfamiliar to them. Brown, Snell, and Lehr (2006) warned that standardized and norm-referenced tools may well underestimate the abilities of students, especially those with the most significant disabilities. A major concern related to assessment findings that suggest limited communication skills is that intervention might engage the students in activities that are not chronologically appropriate or meaningful.

A clear problem with standardized forms of assessment is that they fail to take into account either the demands or supports of the natural environment (Ross & Cress, 2006; Snell, 2002). Rather, the assessment may occur in an isolated environment with the students expected to respond on command to unrelated requests. The assumption is that certain communication skills are needed by everyone. The social environment, however, can have considerable influence on an individual's communication skills, both receptively and expressively. For example, the social environment at recess has expectations for receptive and expressive communication skills among peers as they socially interact. Plus, the environment will be noisy and topics of communication will be unpredictable and varied. In another situation, students are to be quiet and listen when the teacher is reading a story. Receptively they need to understand what the teacher is saying as well as the questions she asks of them. Expressively they need to respond to these direct questions. The environment is quiet and structured, with specific receptive and expressive communication needs and expectations.

Furthermore, the physical condition of the individual may preclude demonstration of a particular skill in a standard developmental sequence. For example, a student may want to direct someone's attention to an item or activity of interest but not have the physical ability to raise his or her arm and point. In addition, due to a severe physical impairment, the individual may have a greater need to request assistance to accomplish various tasks. For example, while other students are taking out their textbooks as directed by the teacher, the student with severe physical disabilities may use this as an opportunity to request help to retrieve the correct textbook. The assessment process needs to identify not only typical communication expectations of students but also opportunities in which students will need to communicate when independent performance is not possible. Standardized assessments typically do not consider such unique situations (Beukelman & Mirenda, 2005).

Therefore, analyzing the social environment to identify expectations and supports for communication is a critically important aspect of assessment. Students' social environments are influenced by their preferences, age, cultural and religious orientation, and type of home and community environment. Analysis of these natural environments should reveal what is expected communicatively so that these expectations can be compared with what students are doing. Therefore, time is not spent teaching developmentally sequenced communication skills that may not be needed or have direct application to immediate needs.

Necessary Accommodations When Using Standardized Assessments

When standardized assessments are used, certain accommodations may be necessary. A greater allotment of time should be considered to accommodate any processing issues, sensory issues, cognitive disabilities, or physical challenges. Furthermore, the test(s) may need to be given over a longer period of time to accommodate both fatigue and motivation on the part of the students. Aspects of the test may need to be interspersed across activities that the students enjoy to gain a clearer understanding of true potential (see Chapter 1).

Because students have limited or no speech, an alternate form of responding will have to be used when speech output is required (e.g., the students are to name a pictured item). Students who do not use speech can point to or reach for the correct picture or object from several options, look at the correct picture or object, or produce a sound or movement when the item of choice is visually or verbally indicated (e.g., "Is this the ball?"). Different options must be presented that are within the students' physical or visual fields. For students with severe physical disabilities, proper positioning must be determined prior to any type of assessment (whether formal or informal) to optimize the students' ability to make a clear selection (Beukelman & Mirenda, 2005). Both physical and occupational therapists can assist in determining the most functional position for the students to best support their controlled movements.

Finally, means of presenting test material will need to be altered. The position of the correct choice will need to be varied so that it is not always in the same place (e.g., middle, last). Also, repetitive presentation of the same stimulus interspersed throughout the assessment may be required to get a more accurate indication of student knowledge.

CHILD-CENTERED APPROACH TO ASSESSMENT

Instead of beginning assessment by comparing students with complex cognitive and communication needs to typically developing peers on standardized tools or on tools specifically designed for populations of children having certain kinds of disabilities, a more child-centered approach is recommended. Children with complex communication needs have unique home and school experiences. Furthermore, each child comes from a family that has specific hopes and dreams for the child. Gaining information from those most closely connected to the children provides a sound foundation for determining the children's abilities and needs (Downing, 2005; Turnbull & Turnbull, 2006).

Determining the unique physical and sensory skills of the children is a critical first step because these skills will have a direct effect on how the children are able to communicate expressively and understand what is said by others. Obtaining information from various team members on how well the students see, hear, and move will be essential for determining both receptive and expressive communication skills. For example, if a student has no functional vision and does not use speech, then an alternate form of expressive communication will probably involve the use of objects, parts of objects, gestures, and perhaps some manual signs. Visual systems for receptive communication will not be appropriate. For a student with physical disabilities, it is imperative to determine the most efficient movements, both in direction and precision, and the range of movements. Such information must be considered when determining the most appropriate forms of AAC for the student to use.

GATHERING INFORMATION FROM
FAMILIES AND OTHER TEAM MEMBERS

Those individuals who are close to the students and have spent years observing the children and inter-acting with them will be able to provide a wealth of information that is highly individualized and reflects the religious and cultural aspects of the children. A critical starting point for meaningful assessment is to talk to family members to obtain information on how the children are communicat-ing in the home (the most comfortable and familiar environment), what the children are communi-cating about, if there are challenges regarding understanding the children or the children making needs understood, and what communication goals they feel would be most critical for the children. See Figure 2.1 for sample questions that can be asked of family members to start the assessment process. Obviously, the preferences and goals of the family for communication must be considered seriously. Family members have different ideas regarding how they would like the children to com-municate (e.g., aided communication via certain types of pictures; unaided communication through the use of gestures, manual signs, and speech when possible). They have the greatest wealth of knowl-edge regarding what procedures have helped the students in the past and where the students demon-strate the most effective communication strategies. They also know situations that appear to cause the greatest frustration and where intervention may be most needed initially. Such information helps pro-vide a baseline for additional information that can be gathered in other less familiar environments.

To obtain the desired information for an individual student, one member of the educational team who has established a rapport with the student's family should initiate the meeting at a time and place convenient for family members. The aim of the meeting is to obtain quality information regarding current communication skills (form and function, whether the student primarily initiates or responds) as well as current and presumed future needs. The team member's role is to encourage detailed responses with which to share with other team members as a starting point for additional assessment. Specific questions can be asked to elicit as much information as possible from those

---

Child: _____   Age: _____

Family member responding: _____   Date: _____

Interviewer: _____

1. How does your child let you know he or she wants something to eat or drink or to play with?
2. How does your child let you know he or she wants to do something different?
3. What does your child do when he or she is happy? When he or she really likes some-thing?
4. What does your child do when he or she is unhappy and does not want something?
5. How does your child tell you he or she is sick or in pain?
6. Does your child initiate interactions with family members? How does he or she do this? For what purposes?
7. How does your child interact with other children? Are there certain activities that your child really seems to enjoy interacting with other children?
8. How does your child ask a question?
9. What does your child do when he or she needs your attention or help?
10. Are there certain things or situations that really seem to frustrate your child? When your child cannot seem to make his or her needs known? How does your child make it clear to you?
11. Are there communication skills that you feel need to be taught right away? Are there skills that you would like your child's educational team to work on?

Figure 2.1.   Parent interview to determine communication skills of students beginning to use AAC.

family members most familiar with the student. See Downing (2005) and Giangreco, Cloninger, and Iverson (1998) for samples of interview questions that can be used as is or adapted to accommodate different situations[1]. The *Behavior Indication Assessment Scale* in Sigafoos et al. (2006) provides a detailed checklist of options that also can be used to assist family members in recalling critical information. Although a face-to-face meeting with family member(s) is recommended, interview information of this nature can also be achieved over the telephone.

Considering the family's culture, religion, values, beliefs, and language is important during a communication assessment. A properly trained interpreter will be needed when gathering information from families who do not speak English (Chen, Chan, & Brekken, 2000). Students who live in households in which English is not spoken or only spoken infrequently will undoubtedly perform more effectively when communicating in their first language. Some individuals will respond to information presented in their native language and use an alternative mode of communication expressively (e.g., pictures, gestures, objects). IDEA 2004 (as well as previous authorizations of this act) clearly mandates the need to assess all children in their native language. Although little research exists on assessment and intervention for learners who have significant disabilities and are learning English (Mueller, Singer, & Carranza, 2006), care must be taken to make sure that any interaction with individuals is respectful of cultural beliefs and that the native language is used by the assessor. Furthermore, respecting cultural beliefs regarding disabilities, intervention, and assessment is critical to developing the trust needed to ensure an exchange of accurate information (Rogers-Adkinson, Ochoa, & Delgado, 2003).

Interviewing other team members regarding the communication skills of the students can serve as a baseline, provide additional information, or confirm information already obtained. Team members, such as teachers, paraprofessionals, related service providers, and friends, can describe communication strengths and needs of the students (Cascella & McNamara, 2004). Examples of communication skills can be given across the day in typical activities. Also, situations in which the students may struggle to convey their thoughts can be identified. Team members can be asked what communicative behavior they would most like the students to attain—what they consider to be most important. This information keeps the focus for intervention on the communicative behavior that should be most useful to the children and socially valid.

OBSERVATIONS OF STUDENTS

Careful observations of children and youth in their natural environments, home, school, and community are recommended to obtain the most reliable authentic information. As stated previously, children need to be observed in natural and age-appropriate activities and routines that are familiar and in which the children feel fairly comfortable. Familiar activities will allow the children to demonstrate optimal communication skills, especially if activities are preferred and there are responsive communication partners (Davern, Schnorr, & Black, 2003; Snell, 2002).

Ecological and Observational Assessment Practices

An ecological and observational assessment procedure is recommended to determine what type of AAC support beginning communicators need (Siegel & Allinder, 2005; Sigafoos et al., 2006). Students need to be observed in a variety of typical activities and environments to get a more complete idea of changing communication demands and needs. Children will be most familiar with the routines in typical environments and more aware of what their communication skills can attain for them. Multiple observations of students in such environments (at home, in school, at parks and

---

[1]The Communication Matrix by Dr. Charity Rowland (available online at http://www.communicationmatrix.org) and the *MacArthur-Bates Communicative Developmental Inventories* by Fenson et al. (2007) can be used by parents and caregivers to document the child's early communication and language content and forms.

swimming pools) can provide a much more thorough and accurate picture of students' communication skills than a checklist of skills that may not relate to any recognizable activity or environment. Therefore, once initial information has been obtained from the families regarding their observations and goals for their children, an in-context observation is recommended.

One way to structure observational assessments that target communication is to create a form that specifies the steps of typical activities and the expected communication skills per step. Figure 2.2 provides an example of a sixth-grade science class with one student who has disabilities and uses AAC. This science class at a local middle school is representative of the majority of class times taught by this teacher. As such, it is a good class to assess.

The first column designates the steps expected of typical sixth graders (e.g., come into classroom, take notes, work cooperatively in a small group to do a project). A team member trained to analyze typical activities can jot down the steps of the activity as they occur. The second column identifies natural cues in the environment and activity that serve to indicate to students the desired behavior (e.g., the teacher talking cues students to listen and take notes). Identifying these natural cues is important so that it can become clear whether the target student is recognizing and responding to such cues or needs additional instructional support. As the person analyzing the activity watches it unfold, natural cues that preceded the expected behavior of the students in the first column can be recorded. At times these cues are easily observable (e.g., the teacher calls on a student), and at other times they can be less clear (e.g., the natural cue for students raising their hands is to get help with some aspect of the lesson). The person documenting these natural cues could list several cues (observed and implied) for each step of the activity.

The third column states whether the step in the first column, which is the desired student behavior, requires or expects communication skills (e.g., while the teacher is talking, students need receptive communication skills sufficient to understand what is being said and should not be engaged in expressive communication). The observer must note per step what the expected communication skills are from the perspective of the student (e.g., to receptively understand the teacher or peer, to expressively make a comment or ask a question). Not every step will have required communication skills, although many will.

The fourth column documents the target student's performance according to each step in the lesson. The recording of data can involve a simple plus sign (+) to represent independent performance and a dash (−) to represent the lack of desired behavior. Another option is to use this column to represent the level of assistance provided (e.g., full assistance, partial assistance). The fifth column identifies the reason for the discrepancy (e.g., why the student did not perform as expected), and the observer makes an educated guess regarding the student and documents potential reasons (e.g., physically cannot use speech, has no alternative form of communication, not motivated to respond).

The final column provides initial suggestions to support the student to learn. The observer writes down brief ideas that could lead to helping the student engage more effectively in the desired communicative behavior (e.g., using a simple pictorial communication system, training peers how to best interact). This final column will be refined as more team members contemplate what could help the student be more successful and as different strategies are tried. The overall goal is to help the child be an active learner in the activity. In this manner, the assessment is linked directly to likely intervention. The assessment stems from the actual social environment of the student (authentic) and leads directly to practical ways to intervene (see Downing, 2005, for additional examples).

Analyzing the Social Environment

The social environment surrounding the students contains critical information that must be determined before a complete assessment can be made. Identifying the communication demands and opportunities of natural environments is a necessary step in the assessment process because no individual exists in a vacuum and the context determines to a large extent the desired communication skills. Determining the people in the students' natural environments who support their commu-

Student: _Blaine_   Age: _11_   Grade: _6_   Class: _Science_   Activity: _Study of rocks_

Steps that peers without disabilities perform	Natural cues that prompt the behavior in Column 1	Communication skills needed (receptive and expressive)	Student performance (+, p, or —)	Discrepancy analysis	Initial intervention ideas
Enter class	Sees door to class, others entering, knows schedule	None	—	Cannot push himself in his wheelchair, unsure of next class	Teach him to request assistance from a peer.
Find seat and sit down	Empty seat, knows seating arrangement	None	—	Cannot push himself in his wheelchair, unsure of where he is to sit	Prompt peer to ask him where he is to go and wait for him to look or gesture in the right direction.
Listen to the teacher	Teacher explaining the lesson, others are listening	Receptive: Understands what the teacher is saying	p	Appears to be listening, but the material may be too abstract	Provide pictorial/object information that goes with the lesson; teach him to use symbol on device to say if he does not understand.
Take notes on information and ask questions if unclear	Hears teacher present information, wants to have a hard copy of what is said, does not understand something stated	Receptive: Understands what is said and questions asked by peers Expressive: States a question as needed	—	Is nonverbal, does not write, does not understand information	Use simplified notes on main ideas with blanks in sentences that he must fill in by choosing the correct picture
Answer questions posed by teacher	Teacher asking questions, knowledge of the information	Receptive: Understands the questions asked and responses from peers Expressive: Responds to questions	—	Is not verbal, material is very abstract and difficult to understand	Have him randomly choose peers to answer questions or choose the questions to ask using a spinner. Teacher asks him a basic question, and he responds using real items or pictures.

		Communication skills	p		
Get into groups of four	Teacher direction, recognizes other members of the group	*Receptive:* Understands what the teacher has said	p	May understand the teacher but cannot physically maneuver into his group	Paraprofessional asks him where his group is and shows him pictures of peers for him to indicate group members. Peer pushes him to his group.
Use computer to investigate properties of type of rock assigned	Teacher assigns type of rock to group, knowledge of how to search the Internet, sees information on the computer screen	*Receptive:* Understands assignment and comments by peers *Expressive:* Makes suggestions to group	—	May not understand the type of rock assigned, cannot physically gain access to the computer, does not know how to type	Use a switch interface that allows him to click on pictures on the Internet or ask his preference regarding pictures to download from the Internet. Provide symbols to allow him to say that it is his turn and to make comments on what peers are doing.
Write report as a group, filling in blanks on a form provided	Blank form, information obtained from the search, having opinions to share	*Receptive:* Understands ideas suggested by others *Expressive:* Gives suggestions	—	Nonverbal, cannot write, information is very abstract	Ask him to make some decisions regarding what illustrations to use. Ask him some simple questions regarding color and size to go in report using pictorial options.
Sign names and turn report into teacher	End of class period, teacher direction, others turning in their reports	*Receptive:* Understands teacher direction	—	Does not write his name, physically difficult to handle paper	Offer him three signature stamps, and ask him to pick the one with his name. Have him collect every group's report on his tray. Ask peer to push him to teacher.

Figure 2.2. Ecological inventory to identify communication expectations and skills of a student in a sixth-grade science class. (Key: +, independent performance; p, performance with partial assistance; — performance with full assistance.)

nicative efforts is important. Obviously, environments containing highly responsive communication partners will provide greater support for the children to attempt exchanges than environments where few or no competent partners exist. Research supports inclusive educational environments in part due to the opportunities for interactions with capable and responsive same-age communication partners (Fisher & Meyer, 2002; McSheehan, Sonnenmeier, & Jorgensen, 2002; vonTetzchner, Brekke, Sjothun, & Grindheim, 2005).

Assessing expectations for communicative competence can be drawn from typical communicative exchanges that occur within typical school environments. What a same-age person in the same activity and environment needs or wants to be able to communicate can be used as a baseline criterion. For instance, in most classrooms students are expected to follow teacher directions (receptive communication skills), ask questions or ask for assistance (expressive communication skill of requesting information or help), discuss a topic with a peer or teacher (expressive communication skill of commenting/sharing information), respond to direct questions from the teacher (expressive communication skill to share information or confirm or deny information), and engage in social interactions with peers. All of the previous expressive communication skills also require receptive communication skills to be able to understand expectations. Once it is clear what communication skills are expected or required in various situations frequented by the students, then observations and interview data from those most familiar with the children can identify what skills the children demonstrate and where there are discrepancies.

A few formal assessment tools have been developed to analyze the communicative environment. Blackstone and Hunt-Berg (2003) developed a tool to gain an understanding of the communication opportunities and partners available to an individual with significant communication difficulties. *Social Networks* stresses the importance of family input in the assessment process and collects information on the skills and abilities of the individual, available communication partners, modes of expressive communication, means of selecting messages, and topics of conversation. Support strategies used with the individual are also documented. The focus of data collection is on the social interactions within typical environments.

Rowland and Schweigert (1993) developed the *Analyzing the Communication Environment (ACE): An Inventory of Ways to Encourage Communication in Functional Activities*. Designed specifically for children with severe and multiple disabilities, including deafblindness, this observational tool provides examples and general guidelines of what to look for with regard to the activity itself, how the student communicates, how the adult interacts, and specific communication opportunities. The presence and role of more competent communicators who can support the target child's emerging communication skills is highlighted. This checklist is designed to help the evaluator consider various components of the communication environment for the child as part of the assessment process.

Finally, the National Joint Committee for the Communication Needs of Persons with Severe Disabilities (NJC; 1998) produced its *Communication Supports Checklist for Programs Serving Individuals with Severe Disabilities*. This tool is designed to help educational teams determine the strengths and limitations of their program with regard to facilitating communication development. The checklist asks a program to consider whether the natural setting is supportive of students' communication development and whether current practices are in line with recommended practice in the field. The focus is on the social and physical environment of the students and whether the team has the knowledge and skills to support those who use AAC. An action plan can be designed to address the limitations identified and enhance the environment for the target students.

Determining How the Student Communicates

It is important to determine how students are communicating when they are not engaging in symbolic forms of communication (e.g., speech, sign). At different times and in different situations, children will use different means of communication to convey their thoughts. Students might use their eyes to look or blink, their heads or hands to gesture, their feet or legs to indicate a need, or any movement they have to confirm or deny what is said or to draw attention. Students also can vocalize (scream, grunt, giggle, whine) to convey a message. They can make use of objects, parts of objects, and/or pictures (Beukelman & Mirenda, 2005; Downing, 2005). Students without disabilities also make use of similar means to express themselves, so these are not abnormal means of communication. Without the use of symbolic communication, however, assessment practices must carefully document the many ways in which students can and do communicate and whether these methods of communication are acceptable and effective in order to determine appropriate intervention.

Students who need AAC engage in multiple forms of communication to express a variety of thoughts and needs. An assessment process should identify how the students demonstrate understanding (receptive communication) as well as how the students convey different purposes of communication (expressive communication). A simple table can be used to document the various ways a particular child communicates (see Figure 2.3). Detailed information can be recorded regarding how a student currently communicates within typical activities and routines. How the student communicates may be effective and socially acceptable at times (e.g., a look or high-five to greet a peer), although at other times the behavior may be socially unacceptable (e.g., kicks or bites to gain attention) or ineffective (e.g., no means to share information about fears or fun experiences). Determining how the student is currently communicating provides a foundation to add other means as needed.

Determining Reasons for the Student to Communicate

Typical activities and environments provide many opportunities for children and youth to communicate. Identifying the ways that children use communicative behavior—for what purposes—will

Behavior purposes	Cries	Kicks or hits	Smiles, laughs	Touches pictures	Moves body toward pre-ferred item or person
Requests a change in position or to eat	X				X
Requests continuation of an action			X (being swung)		X (being tickled by paraprofes-sional)
Requests certain foods or toys				X (computer access)	
Rejects an activity	X (being positioned in a stander)	X (blocks)			
Social (greets someone)			X (peer)		X (Mom)

Figure 2.3.   Documentation of different forms of behavior for communicative intent for a preschool child.

provide not only considerable information regarding skills the students demonstrate but also areas of potential need. Therefore, the many purposes for communication expressed by students must be part of the data collection. Children and youth communicate to request or reject items, people, or actions; confirm or deny information; make comments about things; share information; ask questions; and achieve social closeness (Downing, 2005; Iacono, 2003; Snell et al., 2006).

At times, the individual may be engaging in the same behavior for different reasons. For example, a student may scream for attention and to reject a task being asked of him or her. Without the benefit of symbolic communication, the assessor may need to consider environmental factors (e.g., people present, objects in view, time of day) to determine the communicative function of the student's behavior. This information can be recorded on the form shown in Figure 2.1. Such information highlights any limitations; for example, the student only engages in requesting behavior and very limited other functions of communication such as achieving social closeness, directing attention, and commenting. Such a finding would suggest that the teacher support the student's use of other functions of communication and broaden communicative skills.

Determining Topics of Communication: What Students Converse About

Determining what students typically talk about can provide information regarding motivational factors for the students. Social situations will affect conversational topics, but an individual's interests also play a role. Children may not be motivated to talk about math or chores, but they may be motivated to talk about making cookies, playing with their pet hamster, or swimming. Finding out what are considered appropriate and motivating topics of conversation for a student of a particular age can help guide the assessment in determining what the target student is able to communicate about and where support may be needed. Objects, parts of objects, and pictures with messages attached can all be used to support a student's efforts to communicate regarding different topics of need or interest. Observing the student during social times of the day, such as recess, lunch, or free time, is recommended to document how other students are interacting, how the target student interacts, and where discrepancies exist that need attention.

In addition to obtaining the information on how students communicate (form), why students communicate (function), and what students communicate about (content), observations should also document with whom the students typically engage in conversations (social partners) and whether the students initiate communication interactions or respond to others. The purpose of gathering this information is to determine the breadth of the students' social circles so as to increase that pool as needed and to document the students' initiative in engaging others. It is important to determine if students need support in assuming a more proactive and spontaneous role because many students who use AAC assume the role of a passive participant in most communicative exchanges (Carter, 2002; Halle, 1987). Finally, information from interviewing significant others and observation of students in typical activities across environments should indicate whether the students can repair communication breakdowns and the manner in which that occurs. Communication breakdowns typically occur with students using AAC (Brady & Halle, 2002), and, therefore, it is important to document how the students deal with these breakdowns, how repairs are made, and whether the students need to learn skills in this area. For example, the student will need a way to say, "No, I'm not saying that. Try again." Such messages would need to be added to the device and then taught to the student.

ECOLOGICAL ASSESSMENT
PROCESS: WHAT IS ENOUGH INFORMATION?

Assessment is an ongoing process and with quality intervention should show progress made by students over time. As team members become more familiar with a student's skills in AAC, less comprehensive assessments may be needed. For a student who is new to team members or who has not received any instruction in the area of AAC and is just beginning to make needs known to others, a more time-consuming and comprehensive assessment is recommended. Certainly the team will want to gain information from significant others as described previously in this chapter as a starting point for any assessment procedures. An ecological analysis of as many critical and typical environments for the student as possible (by different team members if needed) is recommended. The main goal, however, is to get at the breadth of different social and physical environments for any given student. Therefore, it would be appropriate to gather information from four or five of the student's critical activities to show the diversity of environmental demands and communication needs, strengths, and limitations of the student. Consideration should be given to opportunities to interact with peers as well as adults, and this variable should be included when activities are assessed. Findings should indicate whether these critical activities are providing sufficient opportunities for the student to develop communication skills as well as how that student performs in those activities.

Once the activities have been analyzed for their communicative potential and for the general involvement of the student, careful observation of exactly what the student is doing communicatively within these activities is needed. Although no rules or regulations exist for the amount of time spent on such observations, perhaps at a minimum a total of 10–15 minutes per activity during a step(s) of the activity that specifically involves interactions with others (e.g., recess, lunch, cooperative learning groups, paired reading) is advisable. Data collected and compiled for these observations should reflect information discussed earlier on form, function, content, initiations, responses, and repair strategies. This data in turn should lead to specific areas of intervention and the development of an IEP to address needs.

Examples of Students with AAC Needs—Assessment

The following examples demonstrate the information provided in this chapter for four students (preschool to high school) within typical classrooms. Despite considerable challenges, these four students have skills that they are using and also have specific areas of need regarding communication within their educational environment. The intent of the assessment of these four students is not to assign a developmental level to their communication skills but to identify what they need to communicate in various settings at school and to begin to identify what supports could be helpful in meeting those needs.

The Preschool Child   Jaiden is a preschool student who uses AAC.

_____   At 4 years old, Jaiden is a happy child who loves music and moving his body to music. His favorite foods are chocolate pudding and applesauce, and he loves to swim in warm water and have his dogs lick his face. Jaiden has no speech and is blind. He communicates with vocalizations, body movements, and actions on objects. He is nonambulatory but is able to bear his weight. Jaiden can hear from his left ear and uses his hands, although in more gross motoric ways, to carefully examine something tactilely (he likes to wave his arms up and down and is particular about what he touches). He attends a typical preschool close to his mother's work and is the only child with severe disabilities at the school, although a few children have other types of disabilities.

Jaiden's assessment began with his family, who gave information regarding his communication at home and activities and items of interest. With this information serving as a baseline of his communication skills, the team, which included the preschool teacher, special educator, paraprofessional, speech-language pathologist (SLP), and vision specialist, observed Jaiden in typical activities of the preschool. They observed Jaiden in small-group activities both indoors and outdoors, playing with one other peer, interacting with an adult, and in preferred as well as nonpreferred activities. Using an ecological inventory that depicts the communication demands and expectations of various activities in the preschool environment, team members observed when Jaiden was able to understand and make his needs and thoughts known to others. Discrepancies were identified, which lead directly into accommodations and adaptations for Jaiden to support his communication efforts. Observations across different activities confirmed parental information regarding his present communicative behavior. Although at times his requesting behavior via the use of touching objects was effective (e.g., he could choose a preferred toy to play with or a preferred food item at lunch using actual items), several times during the day Jaiden needed additional communicative supports to fully participate in typical preschool activities.

Although Jaiden's hearing is functional and he does respond to several communicative actions of others, he needed help on frequent occasions understanding what others were referring to. Expressive communication needs were evident during play times with peers who may not have known how to support his efforts. They will need to be taught how to interact with someone who is blind—how to present options tactilely while also speaking. They will also need to learn how Jaiden expresses his thoughts via the use of hand and arm movements and objects. Because Jaiden rarely initiated interactions and waited until an adult approached him with a question, a communication goal written for Jaiden as a result of the assessment stated, "When Jaiden obviously needs help with something, he will either raise his hand or hold up an object to gain someone's attention 70% of all appropriate opportunities in a 2-week period." Other goals addressed his need to interact effectively with peers. _____

The Elementary Child   Oliver is an elementary school–age student with AAC needs.

_____   Oliver is 9 years old and in the third grade of his neighborhood school. Oliver loves being around people, especially his peers and a particular paraprofessional. Although he wears a helmet for seizures, Oliver likes to move around outside and is ambulatory. He does not use speech to communicate but does use eye gaze, pointing, pictures, and objects. All work in his third-grade class is adapted to meet his cognitive needs. He often will refuse to respond in work situations and is easily distracted by others.

Based on initial information from the family, the assessment of Oliver's communication skills was carried out by the special educator, paraprofessional, and SLP. Structured observations occurred across different classroom activities, such as a language arts whole-class discussion, a social studies small-group activity, a math game with a peer, and a science experiment with three other students. These typical activities were representative of his third-grade class. Oliver was also observed at recess playing with friends and at lunch.

Ecological inventories of these natural environments and activities indicate that Oliver's receptive communication needs include listening to and understanding the teacher's and his peers' comments, questions, and directions. Expressive communication needs included greeting others, asking questions, making comments, sharing information, and requesting items. Observers also documented the communicative behaviors Oliver was using appropriately, such as eye gaze to share a joint referent, pointing to some pictures and items he wants, and occasionally greeting someone with a nod (which all confirmed information attained from his family). Although he had a clear way to reject activities or items (by screaming), a more conventional and appropriate way to reject was needed. Oliver also needed alternate ways to ask questions, share information, and make comments about his life (e.g., a pictorial conversation book). Based on his strengths (present communicative behaviors), intervention could then address communication needs in these environments. One communication goal for Oliver read, "When Oliver wants to reject a person, object, or activity, he will either turn his head to the side and look away or gently push the person or item away for 75% of all such opportunities for 1 week." Another goal for Oliver was "When sitting or standing next to a peer during lunch or recess for 3 minutes, Oliver will hand a picture/message card to a peer asking the peer to play or will point to one picture/message in his conversation book for 10 consecutive lunch or recess periods." _____

The Middle School Student   Rosa is a middle school student who uses AAC.

_____   Rosa was in a special school during her elementary years but is now in seventh grade and in her second year at an inclusive magnet school in her community. Rosa is fascinated by her peers and is very popular. She is very petite for her age, and although she can walk with assistance (personal or a walker), she uses a wheelchair for longer distances. She does not speak but uses eye gaze, reaching to objects, and pictures to convey her thoughts. She looks away from things she does not want. She loves bright colors and to manipulate paper.

Her mother contributed considerable information pertaining to how Rosa communicates at home, which was supported by a paraprofessional who also assists Rosa in her home. Because Rosa attends seventh-grade classes with her peers, all of the classes were assessed as well as lunch and a nutrition break. Classes that Rosa attends include language arts, social studies, science, math, physical education, drama, homeroom, and study skills. Each of these environments offer slightly different communication opportunities for Rosa and require somewhat different communicative expressions from her.

In her middle school academic classes, large-group discussions occurred with question and answer periods throughout. Rosa needed a way to understand what was discussed at her level of understanding and in ways that related to her life (static information needed versus speech). She also needed a way to participate in the discussions (to ask questions and respond to simple questions). Observations of cooperative learning groups in these classes revealed a need to interact with peers, share information, ask questions and ask for help, and make comments regarding the process or final product. In all classes, as well as lunch and nutrition, there were communication needs to follow directions, socially interact with peers (e.g., initiating interactions, responding to others), and make her needs known (e.g., request help, a break, or water).

Although several peers initiated interactions with her throughout the day, Rosa rarely initiated interactions with them, unless it was a specific request to walk. She did smile appropriately to comments made by her peers and could point to objects and some pictures in response to a direct question. Rosa clearly needed a means to allow her to easily initiate interactions and engage her peers in social conversations about her life and interests. As a result of this assessment, a goal written for Rosa stated, "When Rosa has been sitting for 2 minutes and is unsure of what to do in class, she will hand a peer a picture/message card requesting assistance for 9 of 10 consecutive opportunities." Another goal related to her need to make comments read, "When a peer asks Rosa what she thinks of the peer's work, Rosa will use her AAC device to point to one of three possible comments for 12 of 15 consecutive opportunities." _____

The High School Student   Emma is a high school student with AAC needs.

_____   Emma is in 10th grade at her local high school. Through interviewing her grandmother and from observational assessment it was determined that Emma primarily uses eye gaze with objects and a few colored photographs, as well as facial expressions and some gestures, to communicate. She is ambulatory but uses a wheelchair for longer distances. She wears a helmet for her seizure disorder. Emma attends a number of classes including American Sign Language (ASL), photography, chemistry, physical education, ceramics, and keyboarding. These classes were selected by Emma and her educational team based on her interests, communication, social and learning needs, and the style of teaching in these classes.

The special educator and SLP have collaborated to assess all of Emma's classes plus her nutrition break and lunch to determine communication expectations and areas of needed support for Emma. From ecological assessments of the classrooms and other environments that Emma frequents, it is clear that there are many different opportunities for communication, but Emma does not have the necessary communicative supports to actively participate.

All of Emma's classes provided opportunities for her to learn vocabulary, especially the ASL class (even though she is not signing); follow directions; and interact socially with peers. Classes that offered considerable hands-on work (photography, ceramics, chemistry) showed that Emma made use of the objects present to give information and make requests. She primarily relied on a few subtle facial expressions and gestures in other classes, which did not meet all of her communication needs. Students approached her to interact and ask her questions, but she had very limited means of responding to their initiations (primarily facial expressions). She needed an effective means to share information with her peers and ask questions in return. She rarely initiated interactions with others. As a result of her assessment, a goal written for Emma stated, "When asked her opinion of something and shown three pictorial options, Emma will listen to each option as it is pointed out to her and choose within 5 seconds by looking at her choice for 9 of 10 consecutive opportunities." Other goals reflected her need to initiate interactions with others and to share information about herself through the use of pictorial/object conversation books. _____

PRACTICAL APPLICATION OF COMMUNICATION ASSESSMENT

The primary reason to assess communication skills is to support the individual in developing greater skills to more effectively affect his or her environment. Assessment information must be shared with all who are involved in supporting the individual. For the student who uses AAC and has quite unique and subtle behaviors that are used for communicative intent, sharing this identified behavior with all educational team members is a vital concern. Once the assessment process determines the form(s) of communication and intent or purpose for the individual, this information should be recorded for easy access by all who interact with the individual.

Mirenda (2005) referred to this documentation as a *communication dictionary.* In the development of this dictionary, the behavior is described, its intent for the individual is clearly stated, and suggestions are explained for how the communication partners should respond. For example, a student beginning to use AAC may raise his right knee (the form of communication) to agree with a statement made by someone else (the intent of the communicative act is to confirm), and the conversational partner should then respond accordingly. Various behaviors are explained accordingly so that all those interacting with the individual will know what the behaviors mean for the individual and respond in a consistent manner. Consistent responses to unique forms of communicative (or potential communicative) behaviors will help the student recognize that his efforts are being seen and understood and should strengthen (reinforce) those efforts.

IMPLICATIONS FOR THE FIELD

The importance of assessing beginning communication skills in individuals, regardless of age, is apparent. Effective education of these individuals will depend on how well teachers and peers can interact with students who need AAC. We need to ensure that these individuals understand what is being communicated to them and have effective and efficient means of responding as well as initiating interactions. By assessing individuals in their natural environments, which provide motivation to communicate as well as socially responsive partners, the opportunity exists to obtain the most accurate information pertaining to their communicative ability.

Instead of relying on assessment tools that provide equivalent developmental ages of receptive and expressive communication to determine intervention, examining the social-communicative environments focuses more on students' actual needs and abilities within a meaningful context. Students can be given credit for what they are able to communicate and understand under familiar and typical activities and environments versus what they can demonstrate under artificial and out-of-context settings. For the four students described in this chapter, standardized and developmentally based assessments would have indicated very basic and minimal communication skills that would be quite atypical of same-age peers. The resulting assumption might indicate that these students have very limited ability to communicate and should be treated as very young children. The tendency might be to lower expectations of these students as a result and to prevent them from experiencing typical classrooms settings. Low expectations of students with disabilities are not uncommon (Johnston, Stodden, Emanual, Luecking, & Mack, 2002) and must be consistently guarded against to ensure that all students receive an appropriate and challenging curriculum. Placing students in socially stimulating and competent environments can provide the very support these students need to engage in their most efficacious communication. Several studies have demonstrated the increased communicative interactions of students with severe and profound disabilities when educated with their peers who do not have disabilities (Fisher & Meyer, 2002; Foreman, Arthur-Kelly, Pascoe, & Smyth-King, 2004). There is no need to wait for children to demonstrate certain skills, but rather the need is to create meaningful and social environments and then provide the support and instruction that is needed.

Teaming

A team approach is recommended for the most thorough, effective, and time-efficient assessment of these students (Beukelman & Mirenda, 2005; Downing, 2005). Information can be attained from different team members working together to observe the student in a variety of school and home environments. Pooling this information provides the most comprehensive assessment of the student's skills and needs. Therefore, it is not just the SLP who assumes primary responsibility for the assessment but all members of the team who typically support the student across the school day. Furthermore, different members of the team, given their background, training, and experiences, can provide unique suggestions that could serve as effective supports for the student to facilitate optimum communication skills. For example, a physical therapist may be most knowledgeable in determining the most supportive position for the student to increase range of motion and fine motor control that are needed for accurate use of a communication device. Ensuring such support as part of the assessment process (Snell, 2002) provides a more accurate indication of what the student can communicate under optimal conditions.

Team members work cooperatively in the assessment process to identify needs, communicative opportunities, and supports needed to ensure a comprehensive assessment that ties directly to an effective intervention plan. Hunt, Soto, Maier, Müller, and Goetz (2002) stressed the importance of a collaborative teaming model to develop a unified plan of support for three elementary students using AAC in general education classrooms. Although a collaborative team does require planning time and a common vision, the combined knowledge, time, and energy from all team members to effectively assess the student contribute to a more thorough and practical evaluation.

Training Needed

For accurate data to be collected, all those collecting it need to know what to observe, what to look for, and how to identify potential communication opportunities. Once learning opportunities have been identified, assessing the student's ability to make use of such opportunities is needed. All team members will need to know what constitutes a communicative interaction for the individual, how to document that behavior, and how to identify a discrepancy for the individual that will need intervention. Ongoing training and frequent sharing and comparing of assessment data will be needed to ensure consistency and to gather the most comprehensive information on a given student.

The needs of the individual student determine 1) how the team will function, 2) what types of professional development will be needed, and 3) what topics the professional development will cover. As team members change, more training will be needed to keep the team functioning as a united whole. Sharing the responsibility for assessment and data collection not only requires additional planning and training time (Hunt et al., 2002) but also offers a more efficient approach to assessment and greater buy-in from all team members as to the importance of assessment data and effective intervention.

FUTURE RESEARCH NEEDS

The mark of a good assessment is the degree to which it can positively affect quality services for those assessed. Despite numerous recommended assessment procedures, little research exists that targets the outcomes of such procedures. Yet, teachers and other direct service providers need assessment practices that will be efficient in leading to high-quality intervention. Research is needed that compares outcomes from different assessment tools and procedures. For example, Downing and Perino (1992) investigated the perceptions of 38 teachers regarding the benefit of three different types of assessment information for a student with severe to profound multiple disabilities. Using a Likert-type scale and three different assessment packages (standardized, functional-ecological, and a combined package), teachers perceived the functional-ecological approach to be most beneficial for use in educational intervention.

Considering the assessment of the communication skills of students beginning to make use of AAC, information is needed regarding what approach produces the most meaningful outcomes for students. Once assessment information is gathered, what type of information will be most helpful to those responsible for its implementation? Furthermore, do unique characteristics of the child, family, and home environment have an effect on what type of information is most essential to obtain?

Given the importance of recognizing and respecting diverse cultures and families (Hourcade, Pilotte, West, & Parette, 2004), research in assessment of communication skills should carefully look at what types of interactions with family members are the most respectful and effective. As Light and Drager (2007) reported, there is limited research on the perspectives of parents of children who have complex communication needs. They urged that research be done to determine the perspectives and priorities of different families regarding the communication needs of their children. Such perspectives and alliances with family members are critical for a sound assessment procedure in which a child's true abilities will not be overlooked. Strategies for obtaining the most thorough and reliable information regarding a child's communication skills, while taking cultural and linguistic differences into consideration, need to be investigated.

Finally, research is needed to determine the most effective social environments that are supportive of the development of communication skills in those students who are just beginning to use AAC. Questions asked should consider what skills are necessary for communication partners, if differences emerge from having access to a certain number of competent communication partners in a given social context, and what aspects of the social environment tend to support or hinder communication skills development. Determining specific factors of the social environment that are most conducive to enhancing communication skills could lead direct services providers to spend time making the necessary changes as opposed to just focusing on the student's demonstrated skills. Given the social nature of communication, assessment must consider this factor with future research identifying critical variables related to age, culture, familial structure, and ethnicity.

CONCLUSION

This chapter has taken a strength-based approach to the assessment of students just beginning to use AAC (regardless of age) and considered aspects of the assessment process that could prove helpful in determining the most appropriate type of intervention. A systematic observational approach as suggested in this chapter assumes competency of the individual as well as the rights of the person to be a part of typical social environments. Assessment of these students needs to be done in a contextual and meaningful manner so that their strengths can be identified (what they are presently demonstrating) as well as the expectations (and supports) of the social environment for communication and the needs/desires of the student within these environments. Intervention from such an assessment should support the student's active engagement within natural activities and environments and lead to meaningful communicative exchanges. As technological advances continue to be made in the field of augmenting communication skills, supporting the needs of a student just beginning to use AAC may become easier to achieve. Hopefully, the future will hold more possibilities and more accurate ways of truly identifying effective means for each individual to use for communicative purposes.

REFERENCES

Beukelman, D.R., & Mirenda, P. (2005). *Augmentative and alternative communication: Supporting children and adults with complex communication needs* (3rd ed.). Baltimore: Paul H. Brookes Publishing Co.

Blackstone, S.W., & Hunt-Berg, M. (2003). *Social networks: A communication inventory for individuals with complex communication needs and their communication partners.* Monterey, CA: Augmentative Communication.

Brady, N.C., & Halle, J.W. (2002). Breakdowns and repairs in conversations between beginning AAC users and their partners. In D.R. Beukelman & J. Reichle (Series Eds.) & J. Reichle, D.R. Beukelman, & J.C. Light (Vol. Eds.), *Augmentative and alternative communication series: Exemplary practices for beginning communicators: Implications for AAC* (pp. 323–352). Baltimore: Paul H. Brookes Publishing Co.

Brown, F., Snell, M.E., & Lehr, D. (2006). Meaningful assessment. In M.E. Snell & F. Brown (Eds.), *Instruction of students with severe disabilities* (6th ed., pp. 67–111). Columbus, OH: Pearson.

Carter, M. (2002). Communicative spontaneity in individuals with high support needs: An exploratory consideration of causation. *International Journal of Disability, Development, and Education, 49,* 225–242.

Cascella, P.W., & McNamara, K.M. (2004). Empowering students with severe disabilities to actualize communication skills. *TEACHING Exceptional Children, 37*(3), 38–43.

Chen, D., Chan, S., & Brekken, L. (2000). *Conversations for three: Communicating through interpreters* [video and manual]. Baltimore: Paul H. Brookes Publishing Co.

Cress, C.J., & Marvin, C.A. (2003). Common questions about AAC services in early intervention. *Augmentative and Alternative Communication, 19,* 254–272.

Davern, L., Schnorr, R., & Black, J.W. (2003). Planning instruction for the diverse classroom: Approaches that facilitate the inclusion of all students. In D.L. Ryndak & S. Alper (Eds.), *Curriculum and instruction for students with significant disabilities in inclusive settings* (2nd ed., pp. 340–361). Boston: Allyn & Bacon.

Downing, J., & Perino, D.M. (1992). Functional versus standardized assessment procedures: Implications for educational programming. *Mental Retardation, 30,* 289–295.

Downing, J.E. (2005). *Teaching communication skills to students with severe disabilities* (2nd ed.). Baltimore: Paul H. Brookes Publishing Co.

Fenson, L., Marchman, V.A., Thal, D.J., Dale, P.S., Reznick, J.S., & Bates, E. (2007). *MacArthur-Bates Communicative Development Inventories (CDIs).* Baltimore: Paul H. Brookes Publishing Co.

Fisher, M., & Meyer, L.H. (2002). Development and social competence after two years for students enrolled in inclusive and self-contained educational programs. *Research and Practice for Persons with Severe Disabilities, 27,* 165–174.

Foreman, P., Arthur-Kelly, M., Pascoe, S., & Smyth-King, B. (2004). Evaluating the educational experiences of students with profound and multiple disabilities in inclusive and segregated classroom settings: An Australian perspective. *Research and Practice for Persons with Severe Disabilities, 29,* 183–193.

Giangreco, M.F., Cloninger, C.J., & Iverson, V.S. (1998). *Choosing outcomes and accommodations for children (COACH): A guide to educational planning for students with disabilities* (2nd ed.). Baltimore: Paul H. Brookes Publishing Co.

Halle, J. (1987). Teaching language in the natural environment: An analysis of spontaneity. *Journal of The Association for Persons with Severe Handicaps, 12,* 28–37.

Hetzroni, O., & Roth, T. (2003). Effects of a positive support approach to enhance communicative behaviors of children with mental retardation who have challenging behaviors. *Education and Training in Developmental Disabilities, 38,* 95–105.

Hourcade, J., Pilotte, T.E., West, E., & Parette, P. (2004). A history of augmentative and alternative communication for individuals with severe and profound disabilities. *Focus on Autism and Other Developmental Disabilities, 19,* 235–244.

Hunt, P., Soto, G., Maier, J., Müller, E., & Goetz, L. (2002). Collaborative teaming to support students with augmentative and alternative communication needs in general education classrooms. *Augmentative and Alternative Communication, 18,* 20–35.

Iacono, T.A. (2003). Pragmatic development in individuals with developmental disabilities who use AAC. In D.R. Beukelman & J. Reichle (Series Eds.) & J.C. Light, D.R. Beukelman, & J. Reichle (Vol. Eds.), *Augmentative and alternative communication series: Communicative competence for individuals who use AAC: From research to effective practice* (pp. 323–360). Baltimore: Paul H. Brookes Publishing Co.

Individuals with Disabilities Education Improvement Act (IDEA) of 2004, PL 108-446, 20 U.S.C. §§ 1400 *et seq.*

Johnston, D.R., Stodden, R.A., Emanual, E.J., Luecking, R., & Mack, M. (2002). Current challenges facing secondary education and transition services: What research tells us. *Exceptional Children, 68,* 519–531.

Light, J.C., Arnold, K.B., & Clark, E.A. (2003). Finding a place in the "social circle of life": The development of sociorelational competence by individuals who use AAC. In D.R. Beukelman & J. Reichle

(Series Eds.) & J.C. Light, D.R. Beukelman, & J. Reichle (Vol. Eds.), *Augmentative and alternative communication series: Communicative competence for individuals who use AAC: From research to effective practice* (pp. 361–400). Baltimore: Paul H. Brookes Publishing Co.

Light, J., & Drager, K. (2007). AAC technologies for young children with complex communication needs: State of the science and future research directions. *Augmentative and Alternative Communication, 23,* 204–216.

Lund, S.K., & Light, J. (2006). Long-term outcomes for individuals who use augmentative and alternative communication: Part I—What is a "good" outcome? *Augmentative and Alternative Communication, 22,* 284–299.

McSheehan, M., Sonnenmeier, R., & Jorgensen, C.M. (2002). Communication and learning: Creating systems of support for students with significant disabilities. *TASH Connections, 28*(5), 8–13.

Mirenda, P. (2005). Augmentative and alternative communication techniques. In J.E. Downing (Ed.), *Teaching communication skills to students with severe disabilities* (2nd ed., pp. 89–112). Baltimore: Paul H. Brookes Publishing Co.

Mueller, T.G., Singer, G.H.S., & Carranza, F.D. (2006). A national survey of the educational planning and language instruction practices for students with moderate to severe disabilities who are English language learners. *Research and Practice for Persons with Severe Disabilities, 31,* 242–254.

National Joint Committee for the Communication Needs of Persons with Severe Disabilities. (1998). *Communication supports checklist for programs serving individuals with severe disabilities.* Baltimore: Paul H. Brookes Publishing Co.

No Child Left Behind Act of 2001, PL 107-110, 115 Stat. 1425, 20 U.S.C. §§ 6301 *et seq.*

Roach, A. (2006). Influences on parent perceptions of an alternate assessment for students with severe cognitive disabilities. *Research and Practice for Persons with Severe Disabilities, 31,* 267–274.

Rogers-Adkinson, D.L., Ochoa, T.A., & Delgado, B. (2003). Developing cross-cultural competence: Serving families of children with significant developmental needs. *Focus on Autism and Developmental Disabilities, 18,* 4–8.

Ross, B., & Cress, C.J. (2006). Comparison of standardized assessments for cognitive and receptive communication skills in young children with complex communication needs. *Augmentative and Alternative Communication, 22,* 100–111.

Rowland, C., & Schweigert, P. (1993). Analyzing the communication environment to increase functional communication. *Journal of The Association for Persons with Severe Handicaps, 18,* 161–176.

Siegel, E., & Allinder, R.M. (2005). Review of assessment procedures for students with moderate and severe disabilities. *Education and Training in Developmental Disabilities, 40,* 343–351.

Sigafoos, J., Arthur-Kelly, M., & Butterfield, N. (2006). *Enhancing everyday communication for children with disabilities.* Baltimore: Paul H. Brookes Publishing Co.

Sigafoos, J., O'Reilly, M.F., Drasgow, E., & Reichle, J. (2002). Strategies to achieve socially acceptable escape and avoidance. In D.R. Beukelman & J. Reichle (Series Eds.) & J. Reichle, D.R. Beukelman, & J.C. Light (Vol. Eds.), *Augmentative and alternative communication series: Exemplary practices for beginning communicators: Implications for AAC* (pp. 157–186). Baltimore: Paul H. Brookes Publishing Co.

Snell, M.E. (2002). Using dynamic assessment with learners who communicate nonsymbolically. *Augmentative and Alternative Communication, 18,* 163–176.

Snell, M.E., Chen, L., & Hoover, K. (2006). Teaching augmentative and alternative communication to students with severe disabilities: A review of intervention research 1997–2003. *Research and Practice for Persons with Severe Disabilities, 31,* 203–214.

Spooner, F., & Browder, D.M. (2006). Why teach the general curriculum? In D.M. Browder & F. Spooner (Eds.), *Teaching language arts, math, and science to students with significant cognitive disabilities* (pp. 1–14). Baltimore: Paul H. Brookes Publishing Co.

Threats, T.T., & Worrall, L. (2004). Classifying communication disability using the ICF. *Advances in Speech Language Pathology, 6,* 53–62.

Turnbull, A.P., & Turnbull, R.T. (2006). *Families, professionals, and exceptionality: Collaborating for empowerment.* Upper Saddle River, NJ: Prentice Hall.

vonTetzchner, S., Brekke, K.M., Sjothun, B., & Grindheim, E. (2005). Constructing preschool communities of learners that afford alternative language development. *Augmentative and Alternative Communication, 21,* 82–100.

Wacker, D.P., Berg, W.K., & Harding, J.W. (2002). Replacing socially unacceptable behavior with acceptable communication responses. In D.R. Beukelman & J. Reichle (Series Eds.) & J. Reichle, D.R. Beukelman, & J.C. Light (Vol. Eds.), *Augmentative and alternative communication series: Exemplary practices for beginning communicators: Implications for AAC* (pp. 97–122). Baltimore: Paul H. Brookes Publishing Co.

Wehmeyer, M.L., & Agran, M. (2006). Promoting access to the general curriculum for students with significant cognitive disabilities. In D.M. Browder & F. Spooner (Eds.), *Teaching language arts, math, and science to students with significant cognitive disabilities* (pp. 15–38). Baltimore: Paul H. Brookes Publishing Co.

3

Language Assessment for Students Who Use AAC

Lisa A. Proctor and Carole Zangari

Language assessment for students who use augmentative and alternative communication (AAC) is a complex task. Although students with AAC needs require comprehensive evaluations of their hearing, vision, motor, and cognitive skills, school-based practitioners are well aware that the ultimate goal of these individual skill assessments is to assist students to communicate via a rich system of augmentative and alternative means (Beukelman & Mirenda, 2005). Language assessment is a critical component of that process and can help practitioners identify ways to build communicative competence in students with AAC needs. Linguistic proficiency is a significant aspect of communicative competence in AAC and plays a key role in academic success (Corson, 1988; Light, 1989; Lund & Light, 2006). This chapter identifies areas for language assessment and discusses appropriate methods for evaluating skills related to vocabulary, grammar, and discourse. Issues central to the process of planning and implementing comprehensive language assessments are also discussed.

KEY QUESTIONS IN LANGUAGE ASSESSMENT FOR STUDENTS WHO USE AAC

This section addresses important questions that educational teams face in planning and implementing language assessments for their students who need or use AAC.

What Is the Purpose of the Language Assessment?

Identifying a clear purpose for the language assessment is vital. Although comprehensive language assessments are conducted for various purposes, the impetus for linguistic evaluation of students with AAC needs generally relates to 1) selecting, developing, or modifying their AAC systems; 2) creating or adjusting instructional plans; or 3) measuring progress. These assessments are lengthy, require a great deal of effort by both the practitioner and the student, and are conducted infrequently. Language assessments that focus on a single skill or domain area, however, are a more common occurrence. They can be used to identify areas of need, refine intervention programs, relate student skills to curricular demands, and measure growth in a particular area. Though less demanding to complete, domain-specific language testing is, by definition, limited in scope. Whether the need for information about the student's language abilities is broad or quite narrow, articulating a clear purpose for the assessment is an important undertaking for the educational team. Determining a specific purpose of the language assessment will lead to results that can be used to develop meaningful educational goals and plans for instruction.

The order of the authors is alphabetical. Both authors contributed equally to the writing of this chapter.

Who Should Conduct the AAC Language Assessment?

Although AAC is a multidisciplinary field, the language assessment aspect should, in all cases, be driven by speech-language pathologists (SLPs) who are knowledgeable about language development, evaluation practices, and AAC. Ideally, the SLP involved in this process would be qualified not only in terms of his or her academic record, license, and credential, but also in terms of his or her AAC experience. Just as a cancer patient seeks the services of an oncologist, a student with AAC needs should have access to an SLP experienced in AAC. To be qualified to conduct language assessments in AAC, SLPs need to have competencies that exceed the minimum standards set by state licensing boards and educational systems. They should have experience in evaluating language at a level similar to that of the specific student being evaluated and be familiar with technological options appropriate for this type of student. In a field as complex as AAC, it is critical that the evaluator have highly specialized skills. Breast cancer patients do not go to pediatric oncologists. This is not because those physicians are unable to offer some measure of support, but because these patients require doctors with a highly specific set of knowledge and skills that pediatric oncologists do not have. Similarly, students who require AAC should have language assessments by SLPs with relevant AAC experiences who are competent with linguistically based speech-generating devices (SGDs). Consultation with a broader team of stakeholders, including other AAC specialists, plays an important role in this process.

In many cases, a student's educational team may not include an SLP with a great deal of AAC experience because many school-based clinicians serve highly diverse caseloads containing only a small percentage of children requiring AAC modalities (American Speech-Language-Hearing Association, 2006). Teams who do not contain AAC-qualified SLPs should seek them through other school or district resources as they plan the AAC language assessment. If not available at those levels, then teams should obtain them in another fashion. For example, teams may call in the services of a state or regional network or they may contract with private agencies for these services. Although this may be both time consuming and costly, it is not optional—language assessments for students with AAC needs should involve SLPs with demonstrated competence in AAC.

A number of other stakeholders may also be involved in the language assessment, depending on the specific purpose of the evaluation. In some cases, this may be through direct administration of tests, subtests, or informal measures. In other situations, educators, family members, therapists, and/or educational assistants may play a less direct role.

_____ Aliyah's school has a wonderful reading resource teacher who works collaboratively with special educators to support children in inclusive classrooms. Together, the SLP and special educator approached the reading resource teacher about analyzing Aliyah's last four vocabulary tests and asked her to identify any patterns of errors so that they can reteach the concepts that Aliyah has not yet mastered. They also asked the school psychologist to include a vocabulary measure in the psychological testing that has been scheduled for Aliyah. _____

How Should Language Assessments Be Conducted for Students with AAC Needs?

In many respects, language assessment for students who use AAC is quite similar to the processes used for students with other types of disabilities. Practitioners consider the importance of culture, first language, and dialect (Bridges, 2004; McCord & Soto, 2002; Moore-Brown, Huerta, Uranga-Hernandez, & Pena, 2006; Parrette, Blake Huer, & Wyatt, 2002). These professionals reflect on the social validity of specific tools and seek to involve families in appropriate ways (Blackstone & Hunt-Berg, 2003; Crais, 1995). They reflect on the need for language assessment to be multifaceted and include direct testing, observing, and gathering information from individuals who are most important in the child's life. They compare the use of decontextualized testing against the use of observational tools in natural settings and consider the potential for dynamic assessment to improve intervention (Light, 1997; Moore-Brown et al., 2006). Practitioners also measure skills against demands of the curriculum and consider the wide range of skills that must be evaluated (Soto, 2006). They acknowledge that the scope of a language assessment has broadened to include advanced syntactical and semantic structures, nonliteral language, and narratives and recognize that this forms a foundation for any comprehensive assessment for students with AAC needs (Paul, 2007).

Assessment of linguistic knowledge and performance should include both direct and indirect methods of obtaining information (see Figure 3.1). Direct assessment of language abilities should play an important role in this process. When possible, norm-referenced tests should be given according to established protocols (i.e., directions for test administration). When that is not possible, team members may elect to modify the testing process with the understanding that, although not desirable, this may be the best means of obtaining information about the student's language abilities. In some cases, the use of validated instruments is not possible. This is most often the case with students at the earliest levels of language learning, such as those with significant cognitive impairments, and when the purpose for the assessment is tightly linked to the curriculum content. In these cases, direct assessment is still important but will be criterion based (see Paul, 2007, for an extensive discussion of this topic). At this level, the SLP may have to create assessment tasks designed to evaluate the target domain area. Doing this requires a clear understanding of the skill area, the purpose for assessment, and knowledge of the student's skills and challenges.

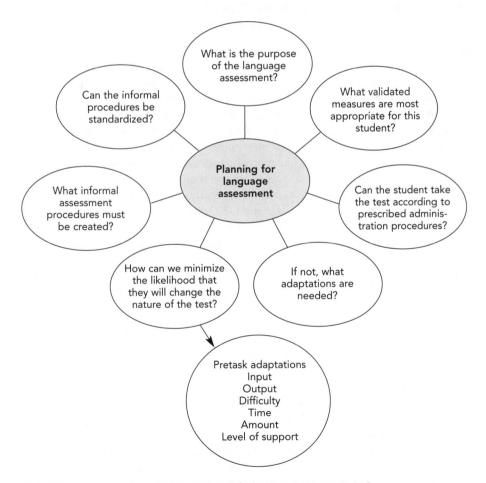

Figure 3.1.   Selecting and/or adapting instruments for language assessment in AAC.

Although direct assessment of linguistic knowledge and skills is critical, it may not yield a complete picture of the students' abilities and communication patterns. Additional information can be gained by observation and discussions with team members. This was certainly the case for Kendra, a sixth-grade student who uses a high-tech SGD, whose situation illustrates the importance of supplemental sources in developing a fuller understanding of the child's word knowledge.

_____ Following an assessment session, the SLP reviewed the data and was puzzled at Kendra's seeming inability to use the correct pronoun in an expressive language task. This was a skill that Kendra had mastered earlier, and she used pronouns spontaneously in interaction. It was not until she spoke with the teacher that a likely explanation presented itself: Kendra's class was nearing the end of a megaunit that emphasized replacing generic terms with more specific alternatives. The knowledge that Kendra had spent the last few weeks learning to replace pronouns with more specific and detailed noun phrases allowed the SLP to reconsider the test results. When she ultimately readministered that subtest, giving explicit instructions to use pronouns rather than elaborated noun phrases, Kendra passed all the items. This gave the team more useful information and guided them toward intervention that was more challenging and appropriate for Kendra. _____

What Should Teams Do When Tests Cannot Be Administered Using Their Standard Protocols?

Despite the differences between students with AAC needs and their peers, whose language development followed a more typical path, language assessment of students with AAC needs should reflect the same components of language as those examined for children who use speech as their primary mode of communication (Beukelman & Mirenda, 2005; Nelson, 1992). Students with AAC needs, however, are often unable to respond to the standardized administration procedures of many tools used to assess language comprehension and production. We recommend that educational teams in these situations first determine the most appropriate ways to test the students using their collective wisdom and experience. Sometimes professionals external to the team are called in to offer special expertise. For example, if the occupational therapist on the team is not experienced in determining the best options for switch access, then the team may call in an occupational therapist at the district level who has more knowledge in this area. The team then uses this information to create a set of testing parameters, or fair testing practices (FTPs), specifically tailored to this student. From that point, any team member testing the student uses his or her personalized FTP as guidelines for the assessment.

Developing individualized FTPs allows the team to answer a large but crucial question: Under what conditions is it fair to assess this student's knowledge and skills? The premise is that once those conditions are identified, team members will use them when they assess the student for a variety of purposes throughout the year. To develop the student's FTP, team members ask themselves a number of guiding questions (see Table 3.1). Student-specific FTPs are designed to ensure that assessments are conducted in ways that optimize the student's ability to demonstrate his or her knowledge and skills. They can be used with norm-referenced tests, curriculum-based assessments, and informal evaluation tasks.

Some professionals choose to adapt standardized tools, though doing so clearly invalidates the use of the normative data (e.g., Soto, Hartmann, & Wilkins, 2006). Nevertheless, giving formal tests in nonstandard ways may yield useful information and be the best option available for understanding the linguistic abilities of a particular student (Lund & Light, 2006; Zangari, 2004). Norm-referenced tests can be modified in several ways, including using preparation activities as well as making changes to the test administration procedures, materials, response mode, and/or feedback

Table 3.1.   Guiding questions for developing individualized fair testing practices (FTPs)

What preparation does the student need in order to participate in the assessment so that we are more likely testing knowledge and skills as opposed to the disability (e.g., seating/positioning, picture schedule of the task, practice with the response mode)?

Can *anyone* test this student, or are there specific skills and characteristics that the evaluator should possess?

How can we ensure that the student understands the expectations and requirements of the test?

How will the student answer forced-choice questions, such as true/false or multiple-choice questions?

How will the student answer open-ended questions, such as fill-in-the-blank or short essays?

How long can the student work before the results reflect fatigue more than knowledge and skills?

Test materials
- What materials are needed (e.g., slant board, sticky notes, marker, augmentative and alternative communication [AAC] device)?
- Who will prepare those materials?
- What vocabulary is needed on the student's AAC device?
- Who will make sure that it is programmed correctly?

Does the student need to be oriented to new vocabulary on the AAC device prior to testing?

What prompts and cues are allowed and are beneficial?

What feedback and reinforcement is allowed and is beneficial?

How will the student indicate that a break is needed?

How will adaptations to standard protocols be documented?

How can we ensure that FTPs are implemented as designed?

---

mechanism (Zangari, 2006). Cole and his colleagues (2000) discussed different types of adaptations, including changes to input (how students receive information), output (how students demonstrate understanding), size (how much of the task will be completed), time (how much time students have for each task), difficulty (how task complexity is addressed), and level of support (how much assistance the students are given). The team must consider how adaptations that are needed may influence results.

In most instances, it is advisable to be conservative in making adaptations as they may alter test validity. Detailed records should be kept to document the ways in which the test was modified when evaluators deviate from standard test administration procedures (Zangari, 2004). This allows the SLP to replicate those test conditions at a later date so that the test can be readministered in the same way. Thus, although we lose the ability to compare a student with AAC needs with students who took the test in a more typical fashion, we retain the ability to compare that student with him- or herself.

ASSESSMENT OF SPECIFIC LANGUAGE DOMAINS

Students who use AAC are an extremely heterogeneous group with varied strengths, needs, and learning profiles. These factors, combined with the specific purpose of the language assessment, suggest the need for highly individualized assessment processes. In most cases, language assessment is ongoing—just as some questions are answered, others emerge. Fortunately, there are an increasing number of language assessment resources and instruments, many of which are useful in evaluating the language of students with AAC needs. The reader is referred to Paul (2007) for a discussion of language assessment tools. These were created for and normed on typically developing children and may require some adaptation for use with students who have motor, visual, or cognitive impairments. Other tools, such as the Test of Aided Communication Symbol Performance (TASP; Bruno, 2006), were specifically designed for children who use AAC. This section discusses receptive and expressive language assessment issues within the domains of semantics and morpho-syntax.

Language Sampling in Students Who Use AAC

SLPs frequently use language sample analysis in addition to formal and criterion-based assessment instruments. Language sampling involves collecting samples of 50–100 utterances under relatively low-structure conditions (see Paul, 2007, for a discussion on obtaining representative language samples). Collecting samples of this size is extremely difficult for most professionals working with students who use AAC because of their slow rate of communication, among other things. In addition, SLPs must ensure that students have access to appropriate communication tools prior to collecting, transcribing, and analyzing the language sample (Light & Drager, 2005; Lund & Light, 2006; Müller & Soto, 2002a, 2002b; Soto & Dukhovny, 2008; Soto, Yu, & Kelso, 2008).

Some SGDs have the capacity to collect data on utterances so that they that can be analyzed for clinical, educational, and/or research purposes. Language Activity Monitoring (LAM) software allows AAC devices to record messages generated on the device and collects data on certain characteristics of the message. For example, it discriminates between messages generated by spelling, individual words, and prestored sentences. This automatic language sample feature can be turned on and off and makes subsequent analysis much easier. Samples can be analyzed using established procedures such as the Systematic Analysis of Language Transcripts (SALT; Miller & Chapman, 2002). Performance Report Tool (PeRT; Hill, 2004; Hill & Romich, 2003) is software designed to analyze AAC interaction using linguistic data from SGDs. It calculates the number of complete utterances, mean length of utterance, number of different word roots, and/or total number of words. Of course, this system emphasizes language via the AAC device and does not address additional communication modalities.

To capture a more complete picture of language and interaction, SLPs can collect additional data from other modalities. Communication sampling includes a full range of AAC modalities. Soto et al. (2006) used communication sampling with specific transcription codes for AAC modalities (e.g., eye gaze) developed by Müller and Soto (2002b). As noted by Soto and Grove (2001), it is often important to tie individual communicative acts to the specific modalities (e.g., sign, pictures) used to convey the idea.

Assessing Vocabulary and Semantic Knowledge and Skills

A thorough assessment of vocabulary knowledge and skills is important because of the critical role that semantics play in linguistic competency and its strong link to academic areas (e.g., reading comprehension; Jitendra, Edwards, Sacks, & Jacobson, 2004). *Semantics* refers to knowledge of vocabulary and the concepts that words represent (Paul, 2007). This section discusses specific areas to be assessed in the receptive and expressive aspects of semantics. Formal and informal assessment instruments are also presented.

Comprehension   A thorough assessment of language comprehension, including vocabulary knowledge, is an important part of the language evaluation process for all children but is particularly important for individuals who use AAC (Romski & Sevcik, 1993; Sevcik, 2006). Assessing language comprehension can provide information about which SGD will be best for which student and can aid in developing appropriate educational goals. Assessing semantic knowledge can also help teachers plan instruction in language arts and other curricular areas and assist them in communicating at levels appropriate for their students. Finally, knowledge about a student's understanding of words can help the educational team plan for appropriate supports and modify instructional practices. Aliyah's team, for example, had many discussions about her reading difficulties and put much effort into remedial programming, most of which was met with limited success.

————   When the SLP's assessment of semantics revealed a deficit far greater than was suspected, Aliyah's team was able to introduce vocabulary instruction and embed opportunities to practice new words throughout the day. By *romping* with her physical therapist, listening to a *satisfying* story in language arts, eating an *enormous* lunch with her friends, and returning *promptly* from gym class, Aliyah experienced a great deal of *accomplishment*. As her rate of learning new words quickened, Aliyah's teachers *delighted* in her progress in decoding, reading comprehension, and other content areas. _____

Areas for Assessment in Vocabulary Comprehension   Semantic assessment can target either the single-word or multiword utterances and should be considered for students of all ability levels. For early language users, the SLP should assess understanding of words in different semantic and grammatical categories and determine the students' abilities to understand progressively longer and more complex speech. For students whose use of language is more robust, formal vocabulary measures, such as the Peabody Picture Vocabulary Test–Third Edition (PPVT-III; Dunn & Dunn, 1997) or Receptive One-Word Picture Vocabulary Test (ROWPVT; Gardner, 2000b), may be used either via standard test administration procedures (when possible) or using response mode modifications (e.g., use of eye gaze or pointing aid to indicate choices). Students with advanced language skills should also be assessed in this area. Though frequently overlooked, semantic assessment of these students may focus on academic language and the development of a "literate lexicon" (Nippold, 1998). In terms of comprehension, semantic assessment should include the ability to infer meaning from linguistic contexts, understand words with multiple meanings (e.g., *beneath* the stairs, behavior that is *beneath* him), and understand verbs that allow for metacognitive and metalinguistic discussion (e.g., *conclude, assume, imply*). Researchers such as Greenhalgh and Strong suggested that "the assessment of literate language is essential for identifying children whose language limitations may hinder their academic and communication success" (2001, p. 115). The extent to which students who use AAC are assessed in the area of literate language is not known. Semantic assessment should also address comprehension of nonliteral language. MacKay and Shaw (2004) suggested that assessment in this area should consider multiple forms of figurative language, such as metaphor, irony, metonymy, rhetorical questions, understatements, hyperbole, and indirect requests.

Receptive Vocabulary Assessment Tools and Strategies   Vocabulary comprehension is one of the easiest aspects of language to assess in students who use AAC because they often use picture-pointing identification tasks that are relatively easy for students who use AAC. All students with AAC needs should have direct assessment in this area, using validated tools whenever possible. Table 3.2 provides information about testing instruments appropriate for this purpose. Tests designed specifically for vocabulary comprehension (e.g., PPVT-III, ROWPVT) can often be administered with little or no modification. Instruments such as these have been administered to students with AAC needs and yielded meaningful results (e.g., Bruno & Trembath, 2006; Light, Roberts, Dimarco, & Greiner, 1998). In addition, many general language batteries, such as the Test for Auditory Comprehension of Language–Third Edition (TACL-3; Carrow-Woolfolk, 1999) and the Miller–Yoder (M-Y) Test of Grammatical Comprehension (Miller & Yoder, 1984), have semantic subtests that can be taken by students who use AAC with little or no modifications. Other times, informal measures and criterion-referenced tests are used to gain insight into vocabulary knowledge. For example, a teacher preparing a science lesson on hypothesis testing may pretest students for vocabulary needed to understand the new material. She may ask the student to sort the words into the following categories: "words I've never heard before," "words I've heard but don't know," "words I know a little about," and "words I know a lot about." This word sort strategy, suggested by Beck, McKeown, and Kucan (2002), can be used initially to identify specific words for instruction and later to measure progress. The reader is referred to Miller and Paul (2000) for further information on the development of criterion-referenced measures to assess comprehension.

An important concept in assessing word knowledge in students who use AAC relates to the role of context. In the context of teaching, language is scaffolded with contextual and other nonlinguistic cues. Getting clear results in vocabulary assessment, however, requires complete decontextualization. Some students attend carefully to subtle cues and have learned to use them effectively to aid in their comprehension. They may follow your gaze, respond to the position/location of test items, or

Table 3.2.   Selected language tests that are appropriate for assessing the grammar of school-age students who use AAC

Test information
Test for Auditory Comprehension of Language–Third Edition (TACL-3) Author: Carrow-Woolfolk Year: 1999 Age range: 3;0 through 9;11
Clinical Evaluation of Language Fundamentals, Fourth Edition Authors: Semel, Wiig, and Secord Year: 2003 Age range: 5;0 through 21;0
Test of Language Development–Primary: Fourth Edition (TOLD-P:4) and Test of Language   **Development–Intermediate: Fourth Edition (TOLD-I:4)** Authors: Hammill and Newcomer Year: 2008 Age range: 4;0 through 8;11 and 8;0 through 17;11
Rice/Wexler Test of Early Grammatical Impairment Authors: Rice and Wexler Year: 2001 Age range: 3;0 through 8;0
Structured Photographic Expressive Language–Test 3 (SPELT-3) Authors: Dawson and Strout Year: 2003 Age range: 4;0 through 9;11

Source: Paul (2007).

listen for changes in loudness or intonation and use this information to select their answers. Students with shallower learning curves can be assessed initially in familiar routines, and, as their skills develop, progress to more decontextualized assessment tasks. A test environment that is free from unplanned cues that may bias the student's response will lead to more accurate findings.

Students at the beginning stages of communication may not be able to take formal tests but may participate in informal vocabulary assessment tasks, particularly if they involve familiar concepts and materials. Tatiana, for example, did attend to the PPVT-III long enough in formal testing to obtain a basal score. Yet, familiar objects and pictures of people and places she knows were used informally to assess word knowledge for the nouns the images depicted, action verbs (*walking, reading*), modifiers (*big, empty, old*), and prepositions (*in, on*). For the earliest language learners, Paul (2007) recommended beginning single-word vocabulary testing with nouns and then verbs and suggested that the evaluator elicit two to three demonstrations of each concept at random intervals to minimize the effect of order.

Information on language comprehension may also be obtained via observations. Light, Roberts, and colleagues (1998) suggested observing receptive language in daily context as well as on informal criterion-referenced tests. Observational data can be used to confirm or clarify findings from direct assessment and is particularly important for students whose scores in formal language testing are below age expectations. For this group, SLPs should probe comprehension of words that are required to succeed in the classroom. Classroom observations will allow the SLP to determine what instructional vocabulary the teachers use so that criterion-referenced testing on these specific words can be conducted. Miller and Paul (2000) provided guidelines for developing criterion-referenced measures of language comprehension tasks at differing developmental levels and for testing students' ability to comprehend specific targets such as actions or following direction.

Production   Assessments of semantic skills also include measures of expressive vocabulary use, although this clearly presents more of a challenge for students who use AAC. This component of the language evaluation yields critical information and should not be overlooked. It may be difficult, however, to assess expressive vocabulary abilities in students with AAC needs particularly if their access to linguistically based AAC tools has been limited. (See Chapter 9 for a discussion of linguistically based AAC systems.) Students who have had access only to communication aids with pre-stored messages, for example, will be unable to respond to test questions that require a generative response. Even students who have access to linguistically based AAC tools may be limited in their ability to demonstrate their true skill level. This is particularly true if 1) they have not yet mastered their system, 2) the system lacks a full complement of grammatical markers, 3) the student is pre-literate, or 4) access to the alphabet is limited. In these situations, students' responses to test items that ask open-ended questions are more reflective of limitations in their AAC tools than their actual skills in vocabulary production. Nevertheless, teams must look for fair and creative ways to gain insight into the semantic expression abilities of students who use AAC.

Areas for Assessment   The expressive portion of semantic assessment looks at the range of words students use and explores their word retrieval skills. *Lexical diversity* refers to the variation in the words children use. Given that lexical diversity has been considered to be an indicator of overall language proficiency (e.g., Zareva, Schwanenflugel, & Nikolova, 2005), it should be examined in students of all ability levels. Performance must be considered, however, in light of the constraints imposed by the students' AAC tools. Consider Jason's situation.

_____   Jason is a first-grade student who appears to have a strong receptive language base and gains access to a high-tech AAC device through two-switch scanning. His spelling skills, although emerging nicely, are not yet sufficient for him to produce most of the words he needs to say. This largely restricts his expressive vocabulary to the words available on his AAC device, which allows some modifications of word forms (e.g., plurals, tenses). Thus, low scores on measures of lexical diversity, such as the number of different words (NDW), are almost certainly an underestimation of Jason's skills. _____

Nonetheless, lexical diversity is an important area for assessment in order to set appropriate goals for instruction and intervention and maximize student access to the general education curriculum.

In addition to lexical diversity, SLPs seek information on students' ability to produce specific words when they are needed. Word retrieval problems, common in students with language learning disabilities, may also be present in students with AAC needs. At times, a student's failure to produce words in his or her repertoire is indicative of true problems with organization and retrieval. Alexandre, a high school student with autism and apraxia of speech, exemplified this situation.

_____   Under low stress conditions (i.e., in a calm environment with familiar partners and no time pressures), Alexandre regularly generated four- to nine-word sentences appropriate to the context. In other circumstances, however, he spoke primarily single-word utterances or used short phrases with highly repetitive language. Alexandre's difficulties with language organization and word retrieval, minimized in calm and familiar situations, were a true challenge for him (as they are for many individuals with autism spectrum disorders [ASDs]) and required specific intervention. _____

In other situations, low performance on word retrieval tasks masks a completely different problem. What appears to be a problem in thinking of the right word may actually be a difficulty in *finding* the word within the AAC system. For example, students who use semantic compaction may have the correct word in mind but err in the process of iconic coding (i.e., using the icon sequence for one word when they were actually trying to say a different word). This frequently happens with students who have sophisticated dynamic displays with words on dozens of different screens. Their ability to say what they mean is hampered by their struggle to find where that word is located. It is important to differentially diagnose a true word retrieval deficit and distinguish that from the difficulties gaining access to a word the student has internally but cannot produce on the AAC device. Both require intervention, but the nature of the instruction will differ significantly depending on the root of the problem.

Assessment Tools and Strategies   The significance of using flexible, precise vocabulary has been noted by Paul (2007) and others. There are two basic approaches to assessing expressive vocabulary: formal testing and language sample analysis. Although challenging to implement and interpret, these are both useful for SLPs working with students who have AAC needs. Table 3.2 lists language assessments that explore semantics from the perspective of language production/expression. If necessary, test administration can be modified. In all cases, though, it should be managed in accordance with the student's FTPs. As noted previously, there are significant challenges in using these tools with students who use AAC. Nonetheless, they may offer important information that cannot be gathered in other ways.

Another approach to assessing semantic production is by obtaining and analyzing language samples. As previously discussed, collecting a representative sample with a sufficient number of utterances can be challenging but extremely useful. Once coded, samples are analyzed for diversity using one or more of the following measures.

- *Type-Token Ratio (TTR)*—Developed by Templin (1957), this traditional measure is used by dividing the total number of words (tokens) by the number of different words (types) in at least a 50-utterance sample. This method is the least sensitive in differentiating students with language disorders from their peers with typical language development (Watkins, Kelly, Harbers, & Hollis, 1995).

- *Number of Total Words (NTW)*—This measure is calculated by adding up the total words used by the student in a language sample. Research (e.g., Klee, 1992) indicated that NTW increases with age and that it can be used effectively to distinguish students with and without language impairments. NTW serves as a useful measure of linguistic productivity.

- *Number of Different Words (NDW)*—This measure is calculated by counting the number of different words in the sample. Repetitions of words used earlier in the sample are not counted. Work by Miller and his colleagues suggested that NDW is the best measure of lexical diversity (Miller, Freiberg, Rolland, & Reeves, 1992).

There are no normative data on students who use AAC using any of these measures. Yet, these analyses can be effective at identifying baseline levels of performance against which future progress can be measured. Soto and Dukhovny (2008) demonstrated the utility of NDW in measuring growth in lexical diversity in language samples of children who use AAC.

There is at least one full test (Tests of Word Finding in Discourse; German, 1991) and several subtests designed to assess challenges in word retrieval that are useful for school-age students. Examples of language batteries with naming/word retrieval tasks include the Language Processing Test (LPT; Richard & Hanner, 1995) and the Clinical Evaluation of Language Fundamentals–4 (CELF-4; Semel, Wiig, & Secord, 2003).

Implications   The assessment of semantic knowledge and skills should address both comprehension (receptive understanding) and production (expressive use). As in other areas, the results from semantic assessment should be used to make educational decisions, such as further refining instruction programs, continuing to customize an SGD, or identifying areas for additional testing. Students whose receptive and expressive vocabularies are at the same level do not need intervention unless those scores fall below chronological age expectancy. If, however, the students do not evidence age-appropriate vocabulary understanding and use, they will likely benefit from and should receive intervention and/or instruction in this area. Idalia's story illustrates some of these points.

———————   Idalia is fifth-grade student who uses a high-tech SGD. She demonstrated somewhat delayed PPVT-III scores and was having increasing difficulty with content area material. Even when the passages and questions were read aloud, she had difficulty answering questions about content in several classes. The SLP noted that Idalia's language was nonspecific and designed an intervention to help Idalia use more variety when talking to adults and peers. Her educational team prioritized new word learning to help Idalia catch up with her peers. _____

Students who use linguistically based, high-tech AAC devices and have semantic knowledge that greatly exceeds their expressive vocabulary require further consideration. Sometimes the discrepancy can be explained by the limited language available on the SGD. In other situations, additional assessment may be needed. If the student's family and teachers report that the range of expressive language in spontaneous conversation is lower than expected, then the SLP may want to administer a formal naming task, such as the Expressive One-Word Picture Vocabulary Test (EOWPVT; Gardner, 2000a). Naming scores that are lower than receptive vocabulary scores indicate that the student knows more words than he or she uses. Clearly, this has a direct implication for both language intervention by the SLP and the teacher's language arts lessons. Additional assessment is needed, however, to elucidate the nature of the problem. Two things that cause lower-than-expected expressive vocabularies in these students are 1) the need for operational competency training to gain access to more words and 2) true difficulties with word retrieval. Students with new or sophisticated AAC systems require systematic instruction to learn to retrieve vocabulary in an efficient way. Periodic training to gain access to new words on their SGDs may also be needed.

What about students whose receptive knowledge is lower than the expressive language they produce? A less common occurrence is when students' scores on expressive measures are higher than their receptive scores. Although we typically expect that understanding precedes expression, for some children, *using* language is an important strategy for learning word meanings.

_____ Laila, a 14-year-old student with autism, uses words that she has been taught to say as part of an applied behavior analysis program. Laila does not understand what a word means until she has used it hundreds of times. For Laila, using a word over and over leads to a gradual understanding of its meaning. Her use of the word gives her a chance to experience the effect of that word in a particular context. Over time, she gains knowledge about the word's connotation. _____

It is important that practitioners recognize and identify this learning profile for two reasons. One, they can exploit this learning strategy—if they want Laila to learn a new word meaning, then they can teach her to say it and coach people in her environment how to respond. As she uses it, Laila's receptive vocabulary expands to include this new semantic element. An even more important reason to recognize this learning pattern relates to vocabulary selection for SGDs and no-tech communication aids. In some situations, practitioners require that students demonstrate understanding of a word or concept before providing access to it via the AAC system. This is clearly counterproductive for some children. The practice of only putting words or messages on an AAC device if the student has demonstrated receptive understanding of them should be avoided, not just for students who learn in this way, but for all students.

Other Issues Related to Assessment of Semantics   Because some AAC systems are organized by semantic categories, it is sometimes useful to obtain information relative to a student's ability to categorize words. Light, Roberts, and colleagues (1998) discussed sorting tasks, pairing, and conducting trial uses of AAC devices as methods for assessing categorization skills. The TASP also provided sorting tasks for determining categorization skills. Wilkinson and Rosenquist (2006) reported on a method for semantic organization that adapted the more traditional match-to-sample task by increasing the number of exemplars that could be selected. Hochstein, McDaniel, and Nettleton (2004) examined how children learn vocabulary that are organized via superordinate categories and noted that children who had difficulty identifying vocabulary stored in categories that were not immediately transparent (e.g., part of speech) were able to improve performance when provided with feedback.

Assessing Grammar and Morpho-Syntax

In addition to learning the meaning of words and how to use these words, students who use AAC must also learn how to combine words and change the structure of words. If individuals do not learn these grammatical/morpho-syntactic skills they will have difficulty clearly conveying messages and will very likely face academic challenges (Binger & Light, 2008). The readers are referred to Binger and Light (2008) for a research review of morphology and syntax for AAC as well as a listing of assessment measures. In the field of speech-language pathology, *syntactical and morphological structure* refers to "inflectional marking of words; sentence components such as the basic noun phrase and verb phrase; and sentence types, such as negative, interrogative, embedded, and conjoined structures" (Paul, 2007, p. 30). *Grammar* is a more generic term that refers to the creation of a structure or set of rules and can be applied to stories as well as syntax and morphology and can be viewed as a more general term to refer to rules that govern both syntax and morphology. The following section will use a combination of the terms *grammar, morphology,* and *syntax* when discussing this aspect of language.

Assessment of grammar comprehension is important for several reasons. First, it allows practitioners to develop appropriate therapeutic and educational goals. Second, it plays an important role in selecting AAC devices and informs decisions about customization (Roth & Cassatt-James, 1989). Finally, it yields information that guides appropriate interaction and instructional methods. Grammar comprehension can be assessed formally with tools designed specifically for that task or with instruments that cover a broader range of skills (e.g., CELF-4; Test of Adolescent Language–Third Edition [TOAL-3], Hammill, Brown, Larson, & Wiederholt, 1994). Multiple measures may be warranted depending on the purpose of the assessment (Light, Roberts, et al., 1998; Roth & Cassatt-James, 1989). Light, Roberts, and colleagues (1998) illustrated this in a case report of an individual with age-appropriate receptive vocabulary scores who had significant difficulties comprehending certain syntactical and morphological structures.

Comprehension   Understanding a child's comprehension of morphological and syntactical structures is important when assessing the language of students with AAC needs and can assist in developing targets for expressive language and selecting and programming AAC devices (Roth & Cassatt-James, 1989). Appropriate selection of informal and standardized tests is needed in order to include assessment of morpho-syntax comprehension because receptive language tests can target a variety of language domains. Assessing grammar comprehension is important for several reasons. First, it allows practitioners to develop appropriate therapeutic and educational goals. Second, it plays an important role in selecting AAC devices and informs decisions about customization (Roth & Cassatt-James, 1989). Finally, it yields information that guides appropriate interaction and instructional methods. Grammar comprehension can be assessed formally with tools designed specifically for that task or with instruments that cover a broader range of skills (e.g., TACL-3). Multiple measures may be warranted depending on the purpose of the assessment (Light, Roberts, et al., 1998; Roth & Cassatt-James, 1989).

Areas for Assessment   Assessment of grammar/morpho-syntax should target a student's understanding of word order and complex syntactical structures as well as his or her understanding of grammatical morphemes and how bound morphemes such as the plural *-s* provide additional information. The reader is referred to Paul (2007) for a comprehensive overview of syntactical and morphological assessment. Although syntax and grammar are integrated components of language form and are often evaluated in combination, assessment methods may include separate subsections for each of these areas. For example, the TACL-3 subtests include one subtest that targets a student's understanding of grammatical morphemes and a separate subtest for examining understanding of elaborated phrases and sentences. Comprehension of grammatical structures should include the range of these skills and can begin with the earliest stages of syntactical development, two-word utterances, and initial grammatical morphemes and continue with understanding of complex syntactical structure and advanced grammatical structures including embedded prepositional phrases, embedded gerunds, and compound sentences with a variety of conjoiners and relative clauses.

Assessment Tools and Strategies   There are a range of tools that can be utilized for assessing syntax and morphology, including standardized and criterion-referenced tests and informal measures. The purpose of the assessment and the skills of the student should guide test selection. If standardized scores are not needed for eligibility, then criterion-referenced tests and more informal measures may provide information about the child's understanding of specific syntactical and morphological structures that can assist in planning goals and intervention as well as device selection. Selected standardized tests, however, may also be used to assess comprehension of syntax and morphology. See Table 3.2 for a list of standardized tests that include receptive and expressive syntax and/or morphology.

For guidance in assessing morphology and syntax at early stages the reader is referred to the Clinical Assessment of Language Comprehension (Miller & Paul, 2000). This tool provides guidelines for evaluating understanding of two-symbol combinations, including action-object, agent-action, possessor-possession, entity-location, and action-location, as well as guidelines for assessing understanding of word-order comprehension for simple sentences and sentences with prepositional phrases. Assessing more advanced morphological and syntactical structures may require probes targeting a particular syntactical or morphological structure, including comprehension tasks as well as judgments of correctness/appropriateness of grammatical structures presented (Binger & Light, 2008; Blockberger & Johnston, 2003). Blockberger and Johnston used a picture-matching paradigm to investigate understanding of three morphological structures. In the same investigation, they also presented children with a series of utterances and asked the children to determine correctness of the utterances. The utterances contained correct and incorrect examples of selected morphological structures. These informal measures can provide information about specific structures that may influence AAC device programming and selection.

Production   Having the ability to produce utterances with more complex grammar/morpho-syntax will allow students who use AAC to convey messages as well as provide the language foundation for written language (Binger & Light, 2008). If individuals do not have the vocabulary and grammatical structures available to them that allow them to produce more complex messages, then they may have to rely on simple or telegraphic messages accompanied by context and communication partner support to convey a message. Individuals using AAC do not have to be limited to incomplete or unclear messages, however, because AAC systems can provide access to more complex syntactical and morphological structures through various means. Preprogrammed messages that contain complex grammar may be made accessible on an individual's AAC system, and in order to "produce" the message, an individual may only be required to activate a single cell. In contrast, words and morphological structures may be made available on the AAC systems, and the individuals will be able to generate messages using grammatical structures using the vocabulary and symbols made available on the device.

Areas for Assessment   Assessment of grammar should provide information on an individual's ability to produce multiword utterances, simple sentences, and compound and complex sentences as well as use grammatical morphemes such as verb tenses, plurals, articles, and prepositions. Analyzing the morphological and syntactical structures produced by an individual using AAC may be based on the same foundation as the analysis for individuals who are speaking (e.g., production of inflectional morphemes, sentence length and complexity); however, specific guidelines for syntactical and morphological production with AAC will need to be developed (Lund & Light, 2006). This is because AAC utterances may lack grammatical structures due to lack of availability of these structures (Beukelman & Mirenda, 2005), may contain preprogrammed messages that do not require generation of grammar (Lund & Light, 2006), and may include multiple modes of communication (Müller & Soto, 2002b). In addition, the desire or need to increase the rate of message production may interfere with an individual's production of some morpho-syntactic structures despite their ability to do so. When transcribing and analyzing the grammar of individuals who use AAC, these unique concerns must be considered in the interpretation of this analysis.

Assessment Tools and Strategies   The most basic method for understanding an individual's use of expressive communication, including grammar, is to record and appropriately analyze the individual's expressive productions during meaningful interactions. Traditional language sampling focuses on unstructured interactions between two or more individuals that are intended to represent the language in daily routines and context of the student being assessed. The communication partner is typically instructed to follow the lead of the student in terms of activities and interests and to facilitate rather than elicit productions. Based on this scenario, parameters for traditional language sampling may be used as a starting point in that students are provided with a conversational or narrative context in which to communicate. The ultimate goal is to converse with students to see what messages they are able to produce spontaneously and with minimal support. Transcription should include modification for recording the modality in which a symbol was produced as well as unique aspects of AAC such as preprogrammed messages, multisymbol messages, and use of multiple modes (Hill, 2004; Lund & Light, 2006; Müller & Soto, 2002a). If the student has a device that contains the messages and vocabulary and symbols to produce messages on a range of topics, as well as the knowledge and skills to utilize all of the messages and symbols on his or her device, then an unstructured language sample may provide accurate information regarding the student's ability to produce grammar via his or her AAC system. It may be difficult, however, to capture the true abilities of students who have had limited exposure to an AAC system that allows for fully generative language. Students whose AAC systems have limited vocabulary and who are not yet literate may have difficulty demonstrating their actual language abilities due to limitations of their communication tools.

Consequently, structured tasks that target and provide appropriate vocabulary for specific syntactical and morphological structures may be useful. For example, both nouns and verbs must be present for a child to produce agent-action two-word productions as well as symbols to represent bound morphemes for present progressive and plural. The TASP includes a subtest for eliciting simple utterances, and children are provided with communication boards with appropriate vocabulary and organization. Children have opportunities to produce simple utterances as well as early-developing grammatical structures (e.g., articles, prepositions, present progressive verb tense) through modeling, open-ended questions, and/or requests for description. Structured tasks may also be used to elicit more complex grammar/morpho-syntax, and specific elicitation tasks have been developed to elicit morphological structures. Blockberger and Johnston (2003) used a cloze procedure to elicit specific morphological structures while at the same time reducing physical requirements to produce utterances. Programming devices with specific vocabulary and symbols and providing opportunities to produce targeted structures can provide important information regarding the student's expressive grammar. For example, for a student not consistently producing subject-verb-object grammatical structures, a device can be programmed to contain agents, actions, and objects in a left-to-right sequence (based on the Fitzgerald Key; Beukelman & Mirenda, 2005; Turkington & Sussman, 1992). The student could then be shown pictures, actions, or books that contain this targeted syntactical structure. The student could be given the opportunity to produce the targeted structure with the appropriate levels of support from communication partners. Similar activities could be developed for specific morphological or syntactical structures with consideration given to the child's communication device and the manner in which messages and symbols are programmed and organized.

Implications   Individuals, including students who use AAC, must be able to either utilize the grammar/morpho-syntax on their AAC system or locate preprogrammed messages in order to generate novel utterances that are specific and clear. Generating novel messages via AAC may pose unique challenges. It is still important, however, in planning language and literacy intervention for these students. Consequently, assessing comprehension and production of grammar/morpho-syntax should be a primary component of AAC language assessment. If assessment is not used to understand a student's receptive and expressive language, then it is likely that grammar will not be targeted as a goal for a student. Without intervention to assist in developing these skills, students will face challenges in developing communication competence as well as being at even greater risk in the area of literacy development. In addition, individuals who do possess a more advanced understanding of morphology and syntax may be forced to try and communicate with AAC systems that do not allow them to express themselves at the level expected for their receptive language.

Other Issues Related to Assessment of Grammar and Morpho-Syntax   The
very nature of AAC systems, such as issues related to modality, rate of communication, and accessibility of specific syntactical and grammatical forms, may alter the production of syntax and morphology. Although there are many challenges associated with complex English syntax and morphology through augmented means, it is important to understand an individual's ability to use these structures via their AAC system (Beukelman & Mirenda, 2005). When collecting a sample from an individual using AAC, we may not be able to know for sure if the language structures produced are equivalent to what the person would be able to produce if he or she were suddenly provided with the ability to produce messages through speech. Despite this limitation, individuals who use AAC are not typically communicating within a setting where there is a specific AAC language. Rather, they are communicating with individuals using the spoken language of the community, and the goal is to have the individual using AAC to communicate within that context. Consequently, it seems important to understand the ability of the individual using AAC to produce the grammar of the language community via AAC in order to fully understand his or her communication abilities.

Finally, assessing morphology and syntax, and particularly production, may vary depending on the individual's exposure to AAC systems containing syntactical and morphological structures as well as the abilities and adaptability of individuals. For students with AAC systems that allow for generative language, it may be possible through one or two sessions to collect a language sample that reflects their skills and potential. For individuals who do not have exposure to AAC systems containing a variety of linguistic structures, the number, length, and intensity of assessment(s) may differ depending on the skills of the student. Some students may need minimal exposure and modeling of targeted structures to demonstrate their syntactical and morphological potential for using a newly introduced AAC system. Other students, however, may need repeated exposure, modeling, and opportunities related to syntactical and morphological structures in order to fully realize their potential to use these structures. Consequently, trial use of AAC devices with appropriate programming, partner training, and data collection are often imperative. Considering the sequential nature of syntactical and morphological acquisition in the language development of typically developing children, the need for exposure and opportunity in order for a student to utilize specific structures on an AAC device is not at all surprising, and it is crucial that these language skills (or lack thereof) not be judged until the appropriate support is provided.

Assessing Pragmatic Knowledge and Skills

In addition to understanding the words and grammar that students with AAC needs comprehend and produce, it is important to see how their language is utilized in conversational contexts. These pragmatic skills consist of "the range of communicative functions (reasons for talking), the frequency of communication, discourse skills (turn-taking, topic maintenance and change), and the flexibility to modify speech for different listeners and social situations" (Paul, 2007, p. 30). Research indicates that individuals who use AAC have pragmatic skills that are impaired (Beukelman & Mirenda, 2005), and, consequently, pragmatics are an important consideration in the language assessment of individuals who use AAC. Assessment and subsequent treatment of pragmatic skills will ensure that an individual's linguistic competence is not limited to specific communication partners and situations but that the individual has the social and strategic competence to successfully interact with communication partners in a variety of contexts (Light, 1989).

Because pragmatic skills involve the exchange between communication partners, they involve aspects of both receptive and expressive language. Certain aspects of pragmatic development, such as the development of communicative functions and frequency of communication, primarily focus on an individual's productive communication skills. Yet, the specific knowledge and skills that are needed to successfully engage in discourse and appropriately modify speech include aspects of both receptive and expressive language. For example, answering a question requires both comprehension of the message produced by a communication partner as well as production of the appropriate response. In the area of pragmatics, measurement tools often address a list of skills, but these skills may not be grouped or identified as receptive and expressive. Consequently, the following sections discuss overall pragmatic skills.

Areas of Assessment in Pragmatics

As previously stated, the development of pragmatics involves communicative functions, discourse skills, and flexibility of communication (Paul, 2007). All of these aspects of pragmatics should be considered in assessment, with the specific items addressed in each area influenced by the individual's level of communication. At the earliest stages of communication development, expected communicative functions might include showing, requesting, commenting, greeting, and protesting. For more developed communicators, communicative functions such as requesting information, providing information, and requesting clarification may be expected. Early discourse skills may involve simple turn-taking skills, whereas in later development, an individual will be expected to introduce, maintain, and/or end a conversation and recognize the needs of the conversation partner. To evaluate the language of young children developing language through AAC, language assessment should provide information on communicative functions expressed as well as turn-taking skills observed in communicative exchanges (Clarke & Kirton, 2003; Light & Drager, 2005; Lilienfeld & Alant, 2005). In addition, communication transcript analysis can provide information regarding discourse structures (Lilienfeld & Alant, 2005).

Pragmatic assessment should also provide information regarding the student's patterns of communication with different groups of communication partners (Blackstone & Hunt Berg, 2003). This will help provide information on the student's communication competence across communication partners. Furthermore, orientations to language disorders have included a systems approach that includes assessing the environment and communication partners in addition to assessing the individual (Paul, 2007), and AAC assessment should include this approach in which both the individual using AAC and the communication partners are part of the assessment process (Light, Roberts, et al., 1998).

Pragmatic Assessment Tools and Strategies

To some extent, obtaining information regarding the pragmatic development of children who use AAC may look similar to obtaining this information for children who are speaking. An interaction between a child using an AAC system and his or her communication partner should be viewed and recorded in order to view the student's skills within meaningful interactions. Investigating the use of AAC in everyday conversations is an essential component of pragmatic assessment (Bloch & Wilkinson, 2004). These interactions can include interactions between students using AAC and their typically developing peers (Clarke & Kirton, 2003; Light, Seligson, & Lund, 1998; Lilienfeld & Alant, 2005). Interactions should be analyzed in order to categorize and understand the student's pragmatic skills. For children with language impairments, coding schemas have been developed to determine the frequency and variety of communicative functions, discourse skills, and responsiveness and assertiveness on the part of the child (Fey, 1986). These coding systems can be used with modifications with children using AAC. The conversation analysis, "the systematic data driven study of naturally occurring talk in interaction," is designed to analyze the interactions between individuals using AAC (Block & Wilkinson, 2004, p. 273). In addition, transcription codes that include codes for eye gaze and head movement have been utilized with individuals using AAC in order to not underestimate the skills of these individuals during conversational interactions (Müller & Soto, 2002a).

Criterion-referenced measures can also be used to record and classify interactions between children who use AAC and their communication partners. For students with emerging language, a tool such as the communication matrix (Roland, 2004) provides a convenient format for recording communication functions and the communication modes used to express those functions.

Structured interviews with the communication partners as well as the individual using AAC can provide information regarding with whom the student communicates as well as the specific communication modes and strategies utilized. The Social Networks Communication Inventory (Blackstone & Hunt Berg, 2003) can assist in analyzing patterns of communication with family, peers, paid workers, and individuals in the community.

Implications   Successful participation is considered to be the primary outcome of AAC intervention (Beukelman & Mirenda, 2005). Consequently, developing pragmatic skills that allow a student using AAC to communicate in daily activities and routines is considered vital for individuals who use AAC. Children are at even greater risk for impaired pragmatic development without appropriate pragmatic assessment and intervention.

Other Issues Related to Assessment of Pragmatics   Individuals using AAC typically are assessed when interacting with individuals who are using speech as their primary mode of communication. It may also be beneficial, however, to consider an individual's conversation patterns with another person using AAC. Müller and Soto (2002a) compared interactions between dyads in which both individuals used AAC versus dyads with an individual using AAC and a "typical" communication partner. The asymmetry that has been noted with "typical" users was not evident in communication interactions between two individuals using AAC.

Assessing Narrative Language

Narrative language is a form of discourse that is inherently different from other types of interaction. It is the language of storytelling, whether those stories are from personal experiences or events that one has seen, heard about, or imagined. Though the use of various genres of narrative language is greatly affected by culture (e.g., Heath, 1986), the ability to construct narratives is an important skill in most traditions and one that develops gradually. It emerges from our experiences in play and conversation, grows in complexity, and reaches toward abstraction throughout our preschool and primary school years. Stories play an important role in social interaction and influence the ways in which we think about ourselves and the world around us. Considering narrative language is particularly important for school-age children given the strong role it plays in academic success and communicative competence (Botting, 2002; Nelson, 1989). It is an area of difficulty for students with language impairments (e.g., Kaderavek & Sulzby, 2000; Scott & Windsor, 2000) and learning disabilities (e.g., Catts, 1993).

Narrative development may pose specific problems for students who use AAC given that skills in this area are built on a foundation of dialogue, conversation, and play. Most students with AAC needs do not have a rich history of extended discourse when they first enter school, and their access to imaginative play routines may have been limited. Many had restricted access to AAC options that allowed them to generate language. Others struggled with physical access and/or word retrieval, making conversation challenging and tiresome. For these reasons, difficulties with narrative development should be anticipated and addressed via a thorough evaluation. Information gleaned from that evaluation should then be used to plan intervention and guide classroom instruction and/or remediation. Narrative language is complex and requires a significant amount of generative language. Because students at the beginning stages of communication may have higher priorities for assessment, narrative language evaluation may be deferred until the student has an appropriate means of using language for conversation. Students with the ability to use language to converse (with or without support) will benefit from narrative language assessment and should participate in periodic evaluations of their narrative skills throughout the school years.

This section looks at assessing comprehension and production of personal, script, and fictional narratives. *Personal narratives* are the earliest genre that children acquire and involve the retelling of a significant personal experience. *Script narratives* require students to recount a routine sequence of actions or events, such as the steps to making a sandwich or explaining what typically happens when people play chess. *Fictional narratives* involve students telling or retelling stories.

To a large extent, the understanding and use of narratives is reflective of linguistic development as a whole. Given the special role narratives play in academic achievement, however, it may be useful to consider narrative assessment somewhat separately from other aspects of language evaluation (Moore-Brown et al., 2006). The next section discusses specific areas for assessment and describes evaluation tools that allow practitioners to consider performance in narrative genres.

Comprehension   Students are exposed to narratives throughout the school day in both academic contexts and social interactions. Careful assessment of students' abilities to comprehend the structural and cohesive elements of narrative structures allows interventionists to construct appropriate instructional plans.

Areas for Assessment   Understanding narrative language is important for academic success and is a part of most test batteries for receptive language, such as the Comprehensive Assessment of Spoken Language (CASL; Carrow-Woolfolk, 1998) and the TOAL-3. Paul (2007) discussed many of the tools appropriate for both younger and older students.

In addition, the SLP may want to assess the students' awareness of their narrative comprehension skills as this is known to be difficult for some students with language learning difficulties. Determining the extent to which students reflect on and accurately evaluate whether they understand what they hear can be very useful. Students with challenges in this area can be provided with strategies to improve comprehension monitoring.

Assessment Tools and Strategies   Assessment of narrative language can be accomplished using both formal test instruments and informal measures. The Test of Narrative Language (TNL; Gillam & Pearson, 2004) is a comprehensive test of oral narratives that tests both comprehension and production using three formats. In the "no picture" format, students listen to a story, answer comprehension questions, then retell the story. In the "multiple picture" format, students listen to a story as the examiner points to a sequence of pictures that illustrate key story elements. They are then given a new sequence of pictures and must produce an appropriate narrative. In the "single picture" format, they listen to a story that corresponds to an illustration, answer comprehension questions, and then produce a narrative about a different (single) picture.

Comprehension monitoring can be assessed through informal means, such as barrier games. Interviews with teachers and family members can also be insightful. For example, parents can contribute insight regarding how their children respond when they do not understand what is being said. Teachers can provide information on whether the student asks appropriate questions when difficult material is presented.

Production   Assessing the construction of narratives is important for all children who use AAC at the conversational level for two reasons. The first is that, as a group, these students are known to 1) have significant difficulties in this area (e.g., Grove & Tucker, 2003; Soto & Hartmann,

2006; Waller et al., 2001) and 2) respond positively to narrative intervention (e.g., Bedrosian, Lasker, Speidel, & Politsch, 2003; Soto, Yu, & Henneberry, 2007). The second rationale for this type of assessment relates to the fact that narrative evaluation tasks are more likely to elucidate specific language problems than communication activities that are primarily conversational in nature (Hadley, 1998). Thus, we can use the results to plan highly focused intervention programs.

Areas for Assessment   There are three main areas to consider in assessing narrative abilities: structure, cohesion, and linguistic richness (see Paul, 2001, for a discussion of these areas). An examination of the narratives of four students who use AAC identified elements that were problematic for these children (Soto & Hartmann, 2006). Soto and Hartmann also identified story elements that were either absent or insufficient, including some of the most common aspects of storytelling—the character and setting—as well as episode structure and evaluative remarks. In addition, they noted significant difficulties with coherence. Their findings are consistent with narrative problems identified in children with language impairments. In this population, researchers noted deficits in grammar and syntax and identified deficiencies in narrative production that include fewer total and different words, diminished use of cohesive devices, and difficulties with story grammar (Swanson, Fey, Mills, & Hood, 2005).

The areas of assessment for narrative skills suggested for students with AAC needs has much in common with narrative assessment suggested for students with language learning difficulties and reading disabilities (e.g., McFadden & Gillam, 1996; Swanson et al., 2005; Westerveld & Gillon, 2008). Paul (2001), for example, recommended evaluating the following areas:

- Using literate language forms (i.e., to regulate thinking, discuss abstract ideas, make inferences; use of low-frequency words, concise syntax, specific vocabulary; Westby, 1991)

- Producing story grammar as it relates to the internal states, plans, and motivations of the characters

- Summarizing stories

Each of these areas should be assessed in students with AAC needs so that instruction and intervention can be adjusted according to specific needs.

Assessment Tools and Strategies   Earlier in this section we discussed the TNL, a formal instrument for assessing the production of narratives. Informal measures such as language sample analysis are also useful. Language samples obtained for the purpose of narrative assessment require thoughtful preparation (Ukrainetz & Gillam, 2006; Ukrainetz et al., 2005). The examiner should prepare materials designed to elicit the type(s) of narratives for which information is sought. Different picture prompts, for example, will be necessary to obtain personal, script, and fictional narratives. The Strong Narrative Assessment Procedure (SNAP; Strong, 1998) is an example of a standardized set of materials and procedures used for eliciting and analyzing narrative language for fictional retelling that may be useful for students who use AAC. Soto et al. (2006) presented a compelling case for the use of another tool, the Narrative Assessment Profile (NAP; Bliss, McCabe, & Miranda, 1998; McCabe & Bliss, 2003). The NAP can be used with any elicitation task. Analysis of narratives generated by these tasks focuses on topic maintenance, event sequencing, explicitness, referencing, conjunctive cohesion, and fluency. To get a comprehensive view of narrative production abilities, SLPs should utilize multiple elicitation tasks. Soto et al. (2006), for example, used personal photo descriptions, familiar book reading and retelling, conversational narrative, story stems, and wordless picture books to generate narratives for analysis.

Analysis of the narrative sample may include considering the semantic, morphological, and syntactic features of language discussed previously in this chapter. In addition, practitioners should gather information regarding complexity and cohesion. Soto and her colleagues (2008) recommended multiple measures, such as those listed next:

- Total number of clauses

- Clausal density (i.e., the amount of dependent clauses in each utterance)

• Cohesiveness at the sentence level (i.e., the frequency with which cohesive markers[1] are used) and with respect to the larger narrative (i.e., story coherence, use of story grammar elements, organization and structure)

CONCLUSION

The importance of good language assessment for students with AAC needs cannot be overstated. It is a complex and lengthy process that is vital in establishing appropriate linguistic goals and for planning appropriate instruction. In addition to all of the language assessment issues we consider for more typically developing children, we are mindful of the special learning, behavioral, cognitive, and physical challenges faced by students who use AAC. These assessments require additional time for planning, creating supportive materials, administrating, analyzing, and documenting. They require specific expertise and challenge even the most experienced professionals. They almost always come with a sense of urgency and responsibility. It is overwhelming under the best of circumstances.

For practical reasons, it often makes sense for the team to make a language assessment plan that considers the student's most urgent needs and prioritizes language assessment activities accordingly. Comprehensive language evaluations (i.e., those that address all components of language from both the receptive and expressive perspectives) are not feasible in most situations. In these instances, the team may prioritize a more narrowly focused assessment on a single component of language. For one student, that may mean an emphasis on receptive language as part of a larger process of SGD selection. Another student may need an in-depth evaluation of lexical diversity to improve his or her capacity to use literate language. Still another child may need a close inspection of how language is used to solve problems or interact with peers. The team may defer assessments of other aspects of language until these more pressing issues are resolved. It is important, however, that over time, the team plan for a systematic assessment of language so that the student has access to appropriate tools, intervention, and instruction.

REFERENCES

American Speech-Language-Hearing Association. (2006). *2006 schools survey. Special report: Caseload trends.* Available at http://www.asha.org/about/membership-certification/member-data/2006SchoolsSurvey.htm.

Beck, I.L., McKeown, M.G., & Kucan, L. (2002). *Bringing words to life: Robust vocabulary instruction.* New York: Guilford Press.

Bedrosian, J., Lasker, J., Speidel, K., & Politsch, A. (2003). Enhancing the written narrative skills of an AAC student with autism: Evidence-based issues. *Topics in Language Disorders, 24,* 305–324.

Beukelman, D.R., & Mirenda, P. (2005). *Augmentative and alternative communication: Supporting children and adults with complex communication needs* (3rd ed.). Baltimore: Paul H. Brookes Publishing Co.

Binger, C., & Light, J. (2008). The morphology and syntax of individuals who use AAC: Research review

and implications of effective practice. *Augmentative and Alternative Communication, 24,* 123–138.

Blackstone, S., & Hunt-Berg, M. (2003). *Social networks: A communication inventory for children with complex communication needs and their communication partners.* Monterey, CA: Augmentative Communication.

Bliss, L.S., McCabe, A., & Miranda, A.E. (1998). Narrative assessment profile: Discourse analysis for school-age children. *Journal of Communication Disorders, 31,* 347–362.

Bloch, S., & Wilkinson, R. (2004). The understandability of AAC: A conversation analysis study of acquired dysarthria. *Augmentative and Alternative Communication, 20,* 272–282.

Blockberger, S., & Johnston, J. (2003). Grammatical morphology acquisition by children with complex communication needs. *Augmentative and Alternative Communication, 19,* 207–221.

---

[1]Cohesive markers include references (words that rely on another source of information for interpretation) and conjunctives (which draw semantic connections and specify relationships between words). Reference markers comprise personal (e.g., *I, its, our, them*), demonstrative (e.g., *a, the, these, here, now*), and comparative (e.g., *another, second, more*) references. They include additives, such as *also, and,* and *besides,* as well as adversatives (e.g., *only, though, but, actually*).

Botting, N. (2002). Narrative as a tool for the assessment of linguistic and pragmatic impairments. *Child Language Teaching and Therapy, 18,* 1–21.

Bridges, S.J. (2004). Multicultural issues in augmentative and alternative communication and language. *Topics in Language Disorders, 24,* 62–75.

Bruno, J. (2006). *Test of Aided Communication Symbol Performance.* Solana Beach, CA: Mayer-Johnson.

Bruno, J., & Trembath, D. (2006). Use of aided language stimulation to improve syntactic performance during a weeklong intervention program. *Augmentative and Alternative Communication, 22,* 300–313.

Carrow-Woolfolk, E. (1998). *Comprehensive Assessment of Spoken Language (CASL).* Circle Pines, MN: American Guidance Services.

Carrow-Woolfolk, E. (1999). *Test for Auditory Comprehension of Language–Third Edition (TACL-3).* Austin, TX: PRO-ED.

Catts, H.W. (1993). The relationship between speech-language impairments and reading disabilities. *Journal of Speech and Hearing Research, 36,* 948–958.

Clarke, M., & Kirton, A. (2003). Patterns of interaction between children with physical disabilities using augmentative and alternative communication and their peers. *Child Language Teaching and Therapy, 19*(2), 136–151.

Cole, S., Horvath, B., Chapman, C., Deschenes, C., Ebeling, D.G., & Sprague, J. (2000). *Adapting curriculum & instruction in inclusive classrooms: A teacher's desk reference* (2nd ed.). Bloomington, IN: Center on Education and Lifelong Learning, Indiana Institute on Disability and Community.

Corson, D. (1988). *Oral language across the curriculum.* Clevedon, UK: Multilingual Matters.

Crais, E. (1995). Expanding the repertoire of tools and techniques for assessing the communication skills of infants and toddlers. *American Journal of Speech-Language Pathology, 4,* 47–59.

Dawson, J., & Strout, C. (2003). *The Structured Photographic Expressive Language Test–Third Edition.* San Antonio, TX: Pearson.

Dunn, L.M., & Dunn, L.M. (1997). *Examiner's manual for the Peabody Picture Vocabulary Test–Third Edition (PPVT-III).* Circle Pines, MN: American Guidance Service.

Fey, M.E. (1986). *Language intervention with young children.* Boston: Allyn & Bacon.

Gardner, M.F. (2000a). *Expressive One-Word Picture Vocabulary Test (EOWPVT).* Navato, CA: Academic Therapy Publications.

Gardner, M.F. (2000b). *Receptive One-Word Picture Vocabulary Test (ROWPVT).* Novato, CA: Academic Therapy Publications.

German, D.J. (1991). *Tests of Word Finding in Discourse.* Allen, TX: DLM.

Gillam, R.B., & Pearson, N. (2004). *Test of Narrative Language.* Austin, TX: PRO-ED.

Greenhalgh, K.S., & Strong, C.J. (2001). Literate language features in spoken narratives of children with typical language and children with language impairments. *Language, Speech, and Hearing Services in Schools, 32,* 114–125.

Grove, N., & Tucker, S. (2003). Narratives in manual sign by children with intellectual impairments. In S. von Tetzchner & N. Grove (Eds.), *Augmentative and alternative communication: Developmental issues* (pp. 229–255). London: Whurr Publishers.

Hadley, P. (1998). Language sampling protocols for eliciting text-level discourse. *Language, Speech, and Hearing Services in Schools, 29,* 132–147.

Hammill, D., Brown, V., Larsen, S., & Wiederholt, J. (1994). *Test of Adolescent and Adult Language–Third Edition (TOAL-3).* Austin, TX: PRO-ED.

Hammill, D.D., & Newcomer, P.L. (2008a). *Test of Language Development–Intermediate: Fourth Edition (TOLD-I:4).* Los Angeles: Western Psychological Services.

Hammill, D.D., & Newcomer, P.L. (2008b). *Test of Language Development–Primary: Fourth Edition (TOLD-P:4).* Los Angeles: Western Psychological Services.

Heath, S.B. (1986). Taking a cross-cultural look at narratives. *Topics in Language Disorders, 7*(1), 84–94.

Hill, K. (2004). Augmentative and alternative communication and language: Evidence-based practice and language activity monitoring. *Topics in Language Disorders, 24,* 18–30.

Hill, K.J., & Romich, B.A. (2003). *Performance Report Tool (PeRT): A computer program for generating the AAC Performance Report.* [Computer software]. Edinboro, PA: AAC Institute.

Hochstein, D.D., McDaniel, M.A., & Nettleton, S. (2004). Recognition of vocabulary in children and adolescents with cerebral palsy: A comparison of two speech coding schemes. *Augmentative and Alternative Communication, 20,* 45–62.

Jitendra, A.K., Edwards, L.L., Sacks, G., & Jacobson, L.A. (2004). What research says about vocabulary instruction for students with learning disabilities. *Exceptional Children, 70*(3), 299–322.

Kaderavek, J.N., & Sulzby, E. (2000). Narrative production with and without specific language impairments: Oral narratives and emergent readings. *Journal of Speech, Language, and Hearing Research, 43,* 34–49.

Klee, T. (1992). Developmental and diagnostic characteristics of quantitative measures of children's language production. *Topics in Language Disorders, 12*(2), 28–41.

Light, J. (1989). Toward a definition of communicative competence for children using augmentative and alternative communication systems. *Augmentative and Alternative Communication, 5,* 137–144.

Light, J. (1997). "Let's go star fishing": Reflections on the contexts of language learning for children who use aided AAC. *Augmentative and Alternative Communication, 13,* 158–171.

Light, J., & Drager, K. (2005, November). *Maximizing language development with young children who require AAC.* Miniseminar presented at the Annual Convention of the American Speech-Language-Hearing Association, San Diego.

Light J., Roberts, B., Dimarco, R., & Greiner, N. (1998). Augmentative and alternative communication to support receptive and expressive communication for people with autism. *Journal of Communication Disorders, 31,* 153–180.

Light, J., Seligson, L., & Lund, S. (1998, August). *Teaching nondisabled peers to interact with children who use AAC.* Paper presented at the biennial conference of the International Society for Augmentative and Alternative Communication, Dublin, Ireland.

Lilienfeld, M., & Alant, E. (2005). The social interaction of an adolescent who uses AAC: The evaluation of a peer-training program. *Augmentative and Alternative Communication, 21,* 278–294.

Lund, S.K., & Light, J. (2006). Long-term outcomes for children who use augmentative and alternative communication–Part I: What is a "good" outcome? *Augmentative and Alternative Communication. 22,* 284–289.

MacKay, G., & Shaw, A. (2004). A comparative study of figurative language in children with autistic spectrum disorders. *Child Language Teaching and Therapy, 20*(1), 13–32.

McCabe, A., & Bliss, L. (2003). *Patterns of narrative discourse: A multicultural, lifespan approach.* Boston: Allyn & Bacon.

McCord, M.S., & Soto, G. (2002). Perceptions of AAC: An ethnographic investigation of Mexican-American families: *Augmentative and Alternative Communication, 20,* 209–227.

McFadden, T.U., & Gillam, R.G. (1996). An examination of the quality of narratives produced by children with language disorders. *Language, Speech, and Hearing Services in Schools, 27,* 48–56.

Miller, J.F., & Chapman, R. (2002). *Systematic Analysis of Language Transcripts* [Computer software]. Madison: University of Wisconsin, Language Analysis Laboratory.

Miller, J.F., Freiberg, C., Rolland, M., & Reeves, M. (1992). Implementing computerized language sample analysis in the public school. *Topics in Language Disorders, 12*(2), 69–82.

Miller, J., & Paul, R. (2000). *The Clinical Assessment of Language Comprehension.* Baltimore: Paul H. Brookes Publishing Co.

Miller, J., & Yoder, D. (1984). *The Miller–Yoder (M-Y) Test of Grammatical Comprehension.* Baltimore: University Park Press.

Moore-Brown, B., Huerta, M., Uranga-Hernandez, Y., & Pena, E.D. (2006). Using dynamic assessment to evaluate children with suspected learning disabilities. *Intervention in School and Clinic, 41,* 209–217.

Müller, E., & Soto, G. (2002a). Capturing the complexity of aided interactions: A conversation analysis perspective. In S. von Tetzchner & J. Clibbens (Eds.), *Understanding the theoretical and methodological bases of augmentative and alternative communication* (pp. 64–83). Proceedings of the Sixth Research Symposium of the International Society for Augmentative and Alternative Communication (ISAAC). Toronto: ISAAC.

Müller, E., & Soto, G. (2002b). Conversation patterns of three adults using aided speech: Variations across partners. *Augmentative and Alternative Communication, 18,* 77–90.

Nelson, K. (Ed.). (1989). *Narratives from the crib.* Cambridge, MA: Harvard University Press.

Nelson, N.W. (1992). Performance is the prize: Language competence and performance among AAC users. *Augmentative and Alternative Communication, 8,* 3–18.

Nippold, M. (1998). *Later language development: The school age and adolescent years.* Austin, TX: PRO-ED.

Parrette, P., Blake Huer, M., & Wyatt, T.A. (2002). Young African American children with disabilities and augmentative and alternative communication issues. *Early Childhood Education Journal, 29,* 201–207.

Paul, R. (2001). *Language disorders from infancy through adolescence* (2nd ed.). St. Louis: Mosby.

Paul, R. (2007). *Language disorders from infancy through adolescence* (3rd ed.). St. Louis: Mosby.

Rice, M.L., & Wexler, K. (2001). *Rice/Wexler Test of Early Grammatical Impairment.* San Antonio, TX. Pearson.

Richard, G., & Hanner, M.A. (1995). *Language Processing Test–Revised.* East Moline, IL: Lingui Systems.

Roland, C. (2004). *Communication Matrix: A communication skills assessment.* Portland, OR: Design to Learn Products.

Romski, M.A., & Sevcik, R.A. (1993). Language comprehension: Considerations for augmentative and alternative communication. *Augmentative and Alternative Communication, 9,* 281–285.

Roth, F.P., & Cassatt-James, L. (1989). The language assessment process: Clinical implications for children with severe speech impairments. *Augmentative and Alternative Communication, 5,* 165–172.

Scott, C.M., & Windsor, J. (2000). General language performance measures in spoken and written narrative discourse and expository discourse of school-age children with language learning disabilities. *Journal of Speech, Language, and Hearing Research, 43,* 324–339.

Semel, E., Wiig, E.H., & Secord, W.A. (2003). *Clinical Evaluation of Language Fundamentals, Fourth Edition (CELF-4).* Toronto, Canada: The Psychological Corporation.

Sevcik, R. (2006). Comprehension: An overlooked component in augmented language development. *Disability and Rehabilitation, 28,* 159–167.

Soto, G. (June, 2006). *Augmentative and alternative communication in children: Issues and strategies.*

Presentation at the Nebraska Summer Conference on Augmentative and Alternative Communication, Lincoln, NE.

Soto, G., & Dukhovny, E. (2008). The effect of shared book reading on the acquisition of expressive vocabulary of a 7 year old who uses AAC. *Seminars in Speech and Language. 29*(2), 133–145.

Soto, G., & Grove, N. (2001). Multi-modal transcription in augmentative and alternative communication: Theoretical and methodological consideration. In S. von Tetzchmer & J. Clibbens (Eds.), *Understanding the theoretical and methodological bases of augmentative and alternative communication* (pp. 12–14). Toronto: International Society for Augmentative and Alternative Communication.

Soto, G., & Hartmann, E. (2006). Analysis of narrative produced by four children who use augmentative and alternative communication. *Journal of Communication Disorders, 39,* 456–480.

Soto, G., Hartmann, E., & Wilkins, D. (2006). Exploring the elements of narrative that emerge in the interactions between an 8-year-old child who uses an AAC device and her teacher. *Augmentative and Alternative Communication, 22,* 231–241.

Soto, G., Yu, B., & Henneberry, S. (2007). Supporting the development of narrative skills of an 8-year-old child who uses an augmentative and alternative communication device: Case study. *Child Language Teaching and Therapy, 23,* 27–45.

Soto, G., Yu, B., & Kelso, J. (2008). Effectiveness of multifaceted narrative intervention on the stories told by a 12 year old girl who uses AAC. *Augmentative and Alternative Communication, 24,* 76–87.

Strong, C.J. (1998). *The Strong Narrative Assessment Procedure.* Madison, WI: Thinking Publications.

Swanson, L.A., Fey, M.E., Mills, C.E., & Hood, L.S. (2005). Use of narrative-based language intervention with children who have specific language impairment. *American Journal of Speech-Language Pathology, 14,* 131–143.

Templin, M. (1957). *Certain language skills in children.* Minneapolis: University of Minnesota Press.

Turkington, C., & Sussman, A. (Eds.). (1992). *The encyclopedia of deafness and hearing disorders.* New York: Facts on File.

Ukrainetz, T., & Gillam, R. (2006, November). *Telling a good story: Children with specific language impairment.* Poster presented at the American Speech-Language-Hearing Association Annual Convention, Miami, FL.

Ukrainetz, T.A., Justice, L.M., Kaderavek, J.N., Eisenberg, S.L., Gillam, R.B., & Harm, H.H. (2005). The development of expressive elaboration in fictional narratives. *Journal of Speech, Language, and Hearing Research, 48,* 1363–1377.

Waller, A., O'Mara, D.A., Tait, L., Booth, L., Brophy-Arnott, B., & Hood, H.E. (2001). Using written stories to support the use of narrative in conversation interactions: Case study. *Augmentative and Alternative Communication, 17,* 221–232.

Watkins, R.V., Kelly, D.J., Harbers, H.M., & Hollis, W. (1995). Measuring children's lexical diversity: Differentiating typical and impaired learners. *Journal of Speech and Hearing Research, 38,* 1349–1355.

Westby, C. (1991). Learning to talk–talking to learn: Oral-literate language differences. In C.S. Simon (Ed.), *Communication skills and classroom success* (pp. 181–218). San Diego: College Hill Press.

Westerveld, M.F., & Gillon, G.T. (2008). Oral narrative intervention for children with mixed reading disability. *Child Language Teaching and Therapy, 24*(1), 31–54.

Wilkinson, K.M., & Rosenquist, C. (2006). Demonstration of a method for assessing semantic organization and category membership in children with autism spectrum disorders and receptive vocabulary limitations. *Augmentative and Alternative Communication, 22,* 242–257.

Zangari, C. (November, 2004). *Adapting standardized tests for children with significant communication impairments.* Paper presented at the American Speech-Language-Hearing Association National Convention, Philadelphia.

Zangari, C. (July, 2006). *Testing children with significant disabilities: Adapting standardized measures.* Paper presented at ASHA Schools 2006 Conference, Phoenix, AZ.

Zareva, A., Schwanenflugel, P., & Nikolova, Y. (2005). Relationship between lexical competence and language proficiency: Variable sensitivity. *Studies in Second Language Acquisition, 27*(4), 567–595.

4

Diagnostic Reading Assessment for Students with AAC Needs

David A. Koppenhaver, Beth E. Foley, and Amy R. Williams

This chapter focuses on describing informal diagnostic reading assessments that may assist educators and clinicians in making more informed instructional decisions as they work with school-age children who have augmentative and alternative communication (AAC) needs. Such children present a challenge to educators because their differences interfere with mainstream reading assessment practices such as miscue analysis, reading fluency measures, timed tests, or reading aloud individual words. As a consequence, teachers find it challenging to identify and address student needs or to monitor progress. This chapter describes a variety of adaptations to common reading assessment tools and processes.

Although scholars have explored reading from many perspectives (e.g., linguistic, psycholinguistic, sociocultural), in this chapter, *reading* refers to the cognitive activity of deriving meaning from text. *Text* refers specifically to words represented by traditional orthography and written to convey meaning through a variety of print and electronic media (e.g., books, blogs, newspapers, digital communication devices). This type of reading and these types of texts have long been the focus of school-based reading instruction and assessment, and this focus has a long history of success in American public schools for many children (see Allington, 2005, for a review). Some children, however, including those who rely on AAC, have not thrived. In order to more appropriately address the needs of these struggling learners, this chapter also addresses reading as a form of situated cognition.

Research in situated cognition, as it applies to schools, takes into account not only cognitive activity but also the ongoing interaction between learners and the social contexts in which they engage in that cognitive activity (Darvin, 2006). Consequently, in order to teach struggling learners more successfully, researchers and teachers must carefully explore both the planned and unplanned effects of their instruction. Schools might, for example, teach children synthetic phonics (i.e., each letter in a word represents a sound that students are taught to blend with other letter sounds in the target word in order to read it) or analytic phonics (i.e., students are taught sounds from words that they know and are taught to compare and contrast them with target words in order to read them). Although both approaches are successful in teaching phonics, they lead to two different strategic approaches when students encounter unfamiliar words in text (National Reading Panel, 2000). That is, even skills taught in isolation are not isolated cognitive activities. In addition to describing the use of assessments for identifying relative cognitive strengths and needs of readers, this chapter also explores assessments for identifying and documenting the effects and effectiveness of the classroom instruction provided to those readers.

ASSUMPTIONS

The first assumption underlying the information presented in this chapter is that all children should be considered candidates for becoming conventionally literate by virtue of being born human. *Conventional literacy* is defined here as the ability to read and write independently using traditional orthography to achieve personal purposes. This view of literacy is neither inclusive of the use of other AAC symbol sets such as picture symbols, nor is it inclusive of other language or media arts such as listening, viewing, or speaking. These are important skills that can and do contribute to literacy learning, but they are not literacy skills in themselves. Converging evidence from research involving a wide variety of populations supports this definition and a belief that 1) children both with and without disabilities have similar literacy learning needs and 2) observed difficulties are a consequence of both individual skill differences and proffered learning opportunities. Recent scholarship has drawn these conclusions from disparate groups such as children with autism spectrum disorders (Nation, Clarke, Wright, & Williams, 2006), specific language impairments (Schuele, Spencer, Barako-Arndt, & Guillot, 2007), and visual impairments (Erickson & Hatton, 2007) and other children who struggle to read (Allington, 2005). In the case of individuals who use AAC, literate adults reported that their schooling experiences match fairly closely with what is known about recommended practices for literacy instruction involving typically developing children (Koppenhaver, Evans, & Yoder, 1991). The design and implementation of reading assessments described in this chapter share these assumptions.

A second set of assumptions has to do with *diagnostic reading assessment* itself, or the careful analysis of the relative strengths and needs of students as they engage in reading texts in a variety of environments. Such assessment is classroom based and most appropriately used to 1) develop profiles of individual student learning strengths and needs, 2) document learning progress or lack thereof, and 3) modify instruction to best meet the learning needs of students. Instructional modifications address changes in 1) frequency, duration, intensity, and type of intervention strategy; 2) presentation or use of materials and assistive technologies; or 3) choice of additional assessment tools and processes to more specifically identify children's learning needs. Diagnostic reading assessment is worth the time it takes only to the extent that the information gained can contribute to the design and delivery of an improved instructional plan. In no case is assessment in isolation a prerequisite to initiating reading instruction. Informal teacher observation during instruction is a critical tool in assessing the effectiveness of instruction and in planning moment-by-moment adjustments to better meet children's needs and interests (Boyd-Batstone, 2004). Most important, informal teacher observation can be accomplished without reducing the precious time allocated to instruction and learning.

WHOLE-TO-PART MODEL OF READING

The whole-to-part model of reading (see Cunningham, 1993; Erickson, Koppenhaver, & Cunningham, 2006) provides the theoretical framework for our assessment of reading as a cognitive process. The underlying premise of the model is that the primary goal of reading instruction is to teach students to read silently with comprehension. This is obvious in the immediate context of high-stakes tests (e.g., imagine a classroom full of typically developing children reading the end-of-grade test out loud) and future adult life (e.g., imagine everyone reading aloud in a library, coffee shop, waiting room, workplace, or airport). To achieve silent reading with comprehension, the reader draws on three cognitive processes simultaneously: word identification, language comprehension, and whole-text print processing. Each of these cognitive processes is a "whole" ability in itself but also a "part" that contributes to the larger instructional goal and "whole" of silent reading with comprehension. Each whole part can be assessed in order to tailor instruction more specifically to a child's relative needs and strengths. Effective teaching results not only in improvement in the whole part (e.g., word identification) but also in the whole (e.g., using sight word knowledge to read text silently with greater comprehension).

The whole-to-part model accounts for each of the five components of scientifically based reading research considered essential to reading acquisition by the National Reading Panel (2000) and required by federal reading initiatives such as Reading First (http://www.ed.gov/programs/readingfirst/index.html). These five components include 1) *phonemic awareness* and 2) *phonics*, both found in the *word identification* component of the whole-to-part model, which also includes *sight word knowledge*; 3) *fluency*, which might be considered a synonym for *print processing* in the whole-to-part model; 4) *vocabulary*, one component of *language comprehension* in the model, which also includes *knowledge of text structure*; and 5) *text comprehension*, or what the model references as *silent reading comprehension*, the goal of reading instruction.

According to the model, *word identification*, the cognitive process of turning print into sound, can be either automatic or mediated. Automatic word identification occurs when words are read effortlessly, without hesitation or conscious attention, and enhances silent reading with comprehension. Mediated word identification requires the reader to apply decoding strategies. Typically, this is accomplished by referencing letter–sound correspondences to produce a plausible phonological representation for the word in beginning reading. Morphological strategies, also referred to as "chunking" by teachers, come into play increasingly in decoding polysyllabic words. In moderation, mediated word identification supports silent reading with comprehension. When a reader has to mediate many words in any given text, however, comprehension declines.

Language comprehension is a second whole part contributing to silent reading with comprehension. Both knowledge of the world and knowledge of text structures contribute to written language comprehension. *World*, or *background*, *knowledge* refers to what the reader knows about the specific topics assumed by a text's author. *Text structure knowledge* refers to what the reader knows about syntax, cohesion, and genres of written language.

The third whole part is *whole-text print processing*, a component that helps explain the reading difficulties experienced by many children with AAC needs. Despite an ability to identify words and to understand text that is read aloud to them, they experience great difficulty in reading text independently (Erickson et al., 2006). Print processing consists of four components—eye-movement strategies, print-to-meaning links, use of inner speech, and projecting prosody—and the integration of these four components. Eye movements are rapid, intermittent movements across and down a text that are cognitively controlled. Print-to-meaning links enable readers to translate print directly to meaning, rather than mediating through sound, and enable both successful reading of homophones and more efficient reading in general. Inner speech involves phonological recoding of text in order to hold text in verbal working memory and monitor understanding. *Projecting prosody* refers to reading with expression, whether done orally or subvocally, by attending to structural features of individual words and text. Integration requires the coordinated application of these cognitive processes.

CLASSROOM LITERACY INSTRUCTION AS SITUATED COGNITION

Classroom literacy instruction is conducted in a variety of ways in a variety of environments. If the instructional settings are not attended to as carefully as the individual's relative strengths and needs, then consistent learning progress is seldom achieved by children with AAC needs (see, e.g., Koppenhaver & Yoder, 1992b; Mike, 1995). Learners are influenced by the nature of the print materials; reading and writing technologies; interactions with teachers, classmates, and volunteers; structure and frequency of learning opportunities; and the expectations of their teachers, related services personnel, and classroom aides (Koppenhaver, Pierce, Steelman, & Yoder, 1994). Children learn not only what we teach, but they also learn by how we teach. Consider the responses of two different teachers after children in each of their classes finished reading a storybook during silent reading time. In the first class, the teacher asked the child to tell her about the story, posed questions about favorite parts, inquired as to whether the child had read any other books on that topic or by that author, asked which classmates she thought might also like to read it, and then encouraged the child to tell a classroom visitor about the book. In the second class, the teacher praised the child for completing the book, encouraged her to reread it a second time, and then sent her to the library to take a computer-based, multiple-choice test on the details of the story. These responses provide quite different opportunities to learn concepts such as the functions of independent reading, the nature of reading as a cognitive activity, the value of reader response, or the importance of classroom community. Although all schools assess children's silent reading comprehension, situated cognition suggests a broader lens that also enables investigation of the degree to which children are able to apply growing silent reading with comprehension skills beyond the classroom and whether they choose to read when it is not required, whether in school or beyond.

KEY ISSUES FOR STUDENTS WITH AAC NEEDS

Learning to read is extremely difficult for students who use AAC (Dahlgren Sandberg, 2001; Koppenhaver & Yoder, 1992a; Vandervelden & Siegel, 1999). The majority of these students, even those with average intelligence, do not attain conventional literacy (Foley & Pollatsek, 1999). Both intrinsic and extrinsic factors contribute to these observed reading difficulties.

Intrinsic Factors

According to Smith (2005), intrinsic factors can be divided into four areas of potential difficulty: physical, sensory/perceptual, linguistic, and cognitive. One additional area is also discussed here—engagement. Difficulties in any of these areas can interfere with reading achievement. When multiple impairments are present, as is the case for the majority of individuals who use AAC, access to conventional literacy may seem out of reach. A number of individuals with multiple impairments have achieved high levels of written language competence (see, e.g., Chapple, 2000; Koppenhaver et al., 1991), however, dispelling the notion that these differences fully explain the literacy problems seen in many individuals who use AAC.

Physical Differences   The majority of individuals with AAC needs have congenital physical impairments, such as cerebral palsy, that limit movement (von Tetzchner & Martinsen, 2000). The severity of these impairments correlates negatively with subsequent reading achievement, at least in part because learning opportunities and interactions with the environment are limited from an early age, as are critical emergent literacy experiences such as independently exploring books (Schonell, 1957). Alternate strategies and adaptations are needed to ensure physical access to books and meaningful participation in reading activities. Even when appropriate alternatives (e.g., adapted or multimedia books, AAC supports) are provided to students with severe physical disabilities, related issues such as poor positioning, limited head control, slow access rates, or fatigue can negatively influence reading performance.

Sensory and Perceptual Differences   Visual and hearing impairments can have a profound impact on learning to read. Visual impairments challenge the development of print processing skills, particularly in children with significant physical impairments, who may not be able to use braille. Hearing impairments negatively affect reading development by limiting access to the sound structure of language, which is critical to learning to read and write in an alphabetic language.

Visual Impairment   Many individuals who use AAC have visual impairments—up to 60% of those with cerebral palsy, for example—and thus have lesser print information available to them as they learn to read (Erhardt, 1990; Smith, 2005). Conditions such as cortical visual impairment can result in both degraded print information and inconsistent performance in visual processing tasks. In order to maximize access to printed words, students with visual impairments may need adaptations such as enlarged print, specific background colors and contrasts, or placement of reading materials at a certain distance or angle. Students who are blind may need supports such as audio or braille books and screen-reader software in order to gain access to text, the computer, or the Internet.

Even individuals with normal visual acuity may have abnormal eye movements that hinder text processing. In a study of reading ability in adults with cerebral palsy, several participants attributed their slow reading rates to frequent involuntary eye movements that caused them to lose their place on the page while reading (Foley & Pollatsek, 1999). For one of these individuals, a standardized reading measure revealed a fourth-grade reading level for extended text. When the same text was presented one line at a time on his computer, however, his reading comprehension score immediately improved to a ninth-grade level. This case underscores the need to carefully consider the potential effect of visual impairments on reading performance and the value of using appropriately adapted reading assessment tools and strategies when visual impairments are a possible concern.

Hearing Impairment The incidence of hearing loss in individuals with cerebral palsy, estimated at 25%–41%, is much higher than in the general population, which is 2.5%–3% (Siegenthaler, 1987). Although the type and severity of hearing impairments among individuals who use AAC vary greatly, even mild hearing loss can significantly delay the acquisition of language and literacy skills (Smith, 2005). With appropriate amplification from hearing aids, classroom FM systems, or other assistive listening devices, the effect of hearing loss can be minimized. Students who are deaf may need sign language interpreting services in the classroom to benefit from reading instruction or fully participate in assessment.

Linguistic Differences Children with AAC needs often struggle to acquire basic language and communication skills, and they frequently exhibit difficulties across multiple language domains (Sturm & Clendon, 2004). Their decreased phonological skills may interfere with acquisition of phonemic awareness, accurate decoding skills, use of inner speech, and, ultimately, text comprehension (Dahlgren Sandberg, 2001; Foley & Pollatsek, 1999; Vandervelden & Siegel, 1999). Restricted vocabulary development and limited background knowledge and experience can make the use of contextual cues during reading more difficult (Light, 1997). Deficits in morphological development impair the ability to recognize meaning changes that are signaled by inflectional (e.g., plural and verb tense markers) and derivational (e.g., prefixes, suffixes) morphemes in written words (Binger & Light, 2002; Sutton, Soto, & Blockberger, 2002). Delays or deviations in syntactic development constrain sentence- and discourse-level text comprehension (Foley & Pollatsek, 1999; van Balkom & Welle Donker-Gimbrère, 1996). Verbal working memory limitations affect integration of cohesive devices (e.g., pronoun references, conjunctions) and ongoing comprehension monitoring during reading of extended text (Foley & Pollatsek, 1999). Impaired pragmatic skills may reduce understanding of different text genres (e.g., narrative versus expository text) as well as the expected participation patterns (e.g., turn taking, requests for clarification) associated with classroom reading routines (von Tetzchner & Martinsen, 2000). By completing a comprehensive language assessment, speech-language pathologists (SLPs) can contribute valuable information to AAC teams regarding the nature of students' receptive and expressive language deficits and their potential effect on reading achievement.

Another linguistic difference gaining attention in the AAC community is that of students who are English language learners. This diverse population shares only a single characteristic in common (i.e., speaking English as a second language; Krashen, 1982). The American Federation of Teachers (2008) noted several critical assessment issues relevant to this population, including 1) the conflict between the testing requirement in the No Child Left Behind (NCLB) Act of 2001 (PL 107-110) and the absence of linguistically modified or native language assessments and 2) the fundamental inconsistency of NCLB's requirement of using valid and reliable assessment and testing English language learners in English. There is widespread professional agreement, however, that using informal, diagnostic assessments, such as those described in this chapter, will support practitioners in more effectively tailoring instruction to individual English language learners' strengths and needs (see, e.g., Cooper & Kiger, 2001; Gillet, Temple, & Crawford, 2004).

Cognitive Differences Because skilled reading requires the application of cognitive and metacognitive resources, there is no question that cognitive impairment affects the ease with which individuals who use AAC acquire reading skills and the extent to which conventional reading skills develop (Smith, 2005). Accurate assessment of cognitive functioning in individuals with severe speech and physical impairments is extremely difficult, however, and, as a result, literacy learning potential is often grossly underestimated. The presence of significant cognitive impairment must not be used as an excuse to exclude students from reading instruction, and legal mandates make it clear that children do not have to prove themselves to be capable of learning to read before appropriate instruction is provided (Downing, 2005). Even individuals diagnosed with severe to profound levels of intellectual impairment have demonstrated the potential for recognizing sight words (Alberto & Fredrick, 2000; Browder & Lalli, 1991; Romski & Sevcik, 1996) and reading for daily living and enjoyment (Lalli & Browder, 1993), with some demonstrating these skills and interests for the first time only as adults (Foley & Staples, 2003).

Engagement   Reading engagement, or student motivation to read, has long been considered a significant contributor to achievement (e.g., Stanovich, 1986) but difficult to measure objectively (McKenna & Kear, 1990). Program for International Student Assessment (PISA) researchers operationally defined *reading engagement* as "the time that students report reading a diversity of material for pleasure and their interest in and attitudes toward reading" (Brozo, Shield, & Topping, 2007/2008, p. 307) and reported that engagement was the student characteristic correlating most highly with reading achievement across the 32 countries studied (Kirsch et al., 2002). *Diversity of reading* referred to six text types: magazines, comics, fiction books, nonfiction books, e-mail, and web pages. *Leisure reading* referred to daily reading by personal choice. *Attitudes toward reading* referred to the extent to which students agreed with statements such as, "I read only if I have to," "Reading is one of my favorite hobbies," or "I cannot sit still and read for more than a few minutes." Of critical importance to educators was the finding that students from the lowest socioeconomic status who were highly engaged readers performed as well on reading achievement measures as 1) highly engaged students from the middle socioeconomic status group and 2) students with medium levels of engagement in the high socioeconomic group. In other words, "keeping students engaged in reading and learning might make it possible for them to overcome what might otherwise be insuperable barriers to academic success" (Brozo et al., 2007/2008, p. 307). Data were not reported on students with disabilities in general or on students with AAC needs specifically.

Summary   The intrinsic factors described previously interact in complex ways to impede literacy development in individuals with AAC needs. Members of AAC teams who assess the physical, sensory/perceptual, linguistic, and cognitive capabilities of students using AAC must collaborate to develop profiles that inform reading assessment and intervention by revealing what students *can* do and how their current strengths can be developed and extended. Similarly, educational teams (and researchers, for that matter) must address greater attention to student reading engagement in selecting assessments and planning interventions.

Extrinsic Factors

Team members must also consider critical extrinsic factors that might be contributing to reported literacy deficits.

Home Environment   It is well known that all children experience greater success in literacy learning when they have engaged in rich language and literacy learning experiences before entering school. Unfortunately, children with AAC needs have far less time available for participation in these types of activities (Light & Kelford Smith, 1993), and the experiences they do have tend to be very different from those of their peers. Children with AAC needs tend to be read to less often and often lack the means to communicate effectively during literacy interactions. Parents and caregivers may not know that reading is an attainable skill for their children, or they may be discouraged by children's short attention spans, difficulty seeing print or pictures, limited feedback, or inability to respond consistently during shared reading activities (Light & Kelford Smith, 1993; Marvin, 1994).

These problems may lead to lower expectations for literacy development. In addition, parental priorities for children who use AAC may emphasize other aspects of development over literacy, such as effective communication, mobility, and feeding (Light & Kelford Smith, 1993; Light & McNaughton, 1993). Research suggests that high parental expectations and priorities for literacy engagement are associated with the development of skilled reading (Koppenhaver et al., 1991). Yet, reduced opportunities for literacy engagement, lower parental expectations, and different priorities may set the stage for later reading problems (Coleman, 1992).

School Environment
Pressley, Mohan, Fingeret, Reffitt, and Raphael-Bogaert (2007) found that in school settings that produce high reading achievement, students reported spending 90% of their time engaged in such meaningful and appropriately challenging reading and writing activities as building background knowledge, reading for a variety of purposes, and talking about books they had read. Reading instruction in these schools was multifaceted, involving explicit teaching and modeling of skills balanced by ample opportunity to apply those skills during real reading and writing activities. Effective teachers provided extensive scaffolding for students as they applied newly learned skills, but they also encouraged students to develop self-regulation, accomplishing as much as they can on their own. Effective classroom environments were consistently positive and motivating and typically overflowed with quality children's literature, student-created texts, and bulletin boards covered with student work.

Most of the literacy experiences of students who use AAC bear little resemblance to these recommended practices in reading instruction (Beukelman, Mirenda, & Sturm, 2005; Mike, 1995). Students with significant disabilities are not always expected to learn to read and write (Erickson & Koppenhaver, 1995; Light & McNaughton, 1993), and literacy goals may not even be considered during educational planning. Unfortunately, literacy goals are too often focused on letter recognition, fill-in-the-blank exercises, or reading "survival" words (Browder & Lalli, 1991; Mike, 1995). This emphasis on isolated skills, one of the least effective strategies for improving literacy, prevents students from engaging in more meaningful instructional activities (Beukelman et al., 2005; Koppenhaver & Yoder, 1992a).

Students with AAC needs typically require more time and practice to acquire literacy skills, and yet they receive significantly less instructional time than their peers (Koppenhaver & Yoder, 1992b). They may spend up to 38% of literacy instructional time on nonliteracy activities, thus losing many critical literacy learning opportunities to activities such as feeding, toileting, and adjusting equipment (Koppenhaver & Yoder, 1993). Students who use AAC typically have limited access to quality children's literature, with few changes or additions made to the reading materials available to them during the school year (Katims, 2000). Unlike their typically developing peers, they frequently receive some or all of their reading instruction from paraprofessionals rather than highly qualified teachers. When students who use AAC do not acquire reading skills during their elementary school years, attempts to teach them to read are often abandoned during their middle school and high school years, despite increasing evidence that their literacy learning can continue across the lifespan (Downing, 2005; Foley & Staples, 2003).

Even when students with AAC needs are provided with opportunities for high-quality reading instruction, they may not be able to communicate sufficiently during these experiences to demonstrate what they know. Because they have limited speech, they cannot read aloud, ask questions, or explain what they are thinking. Access to AAC can reduce these barriers, but only if the available vocabulary is appropriate and the organization of the communication system supports participation in classroom discourse related to core curriculum content and instructional routines (Beukelman & Mirenda, 2005). Unfortunately, most AAC systems provide users with access to only a few hundred concepts, and most children have access to significantly fewer than that (Light, 1997).

Practitioners clearly need reading assessment tools that will help them to identify the individual capabilities of students who use AAC. Identifying intrinsic factors in the absence of addressing extrinsic factors, however, will do little to remediate reading difficulties. Effective reading assessment also must consider carefully the quantity, quality, and effectiveness of reading instruction provided to students with AAC needs.

APPLICATION OF THE DIAGNOSTIC READING ASSESSMENT PROCESS

Informal diagnostic reading assessment is aimed at determining 1) a child's relative strengths and needs with reference to the whole parts of silent reading comprehension and 2) the influences of the instructional environment. This information is then used to shape an intervention plan and document its relative effectiveness.

Adapting Reading Assessments to Individual Differences

Successful application of the diagnostic reading assessment instruments and process described here requires an understanding of the complex array of factors influencing literacy learning in children with AAC needs and an orientation toward problem solving. Children who have AAC needs will likely require individual adaptation of reading assessment materials, presentation modes, and response modes. Because the assessments described in this chapter are informal, such adaptations are encouraged. An understanding of the whole-to-part model of reading, social cognition, and the aims of the specific assessments should guide the decision-making process. Adaptations should be chosen because they make it easier for children to demonstrate what they know, but not at the expense of gaining important information. For example, increasing font size or spacing between words is a reasonable accommodation during silent reading, but reading aloud to children is not because it eliminates the possibility of inferring their print processing capabilities. Partner-assisted scanning with full alphabet arrays is a reasonable accommodation during spelling tasks, but providing only the needed letters in random order is not. See Beukelman and Mirenda (2005) for a more comprehensive discussion of potential adaptations of assessment materials to the individual needs of children. The particular assessment instruments and their application are detailed next.

Assessing Reading as Cognition

Our first assessment aim is to find out how well students read and which aspects of the reading process are their relative strengths or needs. To do so, we first determine whether they are beginning readers or developing readers by informally observing them in classroom literacy tasks, talking with family members and previous teachers, and examining cumulative records. *Beginning readers* are those who know a few sight words and may be able to read or understand very basic texts with a short phrase or sentence per page. With such readers, the focus of assessment is on subprocesses contributing to word identification. The Early Reading Spelling Inventory (ERSI; Morris & Slavin, 2003) and its phonemic awareness subsection are particularly useful for examining the cognitive reading processes of beginning readers. *Developing readers* are those who have a more substantial sight vocabulary, can read text independently, or can understand text that is read aloud to them. With such students, the focus of assessment is on all the components of the whole-to-part model. Informal reading inventories, such as the Qualitative Inventory of Word Knowledge (QIWK; Schlagal, 1982), are useful in assessing the wider array of reading competencies demonstrated by developing readers.

Assessment of Beginning Reading Skills   Beginning reading skills mark a transition from nonconventional emergent literacy understandings and skills. Of particular importance at this earliest stage of conventional literacy are children's understandings and use of letters, sounds, and words.

Administering the Early Reading Spelling Inventory   The ERSI is a collection of informal assessments in four areas (i.e., alphabet knowledge, concept of word, phoneme awareness, and sight word recognition) that contribute to word identification. Originally designed to screen first-grade students who were performing at a low level for intensive tutoring assistance, it is often used by kindergarten and first-grade teachers to provide a comprehensive and detailed picture of beginning reader's word knowledge (Morris, 1998; Morris & Slavin, 2003). The ERSI is a useful assessment to guide instructional decision making for school-age students who are beginning readers and also as a follow-up assessment for students whose word identification level or overall performance is below first grade when tested on an individual reading inventory (IRI).

The *alphabet knowledge* assessment consists of both recognition and production components. For students with AAC needs, the recognition task is adapted from the original so that students are asked to point to the correct choice from letters presented randomly four at a time. All upper- and lowercase letters are assessed. For the production task, the child writes the alphabet letters one by one as the teacher dictates them in random order.

Concept of word refers to the reader's ability to match spoken words to printed words while reading (Morris, 1981). For students with AAC needs, the concept of word task is adapted from the original so that students are asked to point to the text as it is read aloud by someone else slowly but fluently. The teacher models finger-point reading, or pointing by whatever means the child uses, as the teacher reads aloud each of two different short texts, and then the student is asked to point as the text is read aloud a second time. Finally, the student is asked to point to two target words in each sentence. Text presentation may be modified in any way needed to facilitate pointing (e.g., enlarged print).

Assessing *phoneme awareness* in children with AAC needs is facilitated by a body of research demonstrating that typically developing children's invented spellings are a valid assessment of such knowledge (Mann, Tobin, & Wilson, 1987; Morris & Perney, 1984). This assessment requires students to spell 12 target words (i.e., *back, feet, step, junk, picking, mail, side, chin, dress, peeked, lamp, road)* because printed English maps onto spoken English at the phoneme level. Teachers model spelling by sounding out the letters of two short words, thinking aloud through the process as they write each word, "Map...mmmm...aahh...puh...map...mmm...M...aahh...A...puh... P...map...M-A-P." Then each of the 12 target words is spoken aloud by the administrator, and the child is asked to spell it. Words are usually spoken aloud, spoken in a short sentence, and spoken aloud a final time. Unlike the think-aloud models, the administrator does *not* stretch out the pronunciation for the child (e.g., the administrator says *feet*, not *f-f-f-e-e-e-t*). When students spell phonetically, their spellings may be examined for number of phonemes represented logically or accurately. For example, different children might spell *feet* with one logical phoneme (e.g., F, FA), two logical phonemes (e.g., FT, FE), or three (e.g., FETE, FET).

Children also may spell words with strategies other than letter–sound correspondence. If children have keyboard access, then they may spell with random letters. If they have pencil access, then they may scribble. These children understand that print has meaning because they attempt to write something when asked to spell. They understand little about its forms or conventions. Other children will spell with the same few letters, use the same number of letters for every word they write, use a few letters to write words representing small things, or use many letters to write words representing large things. These children are relying on visual cue strategies but do not understand that letters map onto sounds. As children begin to learn rules for spelling, either by inference or direct instruction, they begin to use transitional strategies that are rule based, doubling letters or combining vowels in ways that children spelling with phonetic cues do not (e.g., spelling *light* as *liet*, *play* as *plai*, *steep* as *steap*). Finally, conventional spelling is marked by a majority of words spelled accurately. Most children demonstrate a variety of different strategies across words and writing experiences.

For students with AAC needs, the *sight word recognition* task is adapted from the original so that students are asked to identify five, high-frequency sight words and five short-vowel, decodable words by pointing to each as it presented with three other choices sharing the same number of letters and some of the same letters or sounds.

Interpreting the Early Reading Spelling Inventory and Acting on the Results   In its original form, the ERSI (Morris & Slavin, 2003) is accompanied by a scoring system for within-class student comparison. Most practitioners simply examine the performance of students who use AAC in each of the four sets of tasks and then teach students the skills with which they demonstrate difficulties.

_____   Children with disabilities often require us to adapt assessment protocols if we are to gather instructionally useful information. Tyler was a 10-year-old boy with Down syndrome and limited intelligible speech who appeared to possess beginning reading skills. We administered the ERSI to explore his relative strengths and needs. Because his parents said he used the home computer independently and we wanted to assess his letter name knowledge, we began by asking him to type specific letters. Tyler provided no response to our requests, even after we modeled the task repeatedly. Because his mother said he enjoyed sequencing word cards, we decided letter tiles might be an appropriate alternative. Presenting him with a few letter tiles at a time to make sure he understood the new task, we found he readily responded to our requests to find particular letters. Then, given 5–6 alphabet tiles at a time, Tyler quickly identified 24 uppercase and 7 lowercase letters.

Thinking that context might assist in interpreting Tyler's speech, we decided to assess his concept of word exactly as designed by modeling reading aloud and pointing to the words. Then, we asked Tyler to do the same, followed by pointing to specific target words in the text. Getting little engagement and no desired responses from Tyler, we asked his parents for ideas. They asked him to point to words in the sentence that they were fairly certain he knew. Tyler quickly engaged with the task and soon was pointing in response to any word we requested. He readily demonstrated knowledge of sight words such as *on*, *the*, *dog*, and *is* and even lower-frequency words such as *water* and *walking*.

We still had been unable to get him to demonstrate concept of word by finger-point reading independently. We read one of his favorite books with him, thinking familiarity of text might lead to better engagement and the desired behavior. He still did not read aloud or finger-point to words. What he did begin doing, however, was attempt to move our fingers to get us to continue reading aloud. Finishing one familiar book, we selected another beginning reading text, explained the task to his mother, and asked her to try. She, too, had difficulty eliciting the desired behavior but negotiated with Tyler when he tried to move her hand. She explained that she only would read aloud if he would point to the words for her. She then proceeded to read each word in the text as he pointed to it. In this unconventional way, Tyler demonstrated concept of word by directing his mother's read-aloud behavior.

Remaining tasks were modified to multiple choice, by which means we found that Tyler knew 8 of 10 decodable words (and 50 other sight words) but had limited phonetic spelling skills. By enlisting parent suggestions, guiding parent participation, using familiar books, modeling desired response behaviors in multiple materials, and allowing for multiple-choice responses, we were able to gather a significant amount of information about Tyler's strengths in sight word and alphabet knowledge, concept of word, and concepts about print, as well as his instructional needs in letter–sound relationships.   _____

Administering a Developmental Spelling Assessment   A developmental spelling assessment is a useful and efficient follow-up to guide instructional decision making for school-age students whose word identification level or overall IRI performance is approximately first-grade level. Rather than administering the entire ERSI, as in the case of children whose IRI performance is below first-grade level, practitioners administer just the 12 words of the phoneme assessment described previously in the ERSI administration. The child's spellings provide an indication of beginning word knowledge, within-word letter–sound correspondence, and which strategies the child uses to read or spell unfamiliar words.

Interpreting the Developmental Spelling Assessment and Acting on the Results
For a child who uses random letters or scribbles, practitioners explore using activities such as pairing

texts with nursery rhymes when they are recited, using big books and pointing as they are read aloud to help children become more attuned to the print, reading aloud predictable and patterned texts to help children begin to acquire a few sight words, or using sign-in routines with follow-up modeling as needed so that children learn some letters and how to write their names without engaging in copying tasks. For children writing with phonetic cue strategies, practitioners try to incorporate the use of talking word processors set at the letter and word level, teach children what letters are vowels and that each word they write must have at least one, and try to find additional opportunities for writing throughout the day (e.g., lists of materials needed for activities, letters home, memos to the principal). Cunningham (2004) provided a wide range of additional strategies that may be employed to enhance children's learning of letters, sounds, and words.

Assessment of Developing Reading Skills   As children gain competence in reading words individually and in text, or in understanding texts that are read aloud to them, additional assessments become relevant. Each assessment described next assists in more efficiently fine-tuning reading programs to support student strengths and address student needs.

Administering an Informal Reading Inventory   IRIs enable assessment of the components of the whole-to-part model described previously: word identification, language comprehension, and print processing. After assessing performance in each of the three whole parts, practitioners ask the question, "What is preventing this student from reading silently with comprehension one level higher than present performance?" By comparing performance on IRIs, which yield grade-level performance estimates in each of these three areas, practitioners can then tailor instructional programs and strategies to meet more specifically the needs of particular students. Two IRIs that have been widely used by practitioners and school systems are Johns's (2005) *Basic Reading Inventory* and Leslie and Caldwell's (2005) *Qualitative Reading Inventory–Fourth Edition*. These and other IRIs are similar in structure, consisting of word lists and multiple forms of passages both at increasing degrees of difficulty. All IRIs are informal instruments that are individually administered.

Word Identification   At present, there is no valid and reliable way to assess automatic word recognition (i.e., sight word recognition) in children with AAC needs, although at least one study attempting to develop such a tool is under way (see Erickson et al., 2007, 2008). Mediated word identification (i.e., identifying words by examination, decoding), however, can be assessed by practitioners who select one of the graded word lists from an IRI at a level where they believe the child will be successful. They modify the list by presenting the target word and three other choices that are visually similar. For example, for the target word *bat*, they might also present *bag, bad*, and *dip*. Once the list has been modified, practitioners ask children to "show me *bat*" or "which word is *bat*" while presenting the four visual choices in a format that enables the child to respond by whatever means is most efficient. For example, many children can use finger-pointing to indicate their response, and the adaptation needed might involve adjusting the location of the test items (e.g., closer together, further apart) to make them physically accessible. For children who use an eye-pointing response, test items in an appropriate font size can be attached to the four corners of a Plexiglas eye-gaze board. The child is verbally and physically cued to look at each word choice and then asked to eye-point to the word believed to be correct. For children who cannot use these forms of pointing but who can clearly indicate yes or no through some physical movement (e.g., looking up for yes and down for no), partner-assisted scanning may work well. In this case, the instructor points to each word in sequence and the child indicates yes or no until his or her word choice is clearly identified. The highest graded list in which the child successfully identifies 90% of the words is noted as the word identification level (e.g., second grade).

Note that this adapted assessment requires the child to make a speech-to-print match (i.e., match the assessor's spoken word to its written representation in the four choices) rather than the print-to-speech match (i.e., look at the printed word and pronounce it aloud) required of speaking children, but it provides fewer complications than an alternative that has been used clinically and discussed in the literature—presenting a picture and multiple word choices (see, e.g., Vandervelden & Siegel, 1999). One problem with using pictures is the confusion that they may introduce (e.g., a child may look at a picture and think it represents *chair*, but the intended target is *sit*). A more significant problem is introduced conceptually in that the adaptation confounds word identification assessment with language comprehension task demands. Children with AAC needs must identify the vocabulary item pictured in order to produce its oral language equivalent internally and then match that oral language to the appropriate written word choice.

Language Comprehension   To assess language comprehension, practitioners choose a graded passage from the IRI at the grade level of the child's word identification performance. They read the passage aloud to the child, directing the child to listen carefully so that comprehension questions can be answered. These questions are found accompanying the passages in an IRI. Except in the case of skilled AAC users (i.e., those who have both wide and efficient access to vocabulary), practitioners must adapt most IRIs to provide multiple, plausible, text-based responses of similar length. After the passage is read aloud, practitioners read the first question aloud to the child, read aloud and point to each answer, and then ask the child to indicate which response is believed to be correct (e.g., The practitioner would read aloud while pointing to each, "Where did this story take place? On the water. Under the water. On the beach. On the dock."). Students are not asked to read the questions or the possible responses to themselves in order to keep the assessment as pure a measure of passage comprehension as possible. The process continues for the remaining questions. The highest grade-level passage for which the child answers 80% of the questions correctly (e.g., second grade) is noted as the child's written language comprehension level.

Print Processing   Print processing is not tested directly but rather assumed to be the area of greatest need if the child's performance in reading passages silently with comprehension is at a lower level than the word identification or language comprehension performance. For this assessment, practitioners choose a different graded passage than that used for listening comprehension from the IRI at the level of the child's word identification performance. They direct the child to, "Read the story carefully to yourself, and I will ask you questions about it." Once the child indicates completion of the passage, it is removed. As in the listening comprehension assessment, practitioners read each question aloud to the child, read and point to each answer, and ask the child to indicate which response is correct. Likewise, the highest grade-level passage for which the child successfully answers 80% of the questions (e.g., first grade) is noted as the child's silent reading comprehension level.

Additional Print Processing Assessment   It has been common practice to assess speaking children's reading fluency by calculating words read aloud per minute and comparing it with oral reading fluency tables. This, of course, is not possible for children with AAC needs. Instead, during the silent reading task, practitioners should surreptitiously note the time the child begins and finishes reading the passage and later calculate the words per minute read by the child. This is most easily accomplished by seating children during testing so that a clock is out of their view, typically on the wall behind them. Children should not be aware that the reading is being timed so that they will read at a typical rate and focus on understanding the passage rather than focusing on reading quickly. Student performance can be compared with the silent reading rates generated from the ongoing study of reading fluency of students in second through sixth grade by Morris and colleagues (Frye, Kucan, & Bloodgood, 2007; Morris, Mock, & Perney, 2007) found in Table 4.1. To use these silent reading rates most thoughtfully, practitioners should 1) only calculate words per minute for the highest grade-level passage that the child reads with 80% comprehension or better, not the passage(s) the child struggles with and 2) use the tables to guide intervention decision making in print processing.

Interpreting Performance on the Individual Reading Inventory and Acting on the Results   The child's area of greatest need can be determined once a grade-level estimate for each

Table 4.1.   Silent reading rates of students in Grades 2–6

Grade level	Number of students	Average words per minute
2	126	130
3	257	150
4	234	167
5	219	173
6	105	171

Sources: Frye, Kucan, & Bloodgood, 2007; Morris, Mock, & Perney, 2007.

of the three areas (word identification, language comprehension, silent reading comprehension) is obtained. Obviously, the lowest score is indicative of the child's greatest need. When silent reading comprehension is the lowest score, it is indicative of a print processing need and instructional emphasis on reading fluency. In such a case, higher word identification and language comprehension scores would indicate that they are not the source of greatest difficulty. In the case of ties, however, when listening comprehension is involved, then language is the area of greatest need. Without adequate language comprehension, the child will be unable to read with understanding regardless of word identification or print processing abilities. Children with such a profile of word reading and print processing skills greatly in excess of language abilities often are referred to as hyperlexic (see, e.g., Silberberg & Silberberg, 1967). In the case of a tie between word identification and silent reading comprehension, when language is at a higher level, then word identification is the greatest instructional need. Without an ability to identify words in isolation, processing words in text cannot proceed. Following are a few sample profiles and interpretations:

Luke

Word identification: Grade level 3

Listening comprehension: Grade level 5

Silent reading comprehension: Grade level 2

Luke's lowest performance was in reading passages silently to himself, which he did successfully at the second-grade level. His greatest need then is print processing.

Jackie

Word identification: Grade level 1

Listening comprehension: Grade level 1

Silent reading comprehension: Grade level 1

Jackie performed at the first-grade level on all three assessments. Because listening comprehension performance is involved in the tie for lowest score, her greatest instructional need is language comprehension.

With the resulting profile of reading performance, educators can shift the balance of instruction to more specifically meet the needs of the child. For example, the educator whose student's language comprehension score was lowest on the profile could consult with an SLP, incorporate more guided listening lessons into guided reading instruction, focus more intensively on providing interactive and direct experiences from which to enhance the child's language learning, take extra care to develop background knowledge relevant to specific text-based experiences across the day, and so forth. The educator whose student's word identification score was lowest could examine more closely the success the child is having with the current word-level instruction and supplement it with additional sight word or decoding instruction, use of a talking word processor, or any of a wide variety of child-centered learning activities (e.g., Cunningham, 2004). The educator whose student's print processing performance is interfering with reading progress could increase the quantities of easy reading or repeated readings, employ greater use of partner reading, or encourage reading along with taped books in the home. The profile of grade-level performance estimates in the three whole parts can assist decisions about how to use teaching assistants or volunteers, the kinds of materials to purchase, how to organize the instructional day, and what advice to provide to parents wishing to assist their child's progress.

Administering the Qualitative Inventory of Word Knowledge   The QIWK (Schlagal, 1982) provides additional information as a diagnostic spelling inventory for students who spell most of the words on the developmental spelling assessment correctly or whose overall IRI performance is above a first-grade level. The QIWK is comprised of six graded lists of words. Practitioners should begin assessment with a list that is one grade level below the identified word identification level on the IRI (e.g., if the child scored at the second-grade level in word identification on the IRI, then practitioners would begin QIWK assessment with the first-grade word list). As in the other spelling assessments described previously, practitioners say the target word aloud, say it aloud in a short sentence, and say the word again. The student should write the word only, not the sentence, using any writing tool, including eye-pointing, that enables letter-by-letter spelling.

If a child scores at or below 30% on a word list, then the teacher should move to the next easier list. If the child scores above 30%, then the teacher should continue administering the next more difficult list and continue this process until a frustration level score is reached (i.e., fewer than 30% correct). The results indicate the word level where children are most likely to profit from instruction. Children who work at instructional levels tend to make more sophisticated and predictable errors while learning more efficiently (Morris, Nelson, & Perney, 1986). Word-level instruction can be designed based on the errors in the instructional level list. For instance, if errors indicate a lack of mastery of the distinction between words ending with -ar or -are, then word sort instruction could begin with this feature (e.g., car/care, star/stare, far/fare).

Situated Cognition/Classroom Implementation   Because literacy instruction is an example of situated cognition, practitioners must assess not only student reading performance but also the student's response to instruction, including reading attitudes and interests. Such information can be used profitably to design instruction and instructional environments that teach skills efficiently and build a student's motivation to read.

Administering a Reading Attitude Inventory

Teachers have long used a variety of informal interview procedures and questionnaires to explore students' reading interests. McKenna and Kear (1990), however, have developed a valid and reliable instrument for measuring student attitudes toward reading. Norms for elementary Grades 1–6 have been derived from administration to a national sample of 18,000 children. The test is child friendly in appearance and wording. Students respond to questions such as, "How do you feel about reading during summer vacation?" or "How do you feel about using a dictionary?" by choosing from four pictures of the cartoon character Garfield, who is shown very happy, smiling, frowning, and very unhappy. The multiple-choice student response format makes the assessment easily administered to students with AAC needs. Point totals (4, 3, 2, 1 based on degree of happiness) are added for the items to derive raw scores for the student's interest in recreational, academic, and general reading. A chart is provided by grade level to determine a student's percentiles in these three areas relative to the sample. By administering the assessment early in the school year, educators gain information that may guide instructional planning. By administering the assessment again late in the school year, educators can examine the effect of the instructional program on the student's attitudes toward reading. For example, educators might find that a student loves recreational reading but dislikes academic reading. Providing a strong self-selected reading component in the child's day might create more positive feelings about reading in school.

Systematic Classroom Observation

The systematic observation processes described here are an implementation of the principles of response to intervention (RTI). Designed to address concerns about the definition and identification of students with learning disabilities, RTI has become one of the most popular alternative identification methods (Fuchs, Mock, Morgan, & Young, 2003). Structurally, this dynamic measure involves 1) providing instruction that is generally effective in the classroom, 2) monitoring student progress, 3) providing alternative or additional instruction from the classroom teacher or others to students who struggle, 4) further monitoring student progress, and 5) implementing evaluation for special education services for students who remain unsuccessful despite these steps. There are two primary models of RTI: standard protocol and problem solving. The standard protocol uses empirically validated treatments for all children with similar needs within a particular domain, whereas the problem-solving method is an inductive process that requires evaluating student responsiveness to successive iterations of intervention. Little research conclusively supports the effectiveness of RTI, and the method has yet to be studied in serving or identifying students with severe disabilities.

The systematic observation described here, a version of the problem-solving RTI model, is based on the beliefs that 1) all children can learn and 2) there are an infinite variety of ways to assist their learning. Consequently, if students are not successful, then it is important to systematically modify texts, tasks, technologies, and contexts until more successful outcomes are achieved. Intervention planning draws on empirically validated treatments, research literature involving other struggling readers, clinical observation, teacher experience, and communication between team members. Improved student learning outcomes are the primary goal, and placement or labeling decisions are valued only to the extent that they lead to measurable improvement in literacy learning outcomes. To identify possible interventions, professionals consider not only the recommendations of the National Research Council (1999) and the National Reading Panel (2000) for typically developing children but also the wider array of research-based and practical strategies for struggling readers and children with disabilities such as Allington (2005), Erickson and Koppenhaver (2007), McKenna (2002), or Rasinski and Padak (2004). The ultimate test is whether individual students learn successfully, which can be systematically assessed using the hypothesis-testing procedure described next.

Hypothesis Testing   Ylvisaker et al. (2002) noted that *evidence* should be a factor that practitioners utilize in deciding particular intervention strategies with specific students in their classrooms. The kind of evidence presented in the National Reading Panel (2000) report is one such factor, but teacher observations, student characteristics, and contextual information are others. Although few would challenge the validity of teacher observation in the classroom, many question the reliability. Classroom activity is complex and fleeting, and teachers have multiple responsibilities at any given moment. Hypothesis testing is one way that educators address this concern by systematically recording, organizing, and interpreting their observations.

As applied in the classroom, hypothesis testing consists of a repeated four-step cycle of *observation, interpretation, hypothesis generation,* and *curricular decision making* (Stephens, 1996). During the observation phase, practitioners observe and record what they see that concerns them. The important point is not to leap to interpretations right away (e.g., Jess finds reading difficult) but rather to record observations (e.g., Jess did not volunteer any information when the class was summarizing the reading). Some teachers create forms in which they have spaces to record the child's name, date, texts, tasks, technologies, and contexts of instruction (see, e.g., Afflerbach, 1993). Other teachers use inexpensive and unobtrusive tools (e.g., *Quicktime Pro* software for audio recording a lesson) to gather data for later review. Often, teachers record their observations across three to five lessons before meeting with colleagues or the child's team to brainstorm interpretations. The team attempts to generate many interpretations and then examines them for patterns or most likely possibilities. These are formed into a hypothesis (e.g., If Jess were presented the same activities in a text of first-grade difficulty, then she would volunteer more information during discussion).

A curricular decision follows, is implemented in the next instructional lesson (e.g., an easier book is employed for the lesson), and the hypothesis-testing cycle continues. Beyond addressing learning difficulties, the hypothesis-testing notes form a valuable record for 1) examining the particular utility of various instructional approaches to specific classes or students and 2) reporting on student progress.

Curriculum-Based Measurement   Curriculum-based measurement (CBM) yields another kind of evidence widely used by classroom teachers and clinicians. Originally designed as a method for teachers to gauge the overall effectiveness of their instruction (Deno, 1985), CBM is now used to gauge individual student performance at a point in time or to index student progress over time. CBM is characterized by three features (Fuchs, Fuchs, & Hamlett, 2007): 1) it is standardized (i.e., behaviors to be measured and measurement procedures are specified, 2) test methods and difficulty remain constant, and 3) test content reflects desired end-of-intervention performance. Educators create alternate forms of the assessment and administer them weekly in order to quantify and compare student progress. Unfortunately, the most widely employed CBM assessments are of little use in working with children who have AAC needs. These tasks include passage reading fluency (i.e., a 1-minute oral reading task with alternative forms of passages at a single difficulty level), word identification fluency (i.e., a 1-minute oral reading task with a list sampling from high-frequency words), and letter–sound fluency (i.e., a 1-minute oral naming of sounds that go with randomly ordered letters).

Dynamic Indicators of Basic Early Literacy Skills   Dynamic Indicators of Basic Early Literacy Skills (DIBELS) is a set of CBMs that have become widely used because the measures are: 1) aligned with the recommendations of the National Reading Panel (2000) report, 2) available at no cost online (http://www.dibels.uoregon.edu/index.php), and 3) administered quickly and easily. DIBELS is also one of the more controversial assessments, having been described as "the worst thing to happen to the teaching of reading since the development of flash cards" (Pearson, 2006, p. v), and comes under criticism for many reasons, most notably narrowing the curriculum in schools (see Goodman, 2006, for a review). Professionals serving children with AAC needs may avoid this controversy because the assessments are timed measures of the ability to say aloud initial sounds, alphabet letters, phonemes in words, nonsense words, and words in connected text. These central features, timed and oral performance, eliminate possible application with students with AAC needs.

Maze   The maze task (Guthrie, Siefert, Burnham, & Caplan, 1974) is less controversial and more useful for students with AAC needs. A multiple-choice cloze task, the maze has been used for many years as a CBM of overall reading progress in students who read at or above a first-grade level. In the case of students with AAC needs, the maze has been employed as a proxy measure of reading fluency and to assess the match-of-text difficulty relative to student reading ability. To administer the maze, the teacher selects a passage of approximately 120 words from within an existing text and systematically deletes every fifth word after leaving the first sentence or two intact. For every word that is deleted, three choices are provided. The choices, in addition to the original word, typically include an incorrect word that is the same part of speech as the correct word and an incorrect word that is a different part of speech. The child with AAC needs is then directed to read the passage and point to the word believed to best fill in the blank. In assessing the match of text to reader (e.g., the difficulty of the social studies basal relative to the child's reading ability), the optimal instructional level is considered 60%–70% and an independent level is 85% or higher. A text at instructional level is one that a student can read with understanding with a teacher's assistance (e.g., guided reading experiences should be successful) and one at 85% or higher that the student can read independently with understanding (i.e., independent seat work or homework assignments should be successful). In attempting to match students to appropriate texts for guided reading lessons, teachers seek texts that students achieve instructional level prior to instruction. To enhance and monitor reading fluency, teachers ask students to engage in repeated readings of a text that they can read at an instructional level and then readminister the maze every three to four readings.

Classroom Environment Assessment   Classroom environments play a vital role in all children's learning but particularly for students who struggle to learn to read (Allington, 2005; Pressley, 2002). Assessing the nature of instruction is particularly important in the case of children with AAC needs because the instructional supports provided to them have often been found lacking (see, e.g., Mike, 1995).

The Text Inventory, Text In-Use Observation, and Text Interviews (TEX-IN3) represents one of the few literacy environmental assessment tools that have been validated by growth in student reading achievement (Hoffman, 2004). Consistent with a view of social cognition, the TEX-IN3 views the classroom environment as a dynamic context that affects and is affected by students and their teachers. With the instrument, practitioners can identify and describe the range and quality of texts found in a classroom; observe and record the interactions of teachers and students with texts during reading instruction; and identify and record teacher and student understandings of the forms, functions, and uses of texts in the classroom. The text type inventory includes 17 categories ranging from computers to student written work to textbooks, tradebooks, process charts, and other texts. The overall quality of the text environment is then rated on a scale (ranging from inadequate to extremely rich). For students with AAC needs, additional consideration must be given to the accessibility of the text types relative to the students' individual differences.

The Texts In-Use component requires three observations of 30 minutes each. At the beginning and end of each observation, a snapshot of student engagement is taken, noting which students are engaged with which kinds of text within what sort of context. The observer then surveys three target children identified with the classroom teacher, recording their engagement, texts used, and the context of the engagement.

The Text Interview component is designed to capture the understandings and beliefs of the classroom community (i.e., students and teachers). Teachers rate the importance of each text type while thinking aloud. The observer takes notes on this process and assigns a rating, ranging from enriched/elaborated understanding to little/no knowledge. The students targeted in the Texts In-Use observation are also interviewed about each of the text types, and the same holistic rating is applied to their level of text understanding and knowledge.

CONCLUSION

The diagnostic reading assessments described in this chapter have three primary purposes: 1) developing reading profiles of students that identify relative learning strengths and needs, 2) establishing instructional objectives, and 3) documenting reading growth over time. That is, these assessments allow practitioners to identify where particular students are currently and how much and what kind of progress they have made in the interval since previous assessments and to make more informed decisions about how to assist them in making greater progress in the future. The diagnostic reading assessments shared in this chapter are particularly useful in answering questions about what to teach to children with AAC needs and how to teach it. They have the potential to enable thoughtful practitioners to, as Klenk and Kibby (2000) described it, "re-mediate" intervention planning (i.e., intercede with students in new and different ways based on thoughtful consideration of student performance data). Toward that end, the following guidelines may prove useful in guiding assessment.

First, diagnostic assessments should be administered to any student with AAC needs who reads below grade-level expectations. The older the student, the greater the urgency to meet instructional needs as closely as possible.

Second, the diagnostic assessments described in this chapter do not require frequent administration to be effective as long as practitioners act on the information they obtain. Failure to act will not be remedied by more frequent assessment. Table 4.2 summarizes the frequency and purpose of the assessments described in this chapter.

Table 4.2.   Frequency and purpose of diagnostic reading assessments

Assessments	Frequency and purpose
Early Reading Spelling Inventory (ERSI), developmental spelling test	Early in the year to determine current performance and instructional needs
	Quarterly to document progress and adjust instructional emphases
Individual reading inventory (IRI); Qualitative Inventory of Word Knowledge (QIWK); reading attitude inventory; Text Inventory, Text In-Use Observation, and Text Interviews (TEX-IN3)	Early in the year to document current status and instructional needs
	Late in the year to document growth
Hypothesis testing	Ongoing classroom observation and weekly interpretation and instructional planning
Maze and/or silent reading rate	Monthly to assess appropriateness of text difficulty, progress in reading, and effectiveness of instruction

Third, if practitioners are not prepared to modify instructional strategies, plans, or programs based on assessment results, then there is no reason to administer the assessments, which leads to a final point. Ultimately, the success or failure of the informal diagnostic assessments described in this chapter depend on the most powerful diagnostic assessment instrument—practitioners. There is little purpose to the assessment processes and instruments described here unless practitioners 1) believe in the conventional literacy learning capabilities of their students; 2) understand that the purpose of the assessments is to document learning progress and refine instructional planning; and 3) have a wide understanding of, or a willingness to learn, the breadth of strategies found successful in teaching other struggling readers of various types.

Although designed for informal teacher use, each of the tools and processes has been thoughtfully developed and validated. Each is relatively easy to learn, adapt, use, and interpret. All have been applied by a wide variety of professionals attempting to improve the instruction of children learning to read. Each provides information that will enable thoughtful practitioners to better assist children with AAC needs to successfully learn to read.

REFERENCES

Afflerbach, P. (1993). STAIR: A system for recording and using what we observe and know about our students. *Reading Teacher, 47,* 260–263.

Alberto, P.A., & Fredrick, L.D. (2000). Teaching picture reading as an enabling skill. *Teaching Exceptional Children, 33,* 60–64.

Allington, R.L. (2005). *What really matters for struggling readers* (2nd ed.). Boston: Allyn & Bacon.

American Federation of Teachers. (2008). *English language learners (ELL).* Retrieved February 26, 2008, from http://www.aft.org/topics/nclb/ell.htm

Beukelman, D.R., & Mirenda, P. (2005). *Augmentative and alternative communication: Supporting children and adults with complex communication needs* (3rd ed.). Baltimore: Paul H. Brookes Publishing Co.

Beukelman, D.R., Mirenda, P., & Sturm, J. (2005). Literacy development of children who use AAC. In D.R. Beukelman & P. Mirenda (Eds.), *Augmentative and alternative communication: Supporting children and adults with complex communication needs* (3rd ed., pp. 351–390). Baltimore: Paul H. Brookes Publishing Co.

Binger, K., & Light, J. (2002, November). *Morphology and syntax of individuals who use AAC.* Seminar presented at the American Speech-Language-Hearing Association Convention, Atlanta, GA.

Boyd-Batstone, P. (2004). Focused anecdotal records assessment: A tool for standards-based, authentic assessment. *Reading Teacher, 58,* 230–239.

Browder, D.M., & Lalli, J.S. (1991). Review of research on sight word instruction. *Research in Developmental Disability, 12,* 203–228.

Brozo, W.G., Shield, G., & Topping, K. (2007/2008). Engagement in reading: Lessons learned from three PISA countries. *Journal of Adolescent and Adult Literacy, 51,* 304–315.

Chapple, D. (2000). Empowerment. In M. Fried-Oken & H.A. Bersani, Jr. (Eds.), *Speaking up and spelling it out: Personal essays on augmentative and alternative communication* (pp. 153–159). Baltimore: Paul H. Brookes Publishing Co.

Coleman, P.P. (1992). *Literacy lost: A qualitative analysis of the early literacy experiences of preschool children with severe speech and physical impairments.* Unpublished doctoral dissertation, University of North Carolina, Chapel Hill.

Cooper, J.D., & Kiger, N.D. (2001). *Literacy assessment: Helping teachers plan instruction.* Boston: Houghton Mifflin.

Cunningham, J.W. (1993). Whole-to-part reading diagnosis. *Reading and Writing Quarterly: Overcoming Learning Difficulties, 9,* 31–49.

Cunningham, P.M. (2004). *Phonics they use: Words for reading and writing* (4th ed.). Boston: Allyn & Bacon.

Dahlgren Sandberg, A. (2001). Reading and spelling, phonological awareness, and working memory in children with severe speech impairments: A longitudinal study. *Augmentative and Alternative Communication, 17,* 11–25.

Darvin, J. (2006). "Real-word cognition doesn't end when the bell rings": Literacy instruction strategies derived from situated cognition research. *Journal of Adolescent and Adult Literacy, 49,* 398–407.

Deno, S.L. (1985). Curriculum-based measurement: The emerging alternative. *Exceptional Children, 52,* 219–232.

Downing, J.E. (2005). *Teaching literacy to students with significant disabilities: Strategies for the K–12 inclusive classroom.* Thousand Oaks, CA: Corwin Press.

Erhardt, R.P. (1990). *Developmental visual dysfunction.* Tucson, AZ: Therapy Skill Builders.

Erickson, K.A., Clendon, S.A., Cunningham, J.W., Spadorcia, S., Koppenhaver, D.A., Sturm, J., et al. (2007). *ABC-Link.* Retrieved July 23, 2007, from http://viper.med.unc.edu/abclink/home.cfm.

Erickson, K.A., Clendon, S.A., Cunningham, J.W., Spadorcia, S., Koppenhaver, D.A., Sturm, J., et al. (2008). Automatic word recognition: The validity of a universally accessible assessment task. *Augmentative and Alternative Communication, 24*(1), 64–75.

Erickson, K.A., & Hatton, D. (2007). Literacy and visual impairment. *Seminars in Speech and Language, 28,* 58–68.

Erickson, K.A., & Koppenhaver, D.A. (1995). Developing a literacy program for children with severe disabilities. *Reading Teacher, 48,* 676–684.

Erickson, K.A., & Koppenhaver, D.A. (2007). *Children with disabilities: Reading and writing the Four-Blocks way.* Greensboro, NC: Carson-Dellosa.

Erickson, K.A., Koppenhaver, D.A., & Cunningham, J.W. (2006). Balanced reading intervention and assessment in augmentative communication. In S.F. Warren & M.E. Fey (Series Eds.) & R.J. McCauley & M.E. Fey (Vol. Eds.), *Communication and language intervention series: Treatment of language disorders in children* (pp. 309–345). Baltimore: Paul H. Brookes Publishing Co.

Foley, B., & Pollatsek, A. (1999). Phonological processing and reading abilities in adolescents and adults with severe congenital speech impairments. *Augmentative and Alternative Communication, 15,* 156–173.

Foley, B.E., & Staples, A. (2003). Developing augmentative and alternative communication and literacy interventions for adults with autism in a supported employment setting. *Topics in Language Disorders, 23,* 325–343.

Frye, B., Kucan, L.L., & Bloodgood, J.W. (2007, November). *Norms for reading performance (word recognition, oral and silent reading, and spelling) in grades 2 through 6.* Paper presented at the annual meeting of the National Reading Conference, Austin, TX.

Fuchs, D., Mock, D., Morgan, P.L., & Young, C.L. (2003). Responsiveness-to-intervention: Definitions, evidence, and implications for the learning disabilities construct. *Learning Disabilities Research and Practice, 18,* 157–171.

Fuchs, L.S., Fuchs, D., & Hamlett, C.L. (2007). Using curriculum-based measurement to inform reading instruction. *Reading and Writing, 20,* 553–567.

Gillet, J.W., Temple, C., & Crawford, A.N. (2004). *Understanding reading problems: Assessment and instruction.* Boston: Allyn & Bacon.

Goodman, K.S. (Ed.). (2006). *The truth about DIBELS: What it is. What it does.* Portsmouth, NH: Heinemann.

Guthrie, J., Siefert, M., Burnham, N., & Caplan, R. (1974). The maze technique to assess, monitor reading comprehension. *Reading Teacher, 28,* 161–168.

Hoffman, J.V. (2004). The effective elementary classroom literacy environment: Examining the validity of the TEX-IN3 observation system. *Journal of Literacy Research, 36,* 303–334.

Johns, J. (2005). *Basic reading inventory: Pre-primer through grade twelve and early literacy assessments.* Dubuque, IA: Kendall/Hunt.

Katims, D. (2000). Literacy instruction for people with mental retardation: Historical highlights and contemporary analysis. *Education and Training in Mental Retardation and Developmental Disabilities, 35,* 3–15.

Kirsch, I., de Jong, J., Lafontaine, D., McQueen, J., Mendelovits, J., & Monseur, C. (2002). *Reading for change: Performance and engagement across countries. Results from PISA 2000.* Paris, France: Organization for Economic Co-operation and Development.

Klenk, L., & Kibby, M.W. (2000). Re-mediating reading difficulties: Appraising the past, reconciling the present, constructing the future. In M. Kamil, P. Mosenthal, P.D. Pearson, & R. Barr (Eds.), *Handbook of reading research* (Vol. 3, pp. 667–690). Mahwah, NJ: Lawrence Erlbaum Associates.

Koppenhaver, D.A., Evans, D.A., & Yoder, D.E. (1991). Childhood reading and writing experiences of literate adults with severe speech and motor impairments. *Augmentative and Alternative Communication, 7*(1), 20–33.

Koppenhaver, D.A., Pierce, P.L., Steelman, J.D., & Yoder, D.E. (1994). Contexts of early literacy intervention for children with developmental disabilities. In S.F. Warren & M.E. Fey (Series Eds.) & M.E. Fey, J. Windsor, & S.F. Warren (Vol. Eds.), *Communication and language intervention series: Vol. 5. Language intervention: Preschool through the elementary years* (pp. 241–274). Baltimore: Paul H. Brookes Publishing Co.

Koppenhaver, D.A., & Yoder, D.E. (1992a). Literacy issues in persons with severe physical and speech impairments. In R. Gaylord-Ross (Ed.), *Issues and research in special education* (Vol. 2, pp. 156–201). New York: Teachers College Press.

Koppenhaver, D.A., & Yoder, D.E. (1992b). Literacy learning of children with severe speech and physical impairments in school settings. *Seminars in Speech and Language, 13*(2), 143–153.

Koppenhaver, D.A., & Yoder, D.E. (1993). Classroom literacy instruction for children with severe speech and physical impairments (SSPI): What is and what might be. *Topics in Language Disorders, 13*(2), 1–15.

Krashen, S. (1982). *Principles and practice in second language acquisition.* New York: Pergamon Press.

Lalli, J.S., & Browder, D.M. (1993). Comparison of sight word training procedures with validation of the most practical procedures in teaching reading for daily living. *Research in Developmental Disabilities, 14,* 107–127.

Leslie, L., & Caldwell, J. (2005). *Qualitative reading inventory–Fourth edition.* Boston: Allyn & Bacon.

Light, J. (1997). Communication is the essence of human life: Reflections on communication competence. *Augmentative and Alternative Communication, 13,* 61–70.

Light, J., & Kelford Smith, A. (1993). The home literacy experiences of preschoolers who use augmentative communication systems and their nondisabled peers. *Augmentative and Alternative Communication, 9,* 10–25.

Light, J., & McNaughton, D. (1993). Literacy and augmentative and alternative communication (AAC): The expectations and priorities of parents and teachers. *Topics in Language Disorders, 13*(2), 33–46.

Mann, V., Tobin, P., & Wilson, R. (1987). Measuring phonological awareness through the invented spelling of kindergarten children. *Merrill-Palmer Quarterly, 33,* 365–391.

Marvin, C. (1994). Home literacy experiences of preschool children with single and multiple disorder. *Topics in Early Childhood Special Education, 14,* 436–454.

McKenna, M.C. (2002). *Help for struggling readers: Strategies for grades 3–8.* New York: Guilford Press.

McKenna, M.C., & Kear, D.J. (1990). Measuring attitude toward reading: A new tool for teachers. *Reading Teacher, 43,* 626–639.

Mike, D.G. (1995). Literacy and cerebral palsy: Factors influencing literacy learning in a self-contained setting. *Journal of Reading Behavior, 27,* 627–642.

Morris, D. (1981). Concept of word: A developmental phenomenon in the beginning reading and writing processes. *Language Arts, 58,* 659–668.

Morris, D. (1998). Assessing printed word knowledge in beginning readers: The Early Reading Screening Instrument (ERSI). *Illinois Reading Council Journal, 26*(2), 30–40.

Morris, D., Mock, D., & Perney, J. (2007, November). *The relationship between word recognition automaticity and reading rate: Necessary but not sufficient.* Paper presented at the annual meeting of the National Reading Conference, Austin, TX.

Morris, D., Nelson, L., & Perney, J. (1986). Exploring the concept of "spelling instructional level" through the analysis of error-types. *Elementary School Journal, 87,* 181–200.

Morris, D., & Perney, J. (1984). Developmental spelling as a predictor of first-grade reading achievement. *Elementary School Journal, 84,* 441–457.

Morris, D., & Slavin, R. (2003). *Every child reading.* Boston: Allyn & Bacon.

Nation, K., Clarke, P., Wright, B., & Williams, C. (2006). Patterns of reading ability in children with autism spectrum disorder. *Journal of Autism and Developmental Disorders, 36,* 911–919.

National Reading Panel. (2000). *Teaching children to read: An evidence-based assessment of the scientific research literature on reading and its implications for reading instruction* (NIH Publication No. 00-4769). Washington, DC: National Institute of Child Health and Human Development.

National Research Council. (1999). *Starting out right: A guide to promoting children's reading success.* Washington, DC: National Academies Press.

No Child Left Behind Act of 2001, PL 107-110, 115 Stat. 1425, 20 U.S.C. §§ 6301 *et seq.*

Pearson, P.D. (2006). Foreword. In K.S. Goodman (Ed.), *The truth about DIBELS: What it is. What it does* (pp. v–xix). Portsmouth, NH: Heinemann.

Pressley, M. (2002). *Reading instruction that works: The case for balanced instruction* (3rd ed.). New York: Guilford Press.

Pressley, M., Mohan, L., Fingeret, L., Reffitt, K., & Raphael-Bogaert, L. (2007). Writing instruction in engaging and effective elementary settings. In S. Graham, C. MacArthur, & J. Fitzgerald (Eds.), *Best practices in writing instruction: Solving problems in the teaching of literacy* (pp. 13–27). New York: Guilford Press.

Rasinski, T., & Padak, N. (2004). *Effective reading strategies: Teaching children who find reading difficult* (3rd ed.). Upper Saddle River, NJ: Pearson.

Romski, M.A., & Sevcik, R.A. (1996). *Breaking the speech barrier: Language development through augmented means.* Baltimore: Paul H. Brookes Publishing Co.

Schlagal, R.C. (1982). *A qualitative inventory of word knowledge: A developmental study of spelling, grades 1–6.* Unpublished doctoral dissertation, University of Virginia, Charlottesville.

Schonell, F.E. (1957). *Educating spastic children: The education and guidance of the cerebral palsied.* London: Oliver & Boyd.

Schuele, C.M., Spencer, E.J., Barako-Arndt, K., & Guillot, K.M. (2007). Literacy and children with specific language impairment. *Seminars in Speech and Language, 28,* 35–47.

Siegenthaler, B. (1987). Auditory problems. In E. McDonald (Ed.), *Treating cerebral palsy* (pp. 85–104). Austin, TX: PRO-ED.

Silberberg, N., & Silberberg, M.C. (1967). Hyperlexia: Specific word recognition skills in young children. *Exceptional Children, 34,* 41–42.

Smith, M. (2005). *Literacy and augmentative and alternative communication.* Boston: Elsevier.

Stanovich, K. (1986). Matthew effects in reading: Some consequences of individual differences in the acquisition of literacy. *Reading Research Quarterly, 21,* 360–407.

Stephens, D. (1996). When assessment is inquiry. *Language Arts, 73,* 105–112.

Sturm, J.M., & Clendon, S.A. (2004). AAC, language, and literacy: Fostering the relationship. *Topics in Language Disorders, 24*(1), 76–91.

Sutton, A., Soto, G., & Blockberger, S. (2002). Grammatical issues in graphic symbol communication. *Augmentative and Alternative Communication, 18,* 192–204.

van Balkom, H., & Welle Donker-Gimbrère, M. (1996). A psycholinguistic approach to graphic language use. In S. von Tetzchner & M.H. Jensen (Eds.), *Augmentative and alternative communication: European perspectives* (pp. 153–170). London: Whurr Publishers.

Vandervelden, M., & Siegel, L. (1999). Phonological processing and literacy in AAC users and students with motor speech impairments. *Augmentative and Alternative Communication, 15,* 191–211.

von Tetzchner, S., & Martinsen, H. (2000). *Augmentative and alternative communication* (2nd ed.). London: Whurr Publishers.

Ylvisaker, M., Coelho, C., Kennedy, M., Sohlberg, M.M., Turkstra, L., Avery, J., et al. (2002). Reflections on evidence-based practice and rational clinical decision making. *Journal of Medical Speech Language Pathology, 10*(3), 25–38.

5

Writing Assessment
for Students with AAC Needs

Beth E. Foley, David A. Koppenhaver, and Amy R. Williams

The primary purposes of writing assessment are to identify what writers can do well, what aspects of writing they find difficult, and what instructional strategies are most likely to lead to improvements in writing competence and achievement of state and district core curriculum standards. For students who use augmentative and alternative communication (AAC), writing assessment is typically complicated by the presence of multiple physical, cognitive, and communication impairments that interfere with the writing process. Writing assessment procedures developed for such students must not only reflect recommended practices for analyzing written expression but must also address the unique writing challenges faced by individuals with complex communication needs. This chapter focuses on describing writing assessment strategies and tools intended to fulfill these purposes.

The chapter is divided into four main sections. The first section addresses general considerations for conducting writing assessments with students who use AAC. It includes suggestions for developing student profiles, identifying assistive technology (AT) and instructional support needs, and creating an individualized assessment portfolio. The second section describes the stages of emergent writing development and strategies for assessing emergent literacy skills. The third section provides a model of conventional writing followed by examples of qualitative and quantitative measures of conventional writing abilities. The last section focuses on how to use writing assessment data to develop instructional goals that appropriately reflect general education core curriculum standards.

USING WRITING ASSESSMENTS FOR STUDENTS WITH AAC NEEDS

All writing assessments are based on assumptions about what is being assessed. The assessment framework assumes that writing is first and foremost a form of communication—a social activity requiring the integration of a range of physical, linguistic, and cognitive resources (Nystrand, 1990). It also assumes that writing is a recursive process involving planning, generating text, and revising (Hayes, 2000; Hayes & Flower, 1980). In addition, the assessment assumes that writing is a learned process and used most effectively within meaningful and motivating contexts. Finally, it assumes that writing abilities develop along a continuum from emergent to conventional and that assessment strategies must be appropriately tailored to students' developmental levels.

Given these assumptions, it is clear that writing assessment cannot focus exclusively on the written products that students create. It must also be used to carefully examine the processes used by developing writers as they compose authentic texts for a variety of purposes and audiences. The technological and/or social supports that students need for participation should be considered, as well as the influence of instructional practices and contexts on learning outcomes.

Developing a Student Profile

A detailed student profile can be developed by gathering input about the student's capabilities and needs from a variety of sources, including reviews of past records and individualized education program (IEP) progress reports, teacher and caregiver interviews, as well as observations of structured and unstructured writing activities. Family members, past and current teachers, paraprofessionals, speech-language pathologists (SLPs), and others familiar with the student can provide information on the writing behaviors they have observed in multiple environments. They can describe how and how often the student participates in writing activities, what types of AT supports are most useful (e.g., letter stamps, enlarged writing implements, alternate keyboards, word prediction software, AAC device displays), and what approaches to writing instruction (e.g., teacher modeling, peer-mediated or shared writing, strategy instruction) have or have not led to improved writing outcomes.

Gathering such data enables IEP team members to determine a student's present skill level; capitalize on identified strengths; and target the resources, behaviors, or abilities needing further development. For example, if the profile reveals that a student lacks the fine motor ability required to use standard writing implements, then the team can focus on identifying alternative means for the student to produce text. If the student's current communication system is deemed inadequate for supporting participation in classroom writing activities, then the system can either be modified or more appropriate components for the AAC system can be identified.

Identifying Assistive Technology and Instructional Supports

Access to AT, including AAC devices, minimizes some of the barriers to writing faced by students with complex communication needs. Low-tech AAC supports, such as simple communication boards, can enable students to choose topics to write about, create patterned stories, or make comments about their own or other students' writing (e.g., "I like/don't like that." "That's funny/sad/boring."). Emergent writers may benefit from graphic symbol support for translating ideas into text. Graphic organizers such as story maps, time lines, or cueing charts provide scaffolds for planning and organizing ideas. High-tech AAC devices can provide quick access to prestored generic messages during writing activities (e.g., "I don't know what to write about next." "How do you like my story?") as well as the ability to construct, store, and print out novel text. AT/AAC supports for reviewing text include talking word processors or speech-generating devices that enable students to read text aloud.

The SETT framework (Zabala, 1995) is a simple organizational tool that can be used to assess students' writing needs and the tools and strategies professionals can use to meet those needs. The premise of the SETT framework is that IEP teams must gather information about the *Students*, the *Environments* in which the students spend their time, the *Tasks* required for students to be active participants in teaching/learning processes, and the *Tools* needed to complete those tasks successfully (see Table 5.1 for a simplified example). More detailed information about the SETT framework can be downloaded from http://www.joyzabala.com. Other forms and checklists that describe AT supports for all aspects of the writing process are available on the Georgia Project for Assistive Technology web site (http://www.gpat.org). See the chapter appendix for a list of AT for writing and spelling.

Creating an Assessment Portfolio

In addition to developing detailed student profiles and ensuring access to the AT/AAC supports needed for participation in writing instruction, it is important to keep records of students' responses to a range of instructional activities and approaches. The use of individual portfolios to document student progress has been strongly recommended for students with severe disabilities (Downing, 2005; Kleinhert, Haigh, Kearns, & Kennedy, 2000). In the area of writing, portfolios are used to collect writing samples that are representative of student achievement over time. Samples are typically dated and should include writing produced for different purposes and audiences (e.g., signatures, cards, letters, journal entries, stories), along with descriptions of the contexts under which they were created, the time it took to produce them, and the types of teacher or peer scaffolding provided.

Table 5.1.   Identification of assistive technology and instructional supports using a SETT framework

Student	Environment	Task	Tool
John is 14 years old, has Down syndrome, and does not know how to write his name.	Special education, life skills class	Sign his name on his papers	Name stamp
Maya is 6 years old and can spell grade-level words but does not have legible handwriting.	General education kindergarten classroom	Fill in the blanks of a patterned story	Alphasmart or laptop computer at her desk to fill in a story template
Michael is 10 years old with a cognitive impairment and limited knowledge of print concepts.	Resource room with small-group instruction	Write a story with beginning, middle, and end	Three photos to put in sequence on a story map
Taylor is 8 years old with cerebral palsy and severe dysarthria. He has almost no intelligible speech.	General education second-grade classroom	Read stories aloud during Writer's Workshop so peers can provide feedback	High-tech AAC device: Compose and save stories to device so stories can be read aloud in class

Whenever possible, students should help to decide which samples are included in their portfolios. Encouraging students to select samples of their work for their portfolios helps them develop important self-determination skills that will be beneficial throughout their lives (Downing, 2005). Individualized portfolios can serve as alternative assessments for students with severe disabilities to comply with federal No Child Left Behind (NCLB) Act of 2001 (PL 107-110) mandates for accountability and are more likely than standardized assessment tools to inform and improve instruction (Kleinert et al., 2000).

EMERGENT WRITING DEVELOPMENT

This section describes the stages of writing development that precede conventional writing, which is writing that adheres to sufficient conventions of spelling, grammar, and punctuation that another conventionally literate person can read. Then, the section outlines developmentally appropriate procedures for assessing emergent forms of writing and related skills in students with AAC needs.

Stages of Emergent Writing

Typically developing children engage in a wide range of emergent writing behaviors long before they can write conventionally. Sulzby (1990) proposed the following stages of emergent literacy development, cautioning that writing acquisition in individual students does not always follow an invariant order: drawing, scribble, nonphonetic letter strings, invented spelling, conventional copying, and conventional writing (see Figure 5.1 for representative examples of each stage). According to Sulzby's framework, children first draw and then scribble as they begin to reproduce the characteristics of the writing system in their environment. Then, they begin to use letter-like forms in nonphonetic strings that do not correspond to sounds in the words they are trying to represent. Next, children begin to use invented spelling. Initially, they tend to represent each syllable of a word with a letter—typically the beginning sound in the word. Over time, they demonstrate increasing knowledge of letter–sound correspondences and an awareness of the sounds within syllables. They may also begin to copy words they see in the environment. Finally, as conventional writers, children use letters to indicate all the sounds in words, although words are often still misspelled.

Stage	Representative sample and negotiated message
1. Drawing	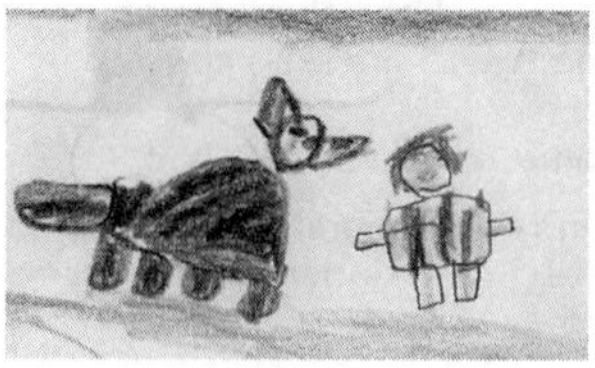 "I like my cat"
2. Scribble	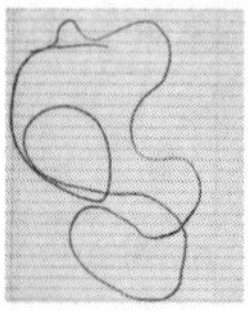 "big snake"
3. Nonphonetic letter strings	Htg "sink"
4. Invented spelling	Weoepndoop "we opened the door"
5. Conventional copying	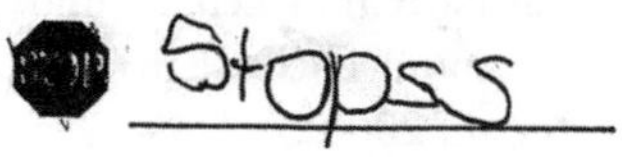 "stop"
6. Conventional writing	I lik The Brn the Kin tie kio of the Brn "I like the bunny. The girl can take care of the bunny."

Figure 5.1.   Stages of emergent writing development.

There is no single identifiable time, text, or task in which a child's emergent writing ceases to be emergent and becomes conventional; rather, there is a gradual increase in the use of convention until not only the child can "read" the writing, but others also can read it. Although a gradual growth in sophistication of understanding of the forms and functions of writing is observable in writing samples across time, a linear hierarchy of emergent writing stages is probably not an accurate conceptualization of the learning process (Sulzby, 1990). Rather, young children continually seem to be reorganizing their repertoire of writing understandings and strategy use; vacillation between emergent and conventional literacy is not unusual.

Most children are writing conventionally by the end of first grade. Students with AAC needs, however, may developmentally be considered emergent writers for a much longer period of time— even into adulthood—depending on their particular disabilities, such as a severe cognitive impairment or limited physical ability, and sociocultural factors, such as limited experience, lack of access to writing tools, or low expectations for literacy development. Of course, one can argue that whenever individuals select AAC symbols to construct messages, they are, in fact, writing. If one takes an emergent literacy perspective, such messages are recognized and reinforced as writing but also contextualized. For example, sometimes we use pictures to tell people what we want, and sometimes we use letters and words. It is important to share the different kinds of written forms, such as messages and text created via pictures or letter stamps, that can be viewed as "writing" with students who use AAC. Frequent experiences with the many forms and functions of print help students develop the understanding that writing can be used to communicate and to function in everyday life.

ASSESSMENT OF EMERGENT WRITING

In keeping with the developmental characteristics of emergent writers, informal observations and structured performance samples are the best means of assessing the emergent writing of students who use AAC. Because observations and performance samples are obtained in the context of actual instructional activities, they can yield theoretically and ecologically valid assessment data that can be used to inform and improve teaching.

Stage of Writing Development

As discussed previously, Sulzby (1990) described a general but complicated pattern of emergent writing development moving from lower-appearing forms, such as drawing, scribbling, and letter-like forms, to letter strings, invented spelling, and finally conventional copying and writing. Writing portfolios containing one or two pieces per week of a student's writing and their meanings provide a valuable resource for assessing progress over time. A checklist of writing stages can be used to document and date the different forms of emergent writing used by the student. For students with AAC needs who cannot physically write, transcriptions of symbol-based messages produced using AAC devices and/or copies of typed text can be included in writing portfolios as evidence of emergent writing development.

Language Level and Message Quality

Clay (2005) developed a three-part rubric focusing on *language levels, message quality,* and *directionality.* This is useful in assessing the early writing of children making the transition from emergent writing into conventional writing. For emerging writers, only the first few levels of each of the six-point scales are relevant.

Language levels are scored as follows:
1. Letters only
2. Words
3. Two-word phrases
4. Simple sentences

Message quality is scored as follows:
1. Concept of signs (e.g., use of letter-like forms, letters, punctuation)
2. Writing that conveys a message
3. Copied messages
4. Repeating sentence patterns (e.g., I like...)
5. Generating own ideas

The child's knowledge of directionality is assessed as follows:
1. No directionality
2. Partial directionality
3. Reversed directionality

4.   Conventional directionality

5.   Conventional directionality with concept of word evident

More important than the scoring, however, is the ability to examine children's relative strengths and needs across these three areas so that instructional materials, learning experiences, and writing tools can be thoughtfully employed in supporting learning. Figure 5.2 contains examples of writing samples with their relevant scoring using this rubric. There is significant overlap in some cases with the emergent writing stages discussed previously.

Learning Environment

As can be seen in Figure 5.2, emergent writing takes on many different forms before an individual writes conventionally. The onset, range, and type of written forms employed seem integrally related to the availability of models of print and print use as well as the availability of tools in the environment (Koppenhaver & Erickson, 2003). It is important, then, that the learning environment be assessed carefully for the relative availability of print, tools, models, and writing opportunities. One widely used tool for such assessment is the Early Language and Literacy Classroom Observation Toolkit (ELLCO), which comes in Pre-K (Smith, Brady, & Anastasopoulos, 2008) and K–3 (Smith, Brady, & Clark-Chiarelli, 2008) versions. The ELLCO uses a literacy environment checklist, classroom observation and teacher interview, and a literacy activities rating scale. The ELLCO is particularly useful in the context of emergent writing because specific items and subsections address the availability of writing materials, experiences, and instructional supports. Although the authors recommend that individuals employing the assessment are experienced educators, it is also important that people employing the assessment in classrooms serving children with AAC needs have relevant AAC experiences. The ELLCO was not developed for use with children with AAC needs and requires careful consideration of individual differences in recording and reporting observations. For example, children without disabilities can handle and talk about any print material they can reach in a classroom. Children with communication, physical, or other impairments will not be able to do so unless the materials are adapted to increase access.

Phonological Awareness

Students with AAC needs have an increased risk of phonological awareness and spelling difficulties (Gillon, 2002). Phonological awareness, the explicit knowledge of the sound structure of words, has consistently proven to be a crucial factor in spelling development (Gillon, 2005). Early spelling requires an understanding of the association between a word's phonological and orthographic representations (Treiman, Sotak, & Bowman, 2001), and many students who use AAC appear to lack a strong foundation for effectively mapping and gaining access to these representations (Vandervelden & Siegel, 1999, 2001). Phonological awareness and spelling difficulties are likely to continue throughout the school years unless they are identified and addressed.

Assessment of phonological awareness in students who use AAC is challenging because traditional assessment tasks usually require a verbal response (e.g., Say *cowboy* without *cow*) and, therefore, must be adapted so that students can respond by nonverbal means such as pointing to pictures or answering yes-no questions. Examples of adaptations to phonological awareness assessment tasks are described next and listed in order of difficulty from relatively early developing (rhyme detection) to later developing skills (segmentation of middle phonemes and phoneme deletion).

Rhyme Detection   Present the student with spoken pairs of rhyming and nonrhyming words (e.g., *dog-log* versus *dog-mat*) and have him or her indicate which word pair rhymes. An alternative and significantly more difficult task is to have the student identify rhyming pairs from a group of visually presented pictures (e.g., dog, dad, log, leg).

Writing sample	Scoring interpretation
CNS Pin o tan ont O Wœ o Kœ rœ Wœ Wœ Si hot bren. "Once upon a time there was a girl. She had a bunny."	*Language level:* 4—simple sentences *Message quality:* 5—generating own ideas *Directionality:* 5—conventional directionality with concept of word evident
me AN d m Y mom R B A E E g "Me and my mom are baking."	*Language level:* 4—simple sentences *Message quality:* 5—generating own ideas *Directionality:* 2—partial directionality
DAD IHPUHDAGDGRP LOVE WILL "Dad, I hope you had a good trip. Love, Will."	*Language level:* 4—simple sentences *Message quality:* 5—generating own ideas *Directionality:* 4—conventional directionality
Lion KiNg FuN "Lion King. Fun."	*Language level:* 3—two-word phrases *Message quality:* 5—generating own ideas *Directionality:* 5—conventional directionality with concept of word evident
A rɔ((rʋ]ɔ]ueea AT MOM AOMO eeɪrɪ duenɪɪeuu uenuɪrɪɔuɪee wMOM.ʃurdy e ɔɪɑrurluɔ uuulɑ "My mom took me out to my grandma's house. We went to see my brother. My dad took me out to eat pizza."	*Language level:* 1–2—letters only and the word *mom* *Message quality:* 1—concept of signs *Directionality:* 4—conventional directionality
B He Sɑt "big snake"	*Language level:* 3—two-word phrases *Message quality:* 5—generating own ideas *Directionality:* 5—conventional directionality with concept of word evident

Figure 5.2.   Assessment of emergent writing using Clay's (2005) three-part rubric.

Syllable Blending   Provide the student with a group of pictures. Then, say the syllables that form one of the words pictured. Ask the student to guess the secret word by blending the spoken syllables (e.g., *ta-ble*). If the student is successfully blending two-syllable words, then present three- and four-syllable words (e.g., *but-ter-fly, cat-er-pil-lar*) for identification.

Syllable Segmenting   Provide the student with a group of pictures representing parts of compound words (e.g., *butter* and *fly* for *butterfly*, *cow* and *boy* for *cowboy*) with foils. Ask the student to identify what word would be left over when part of the word is deleted (e.g., Show me *cowboy* without *cow*).

Phoneme Blending   Provide the student with a group of pictures. Ask the student to blend spoken phonemes and identify the resulting word (e.g., Show me *m-a-t*). Start with words containing two to three phonemes (e.g., *u-p, i-n, b-a-t*). If student is successful, then use target words containing four to five phonemes (e.g., *t-a-b-le, s-t-i-ck, d-r-e-ss-er*).

Phoneme Segmenting   Present the student with sequences of three pictures (e.g., ball, dog, bat). Ask the student to identify which two words start with the same sound. In order of difficulty, assess the student's ability to match initial, final, and middle sounds in words. Alternatives to this task include asking the student to indicate whether or where a target sound is contained in a spoken word (e.g., Is there an /m/ in the word *ham?* Where is the /m/ in the word *ham?*) or to identify the "odd one out" in a picture sequence (bat, mat, cat, cut).

Phoneme Deletion   Provide the student with sequences of four pictures, and ask the student to indicate what word would be left after an initial or final sound is deleted (e.g., show pictures of mice, ice, eye, and dice and say, *"Mice* without /m/ is…" Show pictures of bow, boat, bat, goat and say, *"Boat* without /t/ is…").

Data from the assessment tasks described previously can be used to determine a student's level of phonological awareness and provide a starting point for explicit phonological awareness instruction. Improvements in phonological awareness typically translate into improvements in early spelling development as well. Addressing phonological awareness early will assist emergent writers as they begin to use letters to represent all the sounds they hear in words.

Directed Writing

A particular challenge in assessing emergent writing abilities in students with AAC needs is that they cannot read aloud the nonconventional texts that they produce; this is a central feature of emergent writing assessment with young, typically developing children. Consequently, a variety of directed writing tasks as described next are useful in increasing the interpretability of texts produced by emergent writers.

Name Writing   An individual's name is a particularly useful starting place because it is often the first and most important word that a student learns to write and it is easily integrated into existing learning routines (Bloodgood, 1999). Students can be asked to write their name on artwork, letters to others, their schedules, choices (e.g., hot lunch or cold lunch), class assignments, notes home, and so forth. Each attempt provides a written product that can be assessed relative to the writing tool employed. For example, if a child writes by hand, then left-to-right orientation and letter formation can be examined, whereas a typed sample enables only an examination of the letters typed.

Word Generation   The Test of Writing Vocabulary (Robinson in Clay, 1991) has been widely used with children who speak because it requires only 10 minutes to administer; has simple directions (i.e., "I want to see how many words you can write."); encourages prompts when children are not writing (e.g., "Can you write your name?" "Do you know how to write *the* or *a?*"); and enables assessment of the child's alphabet knowledge, phonemic awareness, concept of word, and written vocabulary.

A reasonable adaptation for emergent writers with AAC needs is to use pictures and/or verbal prompts to elicit interpretable written words. For example, when Jordan wrote *FG BK* underneath the picture of a frog, it was easier to know he was phonetically spelling *frog book*. Yet, when Tracey typed *BB* unprompted in her journal, it required an unsuccessful game of 20 Questions and a telephone call home to learn that she had been listening to a Beach Boys CD in the car on the way to school. Asking students to write dictated words or labels for pictures can help minimize the guesswork that might otherwise be needed to interpret their writing. The Reading A–Z web site (http://www.readinga-z.com) contains a variety of downloadable photo prompts that can be used to elicit word-level writing responses.

Developmental Spelling   When children write known words as in the previous examples, it is possible to assess their developmental understanding of words. A short, developmental spelling test can also be administered. For example, children are asked to spell a list of 12 words of varying spelling patterns such as those as listed in Table 5.2 (e.g., Ferroli & Shanahan, 1987). Students at the emergent literacy level should be encouraged to write as many of the letters/sounds they can hear in the words. Care should be taken first to pronounce the words normally, not stretching the sounds out, and second to encourage the child to attempt to write all the words.

Children's subsequent spellings are examined for evidence of their understanding of how words work. Although a number of different categorical systems exist for examining the progression of children's spelling toward convention (see e.g., Bear, Invernizzi, Templeton, & Johnston, 2008; Ferroli & Shanahan, 1987; Gentry & Gillet, 1993; Schlagal, 2001), there is general agreement that children progress from relatively arbitrary use of letters (e.g., writing *N* for *feet*), to use of letters based on visual strategies that do not reflect an awareness that letters represent sounds (e.g., *WVPOK* for *feet*). Children gradually progress to phonetic spelling in which letters represent sounds typically in initial position first (e.g., *F* for *feet*), then initial plus final (e.g., *FT* for *feet*), and finally initial plus medial plus final (e.g., *FET* for *feet*). As children are placed in instructional environments or acquire more substantial experience with print, they enter a transitional spelling phase and begin increasingly to use morphemes and rules for spelling (e.g., *DRAGIN* for *dragon*, *PEKED* for *peeked*).

Nonword Spelling   A similar assessment task is to ask emergent writers to spell 5–10 simple nonwords (e.g., *fem, bif, zut, heb, rop*). Nonword spelling may tap phonological awareness and knowledge of letter–sound correspondences more directly than spelling of real words that students may have memorized. Scoring involves assigning 1 point to each letter appearing in the correct position in a word (*ffem* = 1 point, *fm/fem* = 2 points, *fim/fem* = 2 points, *fem/fem* = 3 points).

The purpose of all of the directive writing tasks described previously is to determine students' instructional needs. Jennie, for example, typed *S* for *back*, *SS* for *mail*, and *F* for *lake*. She understands that print has meaning and that letters are used to write, but she does not yet understand how the system is organized. She can benefit from having a partner model how to write texts and read them, being given opportunities to write her name, and using environmental print. Alan, however, spelled *do* for *back, sat* for *mail*, and *kid* for *lake*. He is relying on visual strategies, reproducing words he has seen in the environment when asked to write words he does not know how to spell. He can benefit from experiences such as using a word processor that provides auditory feedback at letter and word levels; having simple short texts read aloud where he can see the words as they are spoken; or developing phonological awareness through picture sorts, songs, and games.

Molly demonstrated greater phonemic awareness than the previous two students when she spelled words such as *beca* for *back, ml* for *mail*, and *lac* for *lake*. She would benefit from instructional

Table 5.2.   Developmental spelling word list

back	sink	mail	dress
lake	peeked	light	dragon
stick	side	feet	test

experiences such as developing a sight word vocabulary with word banks, referring to key words representing common spelling patterns during writing activities, and receiving explicit phonemic awareness instruction.

Transitional Spellings Transitional spellings are more characteristic of conventional writing than emergent writing because a child must have begun to infer rules from experience with conventional print or have been taught rules of spelling. Donna demonstrated this type of spelling when she produced *bake* for *back* and *mall* for *mail*. Silent *e* and consonant doubling are highly unusual until rule-based spelling begins. Children at this level can benefit from instructional experiences with word sorts focused on applying rules or spelling by analogy. For example, children might be asked to sort short versus long vowel patterns (*mat/mate*) or sort by word endings (*bat/cat, big/dig*).

Sentence Dictation   Sentence dictation is a final task that is particularly useful in emergent writing assessment of people with AAC needs. By observing what students produce when asked to write a sentence, practitioners can learn whether children understand that print is written left to right (if they use a pencil or pen), whether they have the concept that a word is a group of letters with white space on both sides, whether they know that every word has at least one vowel, or whether they understand conventions such as capital letters and end punctuation.

This section has described a variety of emergent writing assessment tools and strategies that enable practitioners to document progress in various emergent writing domains and to better identify instructional experiences that might move students more efficiently toward conventional writing. Table 5.3 provides a summary of these tools and strategies and the types of information they provide.

CONVENTIONAL WRITING DEVELOPMENT

The next section provides a model of the processes and underlying skills associated with conventional writing, followed by procedures for assessing both writing processes and writing products. Then, the section describes ways to adapt commonly used writing assessment procedures so they can be used more effectively with students who use AAC.

Model of Conventional Writing

Writing is an extremely complex process, and it is not surprising that many students with and without disabilities struggle to become competent writers. In order to compose, writers must recruit, manage, coordinate, and monitor multiple processes simultaneously (Singer & Bashir, 2004). Coordinating these processes makes extensive demands on writers to allocate cognitive resources effectively. Appropriate writing assessments cannot be developed for students who use AAC without understanding these demands and how they affect the writing process. Figure 5.3 represents a model of written language developed by Singer and Bashir (2004) that draws on prior cognitive models of composing processes (Hayes, 2000; Hayes & Flower, 1980) but expands on those models by accounting for critical foundational abilities that underlie skilled writing and the role of executive and self-regulatory functions in the writing process. Although the model was developed to help explain why writing poses such a challenge for students with language-learning disabilities, it also provides a useful framework for understanding the writing problems exhibited by individuals with more severe disabilities, including those who use AAC. The next section describes the basic components of this model as well as key factors affecting conventional writing development in students who use AAC.

Writing Processes The upper portion of the model (see Figure 5.3) specifies four processes involved in composing text: planning, organizing, generating, and revising. When composing, writers need to think of and plan the ideas they wish to express, organize those ideas to convey their meanings, generate linguistic forms that effectively express those meanings, and revise those forms as needed to convey intended meanings according to the writing conventions of the culture

Table 5.3.   Summary of emergent writing assessment domains, tasks, tools, and outcome measures

Domain	Assessment task	Assessment tools	Outcome measures
Writing process	Collect emergent writing samples	Sulzby (1990) checklist	Writing stage assignment
		Clay rubric	Numerical ratings of language level, message quality, and directionality
		Portfolio	Dated writing samples
			Detailed observations of writing in a variety of natural contexts
Writing product	Word-level analyses	Name writing	Left-to-right orientation
		Word dictation	Letter formation
		Photo prompt	Correct letters typed
			Alphabet knowledge
			Concept of word
			Written vocabulary
			Phonemic awareness
		Developmental spelling inventory	Spelling stage assignment
		Spelling in context	Percentage of words spelled correctly in a writing sample
	Sentence-level analyses	Sentence dictation	Directionality
			Concept of word
			Knowledge of vowel rule
			Use of writing conventions (e.g., capital letters, a period)
Phonological awareness	Assess awareness of sound structure of language	Rhyme detection	Percent correct at each level
		• Auditory presentation	
		• Visual presentation	
		Syllable blending	
		Syllable segmentation	
		Phoneme blending	
		Phoneme segmentation	
		Phoneme deletion	

(Singer & Bashir, 2004). Research on typically developing writers suggests that they shift among the processes of planning, organizing, generating, and revising recursively and frequently during all stages of text development. All of these processes are needed and used by effective writers as they compose text, although different processes may be emphasized at any given time based on the purpose and/or audience for a particular piece of writing.

Planning   Planning involves generating and retrieving ideas (Berninger & Swanson, 1994). It is difficult to isolate and examine planning empirically because it is largely an internal process (Singer & Bashir, 2004). Students with language-learning disabilities engage in very little advance planning when they write, averaging 1 minute of planning time prior to writing (MacArthur & Graham, 1987). Although the planning abilities of students with AAC needs have not been examined specifically, such students are more likely to use advance planning when they understand its purpose and when explicit instruction and support are provided (Sturm & Koppenhaver, 2000).

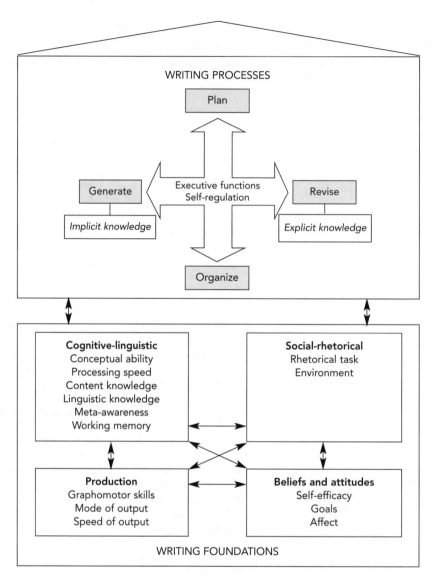

Figure 5.3. A model of written language production. (From Singer, B.D., & Bashir, A.S. [2004]. Developmental variations in writing composition. In C.A. Stone, E.R. Silliman, B.J. Ehren, & K. Apel [Eds.], *Handbook of language and literacy: Development and disorders* [pp. 559–582]. New York: Guilford Press; reprinted by permission.)

Organizing Writing requires the ability to organize one's thoughts and ideas, an ability that draws heavily on linguistic knowledge and content-specific knowledge, as well as knowledge of text schema and genre (Singer & Bashir, 2004). Students who use AAC are disadvantaged in this process because they typically have significant delays in receptive and expressive language development, less world experience and general knowledge than their typically developing peers to draw from (Light, 1997), and less exposure to literate language (e.g., more formal academic language) overall (Koppenhaver & Yoder, 1993; Light & Kelford Smith, 1993; Sturm et al., 2003). As a result, they may lack well-defined schemas for organizing information while composing, instead employing a "knowledge-telling" or "retrieve-and-write" approach to composition, writing whatever comes to mind in whatever order it comes to mind (Bereiter & Scardimalia, 1987). This pattern may persist in students who use AAC well beyond the early elementary school years when such an approach is developmentally appropriate.

Generating   Text generation involves turning the ideas generated in the planning process into language representations within working memory that can then be transcribed into written symbols by handwriting or typing. Writers must draw on knowledge of language meaning, structure, spelling, writing mechanics, and text structure. In face-to-face communication, the preponderance of the utterances produced by students who use AAC are one to two symbols or words in length, with meaning typically co-constructed by the communication partner (Soto, 2006). This telegraphic communication style may be faster and more efficient during conversational interactions, but conventional writing typically requires a more formal communication style, with complete sentences and more explicit vocabulary. Students who use AAC also tend to have significant spelling problems that interfere with the composing process (Hart, 2006). When students who use AAC must devote their attention to the form of their writing (spelling, grammar, punctuation), their rate of text production is reduced and the content of their writing is often diminished.

Revising   Revision involves making changes to text so that it conveys a writer's intended meaning, and this process requires metalinguistic and metacognitive awareness. It requires a writer to draw on knowledge of language at the subword, word, sentence, and discourse levels in order to detect any problems requiring revision (Singer & Bashir, 2004). Students who lack basic linguistic competence—as do most students who use AAC—are likely to struggle with the revision process. In addition, they typically have deficits in decoding, working memory capacity, and comprehending text, all of which make it difficult to effectively evaluate their own writing for meaning, form, and clarity (Foley & Pollatsek, 1999).

Executive Function and Self-Regulation   Executive function and self-regulatory processes overarch all of the writing processes described previously. Within Singer and Bashir's model, executive functions encompass a range of control processes necessary to carry out purposeful and goal-directed behavior. Components of executive function include attentional processes and anticipatory processes. Attentional processes include selective attention (focusing on what you are writing, not pencils dropping or peers talking), sustained attention (sticking with your writing despite distractions), divided attention (paying attention to the *meaning* as well as the *form* of what you are writing), span of attention (how long you can stay focused on your writing), and ability to shift attention (going back to your writing after an interruption). Anticipatory processes include working memory (keeping ideas in mind), planning (deciding how you will approach a writing task), organizing (deciding how to structure and sequence content), and managing affect (motivating yourself to write). These executive functions serve a supervisory function, allowing a writer to prepare, act, and sustain attention to a writing task long enough to complete it (Singer & Bashir, 1999).

Self-regulation refers to behaviors that writers use to monitor, evaluate, and adjust their performance as they compose. They use self-talk to guide themselves through difficult tasks, plan and evaluate their options, and select appropriate strategies to assist their performance. For strategies to be effective, writers must use the executive system to initiate, coordinate, and monitor those strategies. All of these processes are affected when executive functions are compromised (Singer & Bashir, 1999).

Students who use AAC are likely to have deficits across multiple cognitive/linguistic domains. They may fatigue quickly and have difficulty sustaining attention to a physically demanding task. Phonological processing impairments may make the use of "inner speech" less efficient as a self-regulatory mechanism. In the face of such weaknesses, the integrity of executive function and self-regulatory processes may determine how well such students can select, use, and self-monitor the effectiveness of compensatory strategies designed to circumvent or reduce the effect of their domain-specific deficits. Explicit instruction in executive function and self-regulation strategies is likely to benefit students with AAC needs because it addresses the multiple linguistic, cognitive, behavioral, and affective challenges they face by providing them with greater control over the selection and use of compensatory strategies (Foley, 2007).

Writing Foundations   The writing processes described previously rest on the four foundational components illustrated in the lower portion of Figure 5.3. These foundations include the cognitive-linguistic variables, social-rhetorical variables, production variables, and beliefs and attitudes that influence the generation of written text and underlie well-developed composing processes.

Cognitive-Linguistic Variables   Cognitive-linguistic variables include conceptual ability (e.g., verbal intelligence quotient [IQ]), processing speed, prior content knowledge, linguistic knowledge, metalinguistic and metacognitive abilities, and working memory. Verbal conceptual ability, as measured by verbal IQ, accounts for the greatest amount of variance in text generation and quality in school-age students (Berninger, Abbott, Abbott, Graham, & Richards, 2002). Accurate assessment of cognitive functioning in students who use AAC presents a challenge, and little is known about the effect of cognitive impairment on writing development in this population. Available evidence suggests, however, that a relatively high percentage of students who use AAC have cognitive impairments that are likely to increase their risk for writing problems, including difficulties with attention and memory (Koppenhaver & Yoder, 1992).

Processing speed is another critical variable that affects writing, with faster language processing speed thought to support higher-level metacognitive processing during writing tasks (Torgesen, 1994). Research suggests that students with language deficits may process verbal information more slowly than their peers without disabilities, negatively affecting verbal working memory performance (Montgomery, 2002). Similar difficulties have been observed in individuals who use AAC and are likely to constrain their ability to generate and revise text (Foley & Pollatsek, 1999).

Prior content knowledge influences what a writer can write about and what ideas can be retrieved from long-term memory. Students who use AAC are likely to have an impoverished fund of background knowledge due to their restricted life experiences and/or their difficulty acquiring information through reading (Light, 1997; Udwin & Yule, 1990).

Writing is a language-based skill, and linguistic knowledge (i.e., all stored knowledge about the content, form, and use of oral and written language) is necessary for effectively conveying ideas in written form. Linguistic skills at the word, sentence, and text levels play a critical role in the writing process. Students who use AAC are likely to be disadvantaged as writers because they typically struggle with one or more oral and/or written language domains, including semantics (Light, 1997; Udwin & Yule, 1990), morphology (Binger & Light, 2008; Sutton & Gallagher, 1993, 1995; Sutton, Soto, & Blockberger, 2002), syntax (Binger & Light, 2008; Sutton & Gallagher, 1993, 1995; Sutton et al., 2002), pragmatics (Udwin & Yule, 1990; Martinsen & von Tetzchner, 1996), verbal memory (Foley & Pollatsek, 1999), spelling (Dahlgren Sandberg, 2001; Hart, 2006), and reading (Dahlgren Sandberg & Hjelmquist, 2002; Foley & Pollatsek, 1999; Koppenhaver & Yoder, 1992; Sturm & Clendon, 2004).

Social-Rhetorical Variables   Typical writers make lexical, syntactic, and text structure choices based on their purpose(s) for writing, their knowledge of writing genres, and their awareness of their audience (see Table 5.4 for a description of the most common writing genres and their characteristics). A writer's choices are influenced by the desired effect on a reader (e.g., to inform, persuade, entertain) or the need to meet some external standard of performance (e.g., interesting vocabulary, varied sentence types, page limits; Singer & Bashir, 2004). Research indicates that students with language deficits, including those who use AAC, have greater difficulty than their peers managing the rhetorical demands of writing, and they tend to persist in an "oral" style of writing long after their peers without disabilities have adopted more "literate" writing forms and conventions. When rhetorical tasks require a more formal, literate style, writers who lack internal representations

Table 5.4.   Common writing genres and their characteristics

Writing genres	Characteristics
Expository	Genre of writing that informs, describes, or explains with text types that include autobiography, biography, descriptive, essay, informational report, and media article
Narrative	Genre of writing that entertains or tells a story with text types that include adventure, fairy tale, fantasy, historical fiction, mystery, personal narrative, realistic fiction, and science fiction
Persuasive	Genre of writing that attempts to convince readers to embrace a particular point of view with text types that include advertisement, editorial, essay, political cartoon, pro/con, and review
Procedural	Genre of writing that explains the instructions or directions for completing a task with text types that include experiment, how to, and recipe
Transactional	Genre of writing that serves as a communication of ideas and information between individuals with text types that include blog, business letter, friendly e-mail, friendly letter, interview, invitation, and postcard

of critical discourse and text schemas are disadvantaged; individuals with complex communication needs often lack the language and literacy skills and experience needed to develop such schemas (Koppenhaver, Evans, & Yoder, 1991; Light & Kelford Smith, 1993; Udwin & Yule, 1990; von Tetzchner & Martinsen, 1996).

Other issues affecting students who use AAC involve a number of social and physical variables. For example, writing is a social act that involves communication with an unseen reader. A developing writer must learn to create meaning without the support of a conversational partner. This transition from a conversational to a more explicit literate-language style can be challenging for those students with AAC needs who rely heavily on prompts from their communication partners during face-to-face communication. The transition is easier for students who communicate competently using text-based AAC systems. Without the social and time constraints inherent in face-to-face communication, such students are better able to reflect on the content and form of their writing.

Composing can also be influenced by the physical environment and writer preferences. For example, some students who use AAC may be isolated from their peers during writing because they have to write at a computer in the back of the classroom while their peers sit at desks. Some students, especially those with attention deficits, may experience difficulty writing in a noisy environment, whereas others may prefer writing with music in the background. Some may write better using the keyboard on their AAC device than on a computer because it is more familiar or more accessible. Optimal conditions for writing are likely to be highly individualized.

Production Variables   Three production variables interfere with the composing processes: 1) graphomotor skills, which are the processes responsible for transcribing ideas onto a page by hand; 2) mode of output (e.g., whether text is produced with a pen, keyboard, or voice recognition system); and 3) speed of output, which is the degree to which a writer can transcribe text fluently and automatically within a given mode of output. Graphomotor skills affect the writing process because the less fluent and automatic handwriting is, the less attention is available for higher-level text generation processes such as planning and organizing (Berninger, 1999). Difficulties transcribing text to the page interfere with both the quantity and quality of text produced (McCutchen, 1988).

Most students who use AAC have significant graphomotor impairments that constrain the writing process. Although such students may demonstrate better writing skills with one mode of output than another (e.g., word processing versus handwriting), slow speed may be an issue regardless of output mode. In fact, the average rate of composition for individuals who use AAC is less than 4 words per minute (Kelford Smith, Thurston, Light, Parnes, & O'Keefe, 1989) compared with 40–60 words per minute produced by fluent writers. Rate enhancement features available on some

AAC systems (e.g., word prediction, abbreviation expansion) can potentially help increase writing speed; however, for some students, the use of such features may increase cognitive load and thus interfere with higher-level composing processes. Identifying optimal text production methods and strategies should be part of the writing assessment process.

Beliefs and Attitudes   Beliefs and attitudes, or affective variables, include self-efficacy, affect, and the writer's goals (Singer & Bashir, 2004). Self-efficacy is a self-perceived judgment of whether one has the skills and abilities to meet the demands of a writing task and is predictive of interest in writing, motivation to write, and feelings about oneself as a writer. Self-efficacy beliefs can be shaped by external factors (e.g., teacher expectations, instructional approaches, peer feedback) or internal factors (e.g., motivation, interest in a topic, feelings of frustration or failure). Writers with greater self-efficacy set higher writing goals, persist at writing longer, and show more positive affect regarding their writing (Singer & Bashir, 2004). Because they have difficulty managing the many cognitive, linguistic, communicative, and physical demands of writing, students who use AAC are at high risk for developing negative self-efficacy beliefs and lacking motivation to write (Smith, 2005).

Summary

Singer and Bashir's (2004) model of written language production appropriately reflects the complexity of the writing process and the critical foundational abilities that underlie skilled writing. In light of this model, it is easier to understand why learning to write well is challenging for students with AAC needs, most of whom have multiple writing foundation weaknesses. Intrinsic factors alone, however, do not explain the severity of the written language problems observed in this heterogeneous population. Further complicating the picture are a number of extrinsic factors. For example, students who use AAC typically have less experience with and exposure to writing in early childhood than their peers without disabilities (Light & Kelford Smith, 1993). Once in school, they receive a lower quantity and quality of writing instruction than their peers without disabilities, often due to low expectations from teachers or other adults (Koppenhaver, 1991; Koppenhaver & Yoder, 1992, 1993; Mike, 1995). In contrast to recommended practices in writing instruction, students who use AAC are rarely offered opportunities to write on a daily basis (Koppenhaver, 1991). What limited instruction is available is likely to focus on fill-in-the-blank exercises and spelling practice and rarely includes writing beyond the sentence level (Katims, 2001; Ryndak, Morrison, & Sommerstein, 1999). This emphasis on isolated skills keeps students from engaging in more meaningful and effective instructional experiences.

ASSESSMENT OF CONVENTIONAL WRITING

Conventional writing assessment can be accomplished in many different ways, depending on the domain of written language being assessed. These domains generally include

- *Ideas and content*—how the writer develops ideas and relevant details
- *Organization*—how the organization of ideas fits the purpose of a piece
- *Voice*—how the writer engages with the audience
- *Word choice*—the use of a diverse, specific, and content-appropriate vocabulary
- *Sentence fluency*—the use of a variety of sentence types to enhance meaning
- *Conventions*—the correct use of spelling, grammar, and punctuation

For typically developing students and those with language-learning disabilities, these features of writing are assessed using norm-referenced standardized tests, curriculum-based measures (CBMs), rubrics, and informal assessments (e.g., checklists, weekly spelling tests). These methods are described briefly next and the advantages and disadvantages of using them with students who use AAC are discussed.

Norm-Referenced Standardized Tests

Although norm-referenced writing tests provide some information about individual performance, they tend to focus on decontextualized, readily accessed features of language, such as grammatical correctness or punctuation. Such assessments most often reveal what students do wrong but not what they do well; thus, they are of limited use for planning intervention. The use of norm-referenced writing tests with students who use AAC is particularly problematic. Such tools rarely include students with significant disabilities in their standardization samples and often need to be adapted to be accessible to students with significant physical and/or communication impairments. Production rates and physical fatigue may require that testing be completed over a number of test sessions, further compromising the validity of the normative data (Smith, 2005). Overall, norm-referenced tests fail to capture what students with AAC needs know about the writing process and what they can do given appropriate instructional supports. Such tests have limited utility in an assessment process focused on gathering meaningful information for intervention planning and, thus, are not recommended for students who use AAC.

Curriculum-Based Measures

A CBM approach is when generic procedures for measurement are employed with stimulus materials taken directly from the instructional materials used by teachers in their classrooms (Deno, 2003). CBMs are usually composed of a set of standard directions, a timing device, a set of materials, scoring rules, standards for judging performance, and record forms or charts (Hosp, Hosp, & Howell, 2007). CBMs are characterized by several attributes. They are aligned with the general education curriculum because students are tested on the same curriculum they are being taught. The measures are technically adequate, meaning they have established reliability and validity (at least for typically developing students and those with language-learning disabilities), and they are intended to be repeated over time so that progress monitoring can occur. CBMs are criterion referenced and, therefore, more sensitive to instruction than norm-referenced standardized measures. In addition, they can be used to determine when instruction is working and when it should be changed. Several CBM tasks have been developed to quickly assess students' overall writing skills.

Curriculum-Based Measures for Writing
In a typical CBM for writing, students are provided with a story starter, a 1-minute planning period, and 3 minutes to generate their stories without any assistance from the instructor. Student writing samples may be scored according to the 1) number of words written, 2) number of letters written, 3) number of words correctly spelled, and/or 4) number of writing units placed in correct sequence. CBMs for writing, essentially measures of rate and accuracy, have been used successfully with typically developing elementary (Deno, Marston, & Mirkin, 1982), middle school (Espin et al., 2000), and secondary-level students (Espin, Scierka, Skare, & Halverson, 1999), as well as students with language-learning disabilities. Because writing CBM tasks closely resemble those used in district and state writing assessments, proponents argue that experience with such tasks leads to better student outcomes on high-stakes testing (Hosp et al., 2007). There is no evidence to date of any such advantages for students with AAC needs, most of whom will need accommodations to participate in state writing assessments anyway.

Standard administration of the writing CBM is problematic for students with physical impairments. Such individuals are likely to produce written text at a very slow rate and may require extra time to plan and generate a representative writing sample independently. Their writing speed or fluency may not increase significantly, even as the quality and quantity of their writing does. For this reason, the time allotted to these students for completion of writing probes should be extended as needed (e.g., 30 minutes versus 3 minutes), with progress measured against the student's own baseline performance rather than grade-level fluency norms. As is typical in general and special education settings where writing CBM is used, these unscaffolded, extended time CBM probes could be administered three times during the school year (e.g., fall, winter, spring), or even monthly, to monitor changes over time in the quality and quantity of writing the student can produce independently.

Curriculum-Based Measures for Spelling   CBMs for spelling are short, sensitive measures of spelling achievement that have been used successfully with typically developing students and students with language-learning disabilities (Fuchs, Fuchs, & Hamlett, 1989). As with all CBM tasks, the information obtained is intended to provide a database for each student so that appropriate instructional decisions can be made in a timely manner. Spelling CBMs can serve as an alternative to traditional weekly spelling tests, which often do not distinguish between students' actual spelling skill and their ability to memorize or copy words (Loeffler, 2005). Typically, students are required to spell words from alternate forms of grade-level lists and are given 10 seconds to spell each word. Spelling CBMs can be scored for correct letter sequences and the total number of words spelled correctly. Norms are available for Grades 1–12. As with writing CBMs, extending the time limit allowed to spell each word and allowing alternatives to handwriting (e.g., use of a spelling display on an AAC device with word prediction turned off) may enable students who use AAC to more fully demonstrate their understanding of how spelling works. Teachers can create their own grade-level spelling lists, or premade spelling CBM lists for Grades 1–8 can be purchased from http://www.aimsweb.com.

Response to Intervention   Response to intervention (RTI) is an approach used in school settings to evaluate a student's response to an ecological context of instruction and/or intervention. It is a three-tiered approach, with intensity increasing from tier to tier through changes in duration, frequency and time of interventions, group size, and instructor skill level, to meet the needs of all students. Students who need the most intensive interventions (Tier III) have their progress monitored frequently (one to two times per week). CBMs are used within all three tiers; the only thing that really changes is the frequency of assessment. Conclusive research that supports the effectiveness of the RTI model for students with disabilities is needed before any recommendations can be made, but there are at least two potential advantages of using an RTI model for students with AAC needs. First, the model assumes that these students will receive research-based writing instruction that is aligned with core curriculum writing standards, with whatever frequency and intensity is indicated by progress-monitoring measures. Second, it assumes that they will receive daily writing intervention from highly qualified instructors. Research indicates that for the majority of students who use AAC, neither of these conditions is typical in either general or special education settings (Katims, 1991, 2001; Koppenhaver, 1991).

Authentic Assessment   Authentic assessment strategies are used to examine how students learn and what they can achieve with varying degrees and types of scaffolding (Lidz & Pena, 1996; Ukrainetz, Harpell, Walsh, & Coyle, 2000). Thus, they are valuable in assessing writing abilities in students with AAC needs. These strategies provide descriptive information about how students who use AAC function as writers within purposeful contexts, with various AT supports, and in different social and academic environments. Authentic assessment involves hypothesizing, collecting evidence, evaluating the evidence, and determining a course of intervention suited to a particular student (Ukrainetz, 2006). It provides a mechanism for examining both writing products and engagement in the writing process. As discussed previously, the writing development of students who use AAC is affected by a complex interaction of internal factors (e.g., reduced linguistic competence, cognitive impairment, severe physical disability) and external influences (e.g., quality and quantity of writing instruction, availability of AT supports). Authentic assessment appropriately reflects this complexity. It can provide rich descriptions of student abilities and learning needs in a variety of contexts and capture subtle changes in performance in ways that standardized tests and unscaffolded CBM writing probes cannot.

A wealth of information can be gained from observing students as they compose text and analyzing the completed texts. This data can serve as a foundation for writing individualized objectives, determining effective instructional strategies, and measuring change over time (Nelson, Bahr, & Van Meter, 2004). Writing samples representing different genres should be collected because students' writing competence may vary significantly from genre to genre based on experience and prior instruction.

Collecting Writing Samples

As discussed previously, a common writing assessment strategy is to periodically collect brief but complete writing samples or probes in order to see how well students use writing processes such as planning, organizing, drafting, revising, and editing without direct scaffolding. Some students who use AAC, however, may not be able to produce a writing sample at all without considerable scaffolding and encouragement, so the desire to see what students can do independently must be balanced with each student's individual support needs. It makes sense, therefore, to also administer *scaffolded* writing probes during the course of intervention to evaluate the quantity and quality of writing produced when various instructional or AT supports are provided. For example, some students may compose text most efficiently using their AAC devices because they can take advantage of symbol and word prediction features. Students who struggle to retain and maintain content and cohesion when they write may produce higher quality writing samples if they are allowed to brainstorm with teachers or peers first or use graphic organizers for planning and/or keeping track of their ideas. Initially, a high level of teacher modeling and scaffolding may be needed (e.g., generating initial ideas, helping to organize concepts), with less support required as the student gains enough experience and competence to internalize the use of learned writing and self-regulatory strategies.

Prompts for Narratives   There are many methods for eliciting written narratives, including story retelling, picture prompts, and story starters. Nelson, Bahr, and Van Meter (2004) recommend using the following narrative prompt to encourage students to produce a story that has narrative structure, without influencing story content specifically.

- We are interested in the stories students write.
- Your story should tell about a problem and what happens.
- Your characters and your story can be real or imaginary.

Because they often have limited knowledge of narrative text structure, students who use AAC may benefit from prewriting dialogue with a teacher or peer or using story maps that provide additional cues for including required narrative elements (Foley & Staples, 2007). See Figure 5.4 for an example of a narrative story map.

Prompts for Other Genres   Instructions for gathering samples of expository text must be constructed to guide students to think about the key features of the required genres and subgenres (Nelson et al., 2004). For example, a probe for an informational paragraph might prompt a student to choose a topic to write about and to include a topic sentence and three supporting details.

Prompt for informational report

Your beginning sentence tells the topic.

Your sentences make sense and are complete.

You have three facts about the topic.

You write about the facts in your own words.

Your ending sentence tells a feeling about the topic.

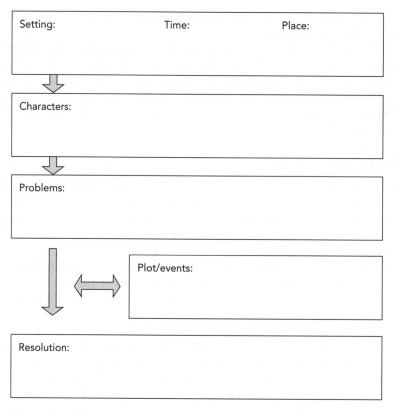

Figure 5.4. Narrative story map.

Different prompts would be required to elicit expository text structures such as descriptions, sequences, or compare/contrast summaries. The characteristics of good writing, however, remain consistent across genres. Whether a student is writing a recipe, a book report, or a paragraph comparing and contrasting butterflies and moths, the fundamental writing skills remain the same. Students must write to an intended audience, maintain focus and organization, develop their ideas, express themselves clearly, and show mastery of English conventions.

Writing Sample Analysis

A student's writing portfolio should contain samples obtained in a variety of contexts, across a range of writing genres. Samples may be obtained through unscaffolded prompts, scaffolded prompts, and unprompted samples produced during the course of classroom writing activities (e.g., writing an informational report on an assigned topic). Once student writing samples have been collected, they can be analyzed using several scoring methods, each with its own advantages and limitations. These include holistic scoring, trait or analytic scale scoring with rubrics, and quantitative measures of specific writing features.

Holistic Scoring Methods   *Holistic scoring* refers to global assessment of written products based on the impression a piece of writing makes as a whole and how it compares with target performance levels for a particular age or grade level (Cooper & Odell, 1977). Although holistic scoring methods may serve as a quick screening method for students who need more comprehensive assessments, they provide no specific information for development of individual goals and objectives. In general, such methods are insensitive to the slower, more subtle progress made by writers who have significant disabilities. Consider, for example, the "global" impression made by the following personal narratives produced by a second-grade student named Taylor using a Dynavox communication device:

Sample 1

I eat applesauce We eat with nana We sleep at night play toys and swing My family goes to grandma eat cake

Sample 2

When I get home I am going to do my homework. And than I am going to play with Courtney. We are going to play babys. Her mom is having a baby. She is having twins that are girls.

Rated by holistic scoring methods, both of Taylor's pieces would receive low scores for her age and grade. Yet, the second sample, produced 2 months after the first one, represents important changes in Taylor's writing development. Taylor wrote the second piece while learning to use word-processing software with word prediction and a new access method (i.e., a trackball). Holistic scoring does not capture her faster typing rate, decreased fatigue, or increased motivation to write. In addition, no points would be awarded for independently using a word wall while writing, increasing sentence length and complexity, or improving her use of writing conventions.

Trait or Analytic Scoring Using Rubrics Trait or analytic scoring approaches modify holistic methods by using rubrics to describe different levels of performance in different writing domains. The 6+1 Trait Analysis is an example that is commonly used in general education settings (http://www.nwrel.org/assessment/department.php?d=1). The 6+1 Trait Analysis is used to evaluate student writing on qualities including ideas and content, organization, voice, word choice, sentence fluency, and conventions. The Writing A–Z web site (http://www.writinga-z.com/razwritingweb/home.do) has a similar trait analysis rubric that can be downloaded and used with students at varying levels from beginning to fluent writing. One advantage of trait analysis over holistic scoring methods is that it yields more than a single numerical value and can be used to evaluate writing at different stages of the writing process; this advantage becomes evident when applied to another of Taylor's writing samples. Sample 3 represents a first draft of a story about a zebra. Sample 4 is the final draft of the story produced after dialogue with teachers and peers resulted in several rounds of revisions and edits.

Sample 3

The zebra was sleeping at the zoo. He role up and run away to vind his flaly. He wolkde to logen and he sor his flaly he was sad bkus his flaly is ded

Sample 4

The Zebras

The zebra was sleeping at the zoo. He woke up and ran away to find his family. He walked to Logan and he saw his family. He was sad because his family was dead. A talking bear was being mean, he was growling "gorr" at them and they ran into the street and a car hit them.

The End

Trait analysis for these two samples using a rubric would result in different scores for content, organization, voice, word choice, sentence fluency, and conventions, as well as an overall assignment to a stage of writing. Comparisons of the ratings for the final draft with those of earlier drafts can be used to demonstrate progress in specific aspects of Taylor's writing. For example, her goal as a writer for this piece was to elicit an emotional reaction from her audience, and she was successful in doing so. Because the trait analysis rubric assigns points not only for content, form, and writing mechanics, but also for connecting with an audience, it can be used to recognize and encourage Taylor's emerging sense of herself as a writer with her own style and voice.

Quantitative Measures of Writing Development   In addition to holistic, trait or analytic scale scoring with rubrics, writing sample analysis can target specific skills at word, sentence, discourse, and writing conventions levels. The next section contains suggestions for assessing students' strengths and needs at each of these levels.

Word-Level Analysis   Word choices greatly influence the quality and clarity of students' writing. Vocabulary diversity (the variety of words a writer uses) and maturity (whether vocabulary use is age appropriate) can be examined to analyze writing skill at the word level. One means of measuring vocabulary diversity is to count the number of different words in a writing sample. A more time-efficient method, however, involves simply looking for evidence of overreliance on simple and/or generic words (e.g., *thing, stuff, good*) in a writing sample. Students who use a restricted number of different words may respond to curriculum-based interventions that explicitly target use of more varied and specific vocabulary.

Spelling assessment is another type of word-level analysis. Spelling errors influence audience perceptions of writing maturity and competence, and numerous errors can render a piece of writing unreadable (Nelson et al., 2004). Spelling assessment can include a count of words spelled incorrectly divided by the total number of words in a writing sample. Another spelling assessment strategy uses a more advanced developmental spelling inventory (e.g., Bear et al., 2008) than described previously for emergent writers. Bear et al.'s *Words Their Way* contains a series of spelling feature analysis inventories and related instructional materials for primary (K–3), elementary, and upper-level (upper elementary, middle, high school, and postsecondary) students. By analyzing spelling patterns and using them to determine stages of spelling development, educators can identify the strategies that students bring to the spelling process and target those not yet in use.

Sentence-Level Analysis   As students' written language develops, a gradual increase occurs in sentence length and complexity. Counting the number of T-units per sentence, defined by Hunt (1970) as "one main clause plus the subordinate clauses attached to or embedded within it" (p. 49), is one way of measuring syntactic complexity. Another measure involves coding and counting different sentence types. Nelson et al. (2004) recommended a system that codes sentences as simple or complex based on the number of verbs in the sentence. Sentences with one verb are rated as simple; those with more than one verb are coded as complex. In addition, sentences are rated as correct or incorrect. Examples from Taylor's writing of each sentence type appear next:

Simple incorrect

They has habitats.

Simple correct

They need food and water.

Complex incorrect

I learn that animal migrate.

Complex correct

Some animals that migrate live in Africa.

Nelson et al. (2004) suggested measuring improved outcomes as advancing proportions of sentences scoring in the higher-level categories along the continuum of simple incorrect, simple correct, complex incorrect, and complex correct.

Other sentence-level analyses include looking for an appropriate variety of sentence types or evidence of noun phrase elaboration (the *big, brown bear* versus *the bear*) and verb phrase elaboration (*He ran quickly* versus *He ran*). If such elements are not present, then appropriate sentence-level interventions, such as sentence combining, can be developed.

Discourse-Level Analysis   Discourse-level analysis considers the global organization of a piece of writing and how well it conveys the writer's intended goals. Subcomponents of assessment at this level include methods for analyzing the following discourse-level skills.

- **Productivity and fluency**
  Productivity is a simple measure of text length that can be calculated by tallying the total number of words in a sample or by counting the total number of sentences or T-units. As sentences become more complex, the mean length of utterance per T-unit increases. Productivity related to a unit of time (e.g., a 30-minute probe) is considered a measure of writing fluency.

  In Taylor's Sample 4, she produced a total of 60 words and a total of 11 T-units. Her sample, produced and revised via word processing over the course of several days, was approximately half the length of stories produced via handwriting by her typically developing peers in 1 or 2 days. The mean length of utterance per T-unit in her sample, however, was comparable with that produced by her peers. This indicates that although writing productivity and fluency are an issue, Taylor is able to demonstrate at least average writing ability given adequate time and appropriate AT supports.

- **Narrative organization and maturity**
  There are several methods for analyzing the organization and maturity of written narratives produced by school-age students, including high-point analysis (McCabe & Peterson, 1991; McCabe & Rollins, 1994). By age 6, typically developing children can tell a well-formed story containing a sequence of events that leads to some sort of climax or high point and then provides a resolution by telling how things turned out after the crisis point.

  Another means of analyzing narrative maturity is through story-grammar analysis (Hedberg & Westby, 1993; Mandler & Johnson, 1977). Narrative writing samples can be analyzed by counting the number of story grammar elements they contain. Taylor's story about Fluffy the cat (Sample 5) contains multiple story grammar elements including characters (Fluffy, owner), character descriptions (grey fur, good cat, doesn't bite), a setting (Africa, the woods), a problem or initiating event (monster), an internal response or plan (scared, ran away), an action (runs to backyard), a resolution/outcome (gets lost in a pail), and an ending/conclusion (was asleep).

Sample 5

Hi I am a cat, my name is fluffy and I have gray fur and my owner is Sarah. We live in Africa. My owner said I am a good cat because I don't bite.

One day when we were walking in the woods all of a sudden there was a monster behind me! It was scary and I ran away. I was yelling aaaaaaaaaaaaaaaaa when I was running. I got lost in a pail in my backyard. I was asleep.

This story was produced after several weeks of explicit classroom instruction relating to the use of story-grammar elements in creative writing. Taylor's earlier stories showed limited awareness and use of these critical elements.

- **Structural organization and maturity for other genres**
  Measures of structural organization and maturity for genres other than narratives must be specific to the required genre. Core curriculum standards often include benchmarks and outcomes for writing development for particular genres at each grade level. These can be used by educators to craft appropriate structural maturity measures that capture critical structural and organizational features. For example, in first grade, students are expected to produce expository text containing a topic sentence with three supporting details, as Taylor did in Sample 6.

Sample 6

I laern that animal Migrate. They has habitats. They need food and water. Some animals that migrate liv in Africa.

Although the sample contains several errors in spelling and noun–verb agreement, it reflects age-appropriate structural organization and maturity.

- **Cohesion measures**
  Cohesion refers to how well a writer connects ideas within and across sentences in a piece of writing. One strategy for assessing cohesion is to count instances in which cohesive ties are either missing (e.g., using a pronoun before establishing its referent) or used incorrectly (e.g., confusing the cohesive conjunctions *because* and *since*). The following example (Sample 7) from Taylor's reading response journal lacks appropriate cohesive ties.

Sample 7

It is about a panda and a man named Messdr po. The panda is ded. They found a baby panda after her mom died. They take the baby panda home.

Problems with cohesion in this sample include using a pronoun without first establishing its referent (they) and making unclear references (i.e., initially the reader does not know which panda died). Taylor correctly uses indefinite and definite articles (a panda, the panda) as cohesive elements.

- **Sense of audience and voice**
  There are qualities of writing that distinguish them as funny, moving, informative, or interesting. Such qualities can be analyzed in a descriptive manner, and examples from a student's writing can be used to document progress. For example, in September of her first grade year, Taylor produced the following narrative (Sample 8) about a traumatic personal experience.

Sample 8

My cat lacey died. She got in the engine. We were going to by new shoes.

In January of her second grade year, Taylor wrote the following piece (Sample 9) on the same topic.

Sample 9

The Saddest Day of My Life

One afternoon we were going to the store to buy me new shoes. My cat Lacey died. She was up in the engine and she was climbing out of the car engine. She died in the engine. Even my dad was crying. My mom and me were crying our eyes out.

In the second version, Taylor described the death of her cat, Lacey, with the explicit goal of eliciting an emotional reaction from her readers. She provided more detailed information about the events leading up to Lacey's death and more elaboration on her family's response to what had transpired. A comparison of this piece to the one written several months earlier shows greater awareness of writing conventions (e.g., story title, capitalization, punctuation) and increased sentence length and complexity, as well as Taylor's developing sense of audience and voice.

Writing Conventions Analysis   Writing conventions include capitalization, punctuation, and formatting. Checklists can be used by instructors and/or students to evaluate the use of writing conventions. Attention to writing conventions, however, should not dominate the composing process. Checklists of conventions taught during the school year are best used in the final stages of editing a text for publication.

Beliefs and Attitudes Foundations Assessment   Often overlooked in writing assessment are what Singer and Bashir (2004) identified as beliefs and attitudes foundations. Given the connection between motivation and literacy learning (see e.g., Turner & Paris, 1995), it is important to systematically explore students' attitudes toward writing. A standardized and student-friendly instrument for such purposes is the Garfield Writing Test (Kear, Coffman, McKenna, & Ambrosio, 2000). The test is easily administered to children who use AAC because it requires only a pointing response to one of four faces of the cartoon character Garfield the cat. Sample items include questions about student feelings when writing about something they have seen or heard, how they would feel about keeping a diary, or how they feel about writing about things they do in science classes. Percentile scores are provided for 1st through 12th grades. Student results can be compared with more informal and observational evidence, suggest the relative need for specific instruction addressing student motivation, or serve as an additional measure of the effectiveness of a student's intervention program if administered pre- and post-intervention.

Integrating Assessment and Intervention

The whole point of conducting writing assessment is to determine how best to help students improve their writing ability. As discussed previously, there are two broad areas to assess: students' engagement in the writing process and the writing products they produce. The information gleaned from ongoing assessment of process and product guide intervention planning in different ways.

Writing Process Intervention   Assessment of a student's participation in the writing process reveals information about how (or whether) the student can plan, organize, generate, revise, and edit text. Intervention planning can target specific changes in student performance that are needed (e.g., more planning prior to writing) or changes in the nature of the student's writing instruction that are deficient (e.g., no models of or strategies for planning are provided). As mandated by NCLB, IEP goals should reflect core curriculum writing standards and be crafted so that they specify the end goal (e.g., the student will engage in planning) and the means by which the goal will be accomplished (e.g., using a graphic organizer). Goals should address each of the planning, organizing, generating, revising, and editing processes that skilled writers use. The goals, however, should be achievable whether students are in emergent or conventional stages of writing development. For example, core curriculum writing standards specify that students write daily to communicate effectively for a variety of purposes and audiences. Carter, a third-grade student with AAC needs who is making the transition from emergent to conventional writing, used the graphic organizer in Figure 5.5 to communicate his understanding of core curriculum content through his selection and organization of pictures and the invented spellings he used to label them. After completing the graphic organizer, he worked with a peer without disabilities to generate, revise, edit, and publish the text in Sample 10.

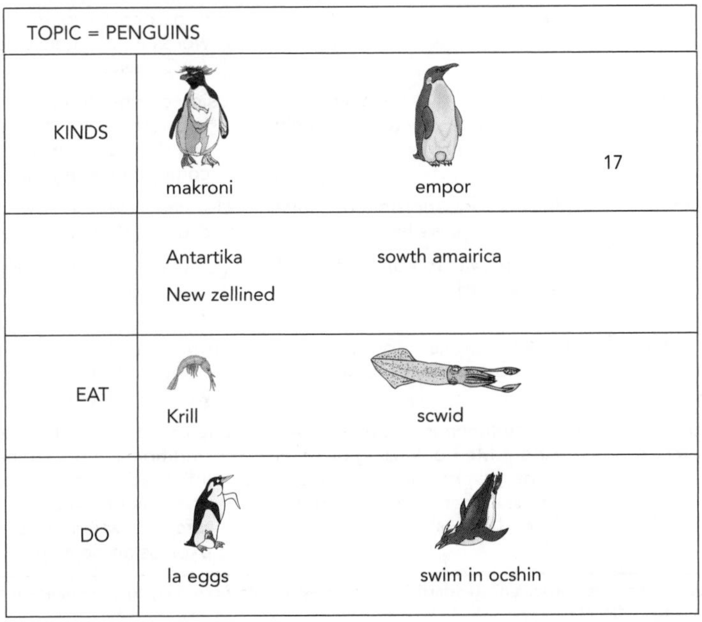

Figure 5.5. Carter's graphic organizer.

Sample 10

Penguins

There are 17 kinds of penguins, like the macaroni penguin and the emperor penguin. Penguins are
birds that live in Antarctica, South America, and New Zealand. They eat krill and squid. They
lay eggs and they like to dive and swim in the ocean.

Carter may not yet be a fully conventional writer, but he is participating daily in all aspects of
the writing process. He is using his AAC device to participate in class discussions, ask and answer
questions, and engage in invented spelling. He is learning new information and communicating
what he knows through emergent writing activities.

Table 5.5 provides additional examples of how core curriculum standards for writing can
be modified for students with AAC needs at both emergent and conventional stages of writing
development.

Writing Product Intervention   At this level, interventions are planned that target
specific features of students' writing (e.g., vocabulary, grammar, spelling) rather than their engagement in the writing process. For example, if assessment reveals an overreliance on general words,
then intervention could be designed around teaching the students to use more varied and specific
vocabulary. Intervention activities might include identifying and using interesting words encoun-
tered during reading or developing a personal word bank. Taylor, for example, used the "describing

Table 5.5.   Examples of modified core curriculum objectives for writing

Objective	Examples of modified objectives for students who use AAC	
	Emergent writers	Conventional writers
Prepare to write by gathering and organizing information and ideas (prewriting)	Generate ideas by drawing or looking at pictures of familiar or favorite activities	Using AAC device, generate a list of topics to write about
		Select a topic from generated list
		Identify audience, purpose, and form of writing
Compose a written draft	Select picture and add label or words	Use graphic organizer to organize draft (e.g., beginning, middle, end) using words and sentences generated with AAC device
Revise by elaborating and clarifying a written draft	Add name to picture in an appropriate way (e.g., scribble, letter stamps, typing)	Using computer and word prediction software, revise draft to add details, use descriptive words, and write in complete sentences
Edit written draft for conventions	Edit name for appropriate capital and lower-case letters	Use checklist to edit writing for correct capitalization and punctuation
	Use word wall to edit spelling of a key word	Use word wall, personal dictionary, or spell-check to correct misspelled words
Use fluent and legible handwriting to communicate	Use AAC device to produce writing using symbols and/or words	Produce legible documents with AAC device, typing, and/or typing using word prediction
Write in different forms and genres	Produce functional text (e.g., All About Me book using pictures, photographs, journal, labels, signs, alphabet books, patterned books)	Use graphic organizers to produce traditional and imaginative stories, informational texts (how-to books, observations, reports), personal letters, and writing to persuade or express an opinion

Note: General education core curriculum standard for writing—students write daily to communicate effectively for a
variety of purposes and audiences.

Key: AAC, augmentative and alternative communication.

words" page of her high-tech AAC device to identify different words, and, by teacher report, her peers often asked her to open to that page so they could use it like a thesaurus. If assessment data show that a student only uses one basic sentence pattern (I have a dog. He is brown. He is small.), then intervention might include minilessons on combining simple sentences to create more complex forms (I have a big, brown dog). The developmental spelling inventories described previously provide data to guide spelling instruction, and there are many useful resources available for this purpose that are linked to core curriculum standards for spelling (e.g., Bear et al., 2008). Students who have difficulty with capitalization and punctuation can learn to use editing checklists to revise their writing. Whether the focus is on vocabulary, grammar, spelling, or other writing conventions, specific intervention targets can be developed and adjusted based on data from ongoing dynamic assessment.

This section of the chapter has presented multiple methods for assessing conventional writing processes and products. Table 5.6 contains a summary of the conventional writing assessment domains, tasks, tools, and outcome measures that have been discussed. Some of the assessment tools are formative in nature (scaffolded writing probes) and others are summative (writing CBMs). Educators must decide which will be most useful for a particular student and how often they should be used.

Table 5.6.   Summary of conventional writing assessment domains, tasks, tools, and outcome measures

Domain	Assessment task	Assessment tools	Outcome measures
Writing process	Administer genre-specific writing probes (unscaffolded) to evaluate the quality and quantity of writing the student can produce independently	Genre-specific rubrics	Numerical ratings relating to content, organization, voice, word choice, sentence fluency, and conventions
		Writing curriculum-based measures (CBMs; extended time)	Total words written (TWW)
			Total letters written (TLW)
		Portfolio	Dated writing samples
			Detailed observations
			Writing process checklists
	Administer genre-specific writing probes (scaffolded) to evaluate the quality and quantity of writing produced when various instructional supports are provided (e.g., graphic organizers)	Genre-specific rubrics	Numerical ratings relating to content, organization, voice, word choice, sentence fluency, and conventions
		Writing CBMs (untimed)	TWW
			TLW
		Portfolio	Dated writing samples
			Completed graphic organizers
			Writing process checklists
			Detailed observations of process writing in natural contexts
Writing product	Word-level analyses	Vocabulary diversity	Number of different words
		Spelling CBMs	Total words correct (TWC)
			Correct letter sequences (CLS)
		Developmental spelling inventory	Spelling stage assignment
		Spelling in context	Percentage of words spelled correctly in a writing sample

(continued)

Table 5.6.   *(continued)*

Domain	Assessment task	Assessment tools	Outcome measures
Writing product *(continued)*	Sentence-level analyses	Syntactic complexity	Number of T-units per sentence
			Percentage of sentence types (e.g., simple, complex)
			Evidence of noun and verb phrase elaboration
	Discourse-level analyses	Productivity and fluency measures per unit of time (e.g., 30-minute probe)	Total number of words
			Total number of sentences
			Total number of T-units
			Mean length of utterance per T-unit
		Story-grammar analysis	Number of story-grammar elements in sample
		Cohesion measures	Number of cohesive ties missing or used incorrectly
	Writing conventions analysis	Developmentally appropriate conventions checklist	Number of errors in punctuation, capitalization, and formatting
Beliefs and attitudes	Explore students' attitudes toward writing	Garfield Writing Test (Kear, Coffman, McKenna, & Ambrosio, 2000)	Numerical rating
			Pre- and postintervention measures of student motivation and interests

CONCLUSION

Educators have many tools and strategies at their disposal to assess critical domains of writing, regardless of where their students who use AAC are on the continuum from emergent to conventional writing development. As educators employ these tools and strategies, however, they must recognize that the real purpose of writing assessment will not be fulfilled unless the data are tied to effective instructional strategies, supports, and learning contexts. Although the writing development of students who use AAC may progress at a slower place than their typically developing peers, these students can continue to grow as writers throughout their lives if given appropriate instructional experiences and opportunities (Foley & Staples, 2003). If writing assessment data are used appropriately, educators can support students' growth throughout their school years and into adulthood.

REFERENCES

Bear, D.R., Invernizzi, M., Templeton, S., & Johnston, F. (2008). *Words their way: Word study for phonics, vocabulary, and spelling instruction* (4th ed.). Upper Saddle River, NJ: Pearson.

Bereiter, C., & Scardimalia, M. (1987). *The psychology of written composition.* Mahwah, NJ: Lawrence Erlbaum Associates.

Berninger, V. (1999). Coordinating transcription and text generation in working memory during composing: Automatic and constructive processes. *Learning Disabilities Quarterly, 22,* 99–112.

Berninger, V.W., Abbott, R., Abbott, S., Graham, S., & Richards, T. (2002). Writing and reading: Connections between language by hand and language by eye. *Journal of Learning Disabilities, 35,* 39–56.

Berninger, V.W., & Swanson, H.L. (1994). Modifying Hayes and Flower's model of skilled writing to explain beginning and developing writing. In J.S. Carlson (Series Ed.) & E.C. Butterfield (Vol. Ed.), *Advances in cognition and educational practice: Children's writing: Toward a process theory of development of skilled writing* (Vol. 2, pp. 57–81). Greenwich, CT: JAI Press.

Binger, C. & Light, J. (2008). The morphology and syntax of individuals who use AAC: Research review and implications for effective practice. *Augmentative and Alternative Communication, 24(2),* 123–138.

Bloodgood, J.W. (1999). What's in a name?: Children's name writing and literacy acquisition. *Reading Research Quarterly, 34(3),* 342–367.

Clay, M.M. (1991). *The early detection of reading difficulties* (3rd ed.). Portsmouth, NH: Heinemann.

Clay, M.M. (2005). *An observation survey of early literacy achievement* (2nd ed.). Portsmouth, NH: Heinemann.

Cooper, C.R., & Odell, L. (Eds.). (1977). *Evaluating writing: Describing, measuring, judging.* Urbana, IL: National Council of Teachers of English.

Dahlgren Sandberg, A. (2001). Reading and spelling, phonological awareness, and working memory in children with severe speech impairments: A longitudinal study. *Augmentative and Alternative Communication, 17,* 11–25.

Dahlgren Sandberg, A., & Hjelmquist, E. (2002). Phonological recoding problems in children with cerebral palsy: The importance of productive speech. In A.F.E. Witruk & T. Lachmann (Eds.), *Basic mechanisms of language and language disorders* (pp. 315–327). Dordrecht, The Netherlands: Kluwer Academic.

Deno, S.L. (2003). Developments in curriculum-based measurement. *Journal of Special Education, 37,* 184–192.

Deno, S.L., Marston, D., & Mirkin, P. (1982). Valid measurement procedures for continuous evaluation of written expression. *Exceptional Children Special Education and Pediatrics: A New Relationship, 48,* 368–371.

Downing, J.E. (2005). *Teaching literacy to students with significant disabilities: Strategies for the K–12 inclusive classroom.* Thousand Oaks, CA: Corwin Press.

Espin, C.A., Scierka, B.J., Skare, S., & Halverson, N. (1999). Criterion-related validity of curriculum-based measures in writing for secondary school students. *Reading and Writing Quarterly: Overcoming Learning Difficulties, 15,* 5–27.

Espin, C., Shin, J., Deno, S.L., Skare, S., Robinson, S., & Benner, B. (2000). Identifying indicators of written expression proficiency for middle school students. *Journal of Special Education, 34,* 140–153.

Ferroli, L., & Shanahan, T. (1987). Kindergarten spelling: Explaining its relationship to first-grade reading. In J.E. Readence & R.S. Baldwin (Eds.), *Research in literacy: Merging perspectives* (pp. 93–99). Rochester, NY: National Reading Conference.

Foley, B.E. (2007). Integrating process writing and self-regulatory strategy development with a written

narrative intervention. In *Proceedings of the 12th Biennial International Conference of the International Society for Augmentative and Alternative Communication, Düsseldorf, Germany, August 2006.* Toronto, Ontario: ISAAC.

Foley, B.E., & Pollatsek, A. (1999). Phonological processes and reading abilities in adolescents and adults with severe congenital speech impairments. *Augmentative and Alternative Communication, 15(2),* 153–162.

Foley, B.E., & Staples, A. (2003). Developing augmentative and alternative communication and literacy interventions for adults with autism in a supported employment setting. *Topics in Language Disorders, 23(4),* 325–343.

Foley, B., & Staples, A. (2007). Supporting literacy development with assistive technology. In S.R. Copeland & E.B. Keefe (Eds.), *Effective literacy instruction for students with moderate or severe disabilities* (pp. 127–148). Baltimore: Paul H. Brookes Publishing Co.

Fuchs, L.S., Fuchs, D., & Hamlett, C.L. (1989). Effects of instructional use of curriculum-based measurement to enhance instructional programmes. *Remedial and Special Education, 10(2),* 43–52.

Gentry, J.R., & Gillet, J.W. (1993). *Teaching kids to spell.* Portsmouth, NH: Heinemann.

Gillon, G.T. (2002). Follow-up study investigating the benefits of phoneme awareness intervention for children with spoken language impairment. *International Journal of Language and Communication Disorders, 37,* 381–400.

Gillon, G.T. (2005). Facilitating phoneme awareness development in 3- and 4-year-old children with speech impairment. *Language, Speech, and Hearing Services in Schools, 36,* 308–324.

Hart, P. (2006). Spelling considerations for AAC intervention. *Perspectives on Augmentative and Alternative Communication, 15(2),* 12–14.

Hayes, J.R. (2000). A new framework for understanding cognition and affect in writing. In J.R. Squire (Ed.), *Perspectives on writing: Research, theory, and practice* (pp. 6–44). Newark, DE: International Reading Association.

Hayes, J., & Flower, L. (1980). Identifying the organization of the writing process. In L.W. Gregg & E.R. Steinberg (Eds.), *Cognitive processes in writing* (pp. 3–10). Mahwah, NJ: Lawrence Erlbaum Associates.

Hedberg, N.L., & Westby, C.E. (1993). *Analyzing story telling skills: Theory to practice.* Austin, TX: PRO-ED.

Hosp, M.K., Hosp, J.L., & Howell, K.W. (2007). *The ABCs of CBM: A practical guide to curriculum-based measurement.* New York: Guilford Press.

Hunt, K.W. (1970). Syntactic maturity in school children and adults. *Monographs of the Society for Research in Child Development* (No. 134).

Katims, D.S. (1991). Emergent literacy in childhood special education: Curriculum and education.

Topics in Early Childhood Special Education, 11(1), 69–84.

Katims, D.S. (2001). Literacy assessment of students with mental retardation: An exploratory investigation. *Education and Training in Mental Retardation and Developmental Disabilities, 36*, 363–372.

Kear, D.J., Coffman, G.A., McKenna, M.C., & Ambrosio, A.L. (2000). Measuring attitude toward writing: A new tool for teachers. *Reading Teacher, 54*, 10–23.

Kelford Smith, A., Thurston, S., Light, J., Parnes, P., & O'Keefe, B. (1989). The form and use of written communication produced by physically disabled individuals using microcomputers. *Augmentative and Alternative Communication, 5*, 115–124.

Kleinhert, H.L., Haigh, J., Kearns, J.F., & Kennedy, S. (2000). Alternate assessments: Lessons learned and roads to be taken. *Exceptional Children, 67*, 51–66.

Koppenhaver, D.A. (1991). *A descriptive analysis of classroom literacy instruction provided to children with severe speech and physical impairments*. Chapel Hill: University of North Carolina.

Koppenhaver, D.A., & Erickson, K.A. (2003). Natural emergent literacy supports for preschoolers with autism and severe communication impairments. *Topics in Language Disorders, 23*, 283–292.

Koppenhaver, D.A., Evans, D., & Yoder, D. (1991). Childhood reading and writing experiences of literate adults with severe speech and motor impairments. *Augmentative and Alternative Communication, 7*, 20–33.

Koppenhaver, D., & Yoder, D. (1992). Literacy issues in persons with severe speech and physical impairments. In R. Gaylord-Ross (Ed.), *Issues and research in special education* (Vol. 2, pp. 156–201). New York: Teachers College Press.

Koppenhaver, D., & Yoder, D. (1993). Classroom literacy instruction for children with severe speech and physical impairments (SSPI): What is and what might be. *Topics in Language Disorders, 13*(2), 1–15.

Lidz, C.S., & Pena, E.D. (1996). *Dynamic assessment: The model, its relevance as a nonbiased approach, and its application to Latino American preschool children* (NCTE Research Report No. 1). Urbana, IL: National Council of Teachers of English.

Light, J. (1997). Communication is the essence of human life: Reflections on communication competence. *Augmentative and Alternative Communication, 13*, 61–70.

Light, J., & Kelford Smith, A. (1993). The home literacy experiences of preschoolers who use augmentative communication systems and their nondisabled peers. *Augmentative and Alternative Communication, 9*, 10–25.

Loeffler, K.A. (2005). No more Friday spelling tests? An alternative spelling assessment for students with learning disabilities. *Teaching Exceptional Children, 37*(4), 24–27.

MacArthur, C.A., & Graham, S. (1987). Learning disabled students composing under three methods of text production: Handwriting, word processing, and dictation. *Journal of Special Education, 21*, 22–42.

Mandler, J., & Johnson, N. (1977). Remembrance of things parsed: Story structure and recall. *Cognitive Psychology, 9*, 111–151.

Martinsen, H., & von Tetzchner, S. (1996). Situating augmentative and alternative communication intervention. In S. von Tetzchner & M. Hygum-Jensen (Eds.), *Augmentative and alternative communication: European perspectives* (pp. 49–64). London: Whurr.

McCabe, A., & Peterson, C. (Eds.). (1991). *Developing narrative structure*. Mahwah, NJ: Lawrence Erlbaum Associates.

McCabe, A., & Rollins, P.R. (1994). Assessment of preschool narrative skills. *American Journal of Speech Language Pathology, 3*(1), 45–56.

McCutchen, D. (1988). "Functional automaticity" in children's writing: A problem of metacognitive control. *Written Communication, 5*, 306–324.

Mike, D.G. (1995). Literacy and cerebral palsy: Factors influencing literacy learning in a self-contained setting. *Journal of Literacy Research, 27*, 627–642.

Montgomery, J. (2002). Understanding the language difficulties of children with specific language impairments: Does working memory matter? *American Journal of Speech-Language Pathology, 11*, 77–91.

Nelson, N.W., Bahr, C.M., & Van Meter, A.M. (2004). *The writing lab approach to language instruction and intervention*. Baltimore: Paul H. Brookes Publishing Co.

No Child Left Behind Act of 2001, PL 107-110, 115 Stat. 1425, 20 U.S.C. §§ 6301 *et seq.*

Nystrand, M. (1990). Sharing words: The effects of readers on developing writers. *Written Communication, 7*(1), 3–24.

Ryndak, D.L., Morrison, A.P., & Sommerstein, L. (1999). Literacy before and after inclusion in general education settings: A case study. *Journal of The Association for Students with Severe Handicaps, 24*, 5–22.

Schlagal, B. (2001). Traditional, developmental, and structured language approaches to spelling: Review and recommendations. *Annals of Dyslexia, 51*, 147–176.

Singer, A.S., & Bashir, A.S. (1999). What are executive functions and self-regulation and what do they have to do with language-learning disorders? *Speech, Language, and Hearing Services in the Schools, 30*, 265–273.

Singer, B.D., & Bashir, A.S. (2004). Developmental variations in writing composition. In C.A. Stone, E.R. Silliman, B.J. Ehren, & K. Apel (Eds.), *Handbook of language and literacy: Development and disorders* (pp. 559–582). New York: Guilford Press.

Smith, M. (2005). *Literacy and augmentative and alternative communication.* Boston: Elsevier Academic Press.

Smith, M.W., Brady, J.P., & Anastasopoulos, L. (2008). *Early Language and Literacy Classroom Observation (ELLCO) Tool Pre-K.* Baltimore: Paul H. Brookes Publishing Co.

Smith, M.W., Brady, J.P., & Clark-Chiarelli, N. (2008). *Early Language and Literacy Classroom Observation (ELLCO) Tool K–3* (Research ed.). Baltimore: Paul H. Brookes Publishing Co.

Soto, G. (2006). Supporting the development of narratives skills in children who use AAC. *Perspectives on Augmentative and Alternative Communication, 15*(2), 7–11.

Sturm, J.M., & Clendon, S.A. (2004). AAC, language, and literacy: Fostering the relationship. *Topics in Language Disorders, 24*(1), 76–91.

Sturm, J., Spadorcia, S., Cunningham, J., Cali, K., Staples, A., Erickson, K., et al. (2003). What happens to reading between first and third grade? Implications for students who use AAC. *Augmentative and Alternative Communication, 22*(1), 21–36.

Sturm, J., & Koppenhaver, D.A. (2000). Supporting writing development in adolescents with developmental disabilities. *Topics in Language Disorders, 20*(2), 73–92.

Sulzby, E. (1990). Assessment of emergent writing and children's language while writing. In L.M. Morrow & J.K. Smith (Eds.), *Assessment for instruction in early literacy* (pp. 83–109). Upper Saddle River, NJ: Prentice Hall.

Sutton, A., & Gallagher, T. (1993). Verb class distinctions and AAC language-encoding limitations. *Journal of Speech and Hearing Research, 36*, 1216–1226.

Sutton, A., & Gallagher, T. (1995). Comprehension assessment of a child using an AAC system. *American Journal of Speech-Language Pathology, 4*, 60–69.

Sutton, A., Soto, G., & Blockberger, S. (2002). Grammatical issues in graphic symbol communication. *Augmentative and Alternative Communication, 18*, 192–204.

Torgesen, J.K. (1994). Issues in the assessment of executive function: An information-processing perspective. In G.R. Lyon (Ed.), *Frames of reference for the assessment of learning disabilities* (pp. 143–162). Baltimore: Paul H. Brookes Publishing Co.

Treiman, R., Sotak, L., & Bowman, M. (2001). The role of letter names and letter sounds in connecting print and speech. *Memory & Cognition, 29*, 860–873.

Turner, J., & Paris, S. (1995). How literacy tasks influence children's motivation for literacy. *Reading Teacher, 48*, 662–673.

Udwin, O., & Yule, W. (1990). Augmentative communication systems taught to cerebral palsied children: A longitudinal study: I. The acquisition of signs and symbols, and syntactic aspects of their use over time. *British Journal of Disorders of Communication, 25*, 295–309.

Ukrainetz, T.A. (Ed.). (2006). *Contextualized language intervention: Scaffolding preK–12 literacy achievement.* Eau Claire, WI: Thinking Publications.

Ukrainetz, T.A., Harpell, S., Walsh, C., & Coyle, C. (2000). A preliminary investigation of dynamic assessment with Native American kindergartners. *Language, Speech, and Hearing Services in Schools, 31*, 142–153.

Vandervelden, M., & Siegel, L. (1999). Phonological processing and literacy in AAC users and students with motor speech impairments. *Augmentative and Alternative Communication, 15*, 191–211.

Vandervelden, M., & Siegel, L. (2001). Phonological processing in written word learning: Assessment for children who use augmentative and alternative communication. *Augmentative and Alternative Communication, 17*, 37–51.

von Tetzchner, S., & Martinsen, H. (1996). Words and strategies: Communicating with young children who use aided language. In S. von Tetzchner, & M.H. Jensen (Eds.), *Augmentative and alternative communication: European perspectives* (pp. 65–88). London, UK: Whurr.

Zabala, J.S. (1995) *The SETT framework: Critical areas to consider when making informed assistive technology decisions.* Houston, TX: Region IV Education Service Center. (ERIC Document Reproduction Service No. ED381962)

Appendix

Assistive Technology Devices for Writing and Spelling

This appendix contains information on the range of assistive technology devices that can be used by struggling writers to increase the legibility, complexity, and accuracy of their written products. Many of these devices also support increased efficiency, productivity, and independence. In most instances, students use a combination of assistive technology devices to meet their writing needs. The types of assistive technology devices used to support writing are determined by individual student abilities and needs as well as the required writing tasks across all instructional environments.

In this appendix, assistive technology devices are organized into various categories based on the primary features or applications of the technology. Moreover, the age ranges for which the devices are appropriate are identified in the following categories: elementary, middle, and high school. Lastly, tools are linked to the various writing skills addressed in the Georgia Performance Standards. The skills areas are briefly defined next. It is recommended that individuals utilizing this appendix refer to the standards to determine the specific skills that are addressed at each grade level.

WRITING PROCESS

- *Organizational structure*—Ideas are organized due to purpose (cause–effect, chronological) or genre (type of writing: persuasive, narrative, technical).
- *Prewriting and brainstorming*—Ideas are generated based on the provided topic. In order to facilitate retention of these ideas, notes, outlines, or concept maps may be used.
- *Drafting*—The ideas generated in the prewriting and brainstorming process are recorded by the student.
- *Editing*—The student's work is checked for spelling, grammar, and mechanics errors. These errors are corrected.
- *Revising*—The draft is revised, and this revision may include rewording sentences, adding details, and/or adding more content.
- *Use of resources*—The student uses a variety of resources to obtain facts related to the writing topic. This may include informational resources such as encyclopedias, Internet resources, literary books, or reference books such as dictionaries or thesauruses.

CONVENTIONS

- *Grammar*—includes subject–verb agreement, sentence structure and complexity, parts of speech, and word usage
- *Mechanics*—includes punctuation (commas, semicolons, end marks), capitalization, and paragraph indentations

---

This document was developed by the Georgia Project for Assistive Technology, a project of the Georgia Department of Education, Division for Special Education Supports. Copyright May 2008.

- *Spelling*—includes correct spelling of words used in the written product
- *Legibility*—refers to spacing, letter formation, and size and the reader's ability to read the written product

Additional information about the assistive technology devices referenced in this document is available on the Georgia Project for Assistive Technology's web site at http://www.gpat.org. Additional information about the Georgia Performance Standards is available on the Georgia Department of Education's web site at http://doe.k12.ga.us.

Device category	Examples	Legibility	Spelling	Mechanics	Grammar	Use of resources	Editing	Revising	Drafting	Prewriting	Organizational structure	High school	Middle school	Elementary
Positioning aids	Slant boards, page holders (Pocket Full of Therapy, Therapy Shoppe)	X										X	X	X
	Dycem, book stands (Sammons Preston Rolyan, Onion Mountain Technology)	X										X	X	X
	Shelf liner/nonslip mat (discount stores)	X										X	X	X
	Clipboards (office supply stores, discount stores)	X										X	X	X
Contrast aids	Highlighter tape, pens (Crystal Springs Books, office supply)		X									X	X	X
	EZC Reader/Reading Helper (Really Good Stuff)		X									X	X	X
	Colored overlays (National Reading Styles Institute, See It Right, Onion Mountain Technology)	X	X									X	X	X
Adapted writing utensils	Pencils, pens, pencil grips (Onion Mountain Technology, Pocket Full of Therapy, Sammons Preston, Beacon Ridge)	X										X	X	X
Adapted paper/writing guides	Paper: bold and raised lined (Onion Mountain Technology, Sammons Preston, Beacon Ridge, Pocket Full of Therapy)	X										X	X	X
	Dry erase boards (Really Good Stuff)	X										X	X	X
	Writing guides (Independent Living Aids)	X										X	X	X
Personal vocabulary/ spelling dictionaries	Notebook (office supply stores, discount stores)		X									X	X	X
	Quick Word Handbooks (Curriculum Associates)				X							X	X	X
Handheld spellcheckers/ dictionaries	Children's Talking Dictionary & Spell Corrector (Franklin)	X	X		X	X								X
	Merriam-Webster Speaking Dictionary & Thesaurus (Franklin)		X		X	X						X	X	X
	Speaking Language Master (Franklin)		X	X	X	X							X	X
Recorders	Handi-Cassette II (American Printing House for the Blind)	X								X		X	X	X
	Digital recorder (office supply store)	X								X		X	X	X

Category	Product													
Handheld scanners	Notetaker (Don Johnston)	X	X	X										X
	Iris Pen (Onion Mountain Technology)	X	X											X
Interactive whiteboard	SmartBoard (Smart Technologies Incorporated)	X	X	X										X
	Mimio (Virtual Ink)	X	X	X										
Printed graphic organizers	Teacher-made graphic organizers	X	X	X	X	X								
	Microsoft Word (Microsoft)	X	X	X	X								X	X
	Kidspiration (Inspiration)	X	X	X	X								X	X
	Inspiration (Inspiration)	X	X	X	X								X	X
Portable word processor	AlphaSmart 3000 (AlphaSmart)	X	X	X			X	X				X		X
	Neo (AlphaSmart)	X	X					X						X
	Dana (AlphaSmart)	X	X	X			X	X				X		X
	Personal digital assistant—PDA (office supply stores)	X	X					X						X
	Laser PC6 (Perfect Solutions)	X	X	X				X				X		X
	CalcuScribe (CalcuScribe)	X	X					X						X
Concept/webbing applications	Inspiration (Inspiration)	X	X	X	X	X	X	X				X		X
	Kidspiration (Inspiration)	X	X		X	X		X						X
	Draft:Builder SOLO (Don Johnston)	X	X	X	X	X	X	X	X			X		X
Electronic dictionary thesaurus	WordWeb Dictionary Thesaurus (WordWeb Software)	X	X					X	X			X		
Standard word processing software	Microsoft Word (Microsoft)	X	X	X	X	X	X	X	X	X		X	X	X
	WordTalk (www.wordtalk.org.uk)	X	X		X	X	X	X	X	X	X		X	X
	WordPerfect (Corel)	X	X	X	X	X	X	X	X					
Graphic word processing software	Writing with Symbols 2000 (Mayer Johnson)	X	X	X	X	X	X	X				X	X	X
	Classroom Suite (IntelliTools)	X	X	X	X	X	X	X				X	X	X
	Clicker (Crick)	X	X	X	X	X	X	X					X	X
	PixWriter (Slater Software)	X	X	X	X	X	X	X				X	X	X
Talking word processing software	Write:OutLoud SOLO (Don Johnston)	X	X	X	X	X	X	X	X		X	X	X	X
	Classroom Suite (IntelliTools)	X	X	X	X	X	X	X	X		X	X	X	X
	Cast eReader (Don Johnston)	X	X	X	X	X	X	X	X		X	X	X	X

Appendix 5.1. Assistive technology devices for writing and spelling. (Reprinted from the Georgia Project for Assistive Technology, a project of the Georgia Department of Education, Division for Special Education Supports. Copyright May 2008.)

(continued)

Appendix 5.1. *(continued)*

Device category	Examples	Age range			Writing process						Conventions of writing			
		Elementary	Middle school	High school	Organizational structure	Prewriting	Drafting	Revising	Editing	Use of resources	Grammar	Mechanics	Spelling	Legibility
Talking word processing software *(continued)*	Talking word processor (Premier Assistive Technology)	X	X	X		X	X	X	X		X		X	X
	Tex-Edit Plus (Trans-Tex Software)	X	X	X		X	X	X	X		X		X	X
	Writing with Symbols (Mayer Johnson)	X	X	X		X	X	X	X		X		X	X
Word prediction software	Co:Writer 4000 SOLO (Don Johnston)	X	X	X			X	X	X		X		X	X
	Read & Write (TextHelp)	X	X	X			X	X	X				X	X
	Aurora Prediction 3.0 for Windows (Aurora Systems)	X	X	X			X	X	X		X		X	X
	Word Q2 (Quillsoft)	X	X	X				X	X				X	X
	SoothSayer (Applied Human Factor)	X	X	X			X	X	X		X		X	X
Electronic worksheets	PaperPort (Nuance Communications)	X	X	X										X
	OmniForm (Nuance Communications)	X	X	X									X	X
	TestTalker (Freedom Scientific)	X	X	X										X
Advanced reading and writing aid software	SOLO (Don Johnston)	X	X	X	X	X	X	X	X				X	X
	Kurzweil 3000 (Kurzweil Educational Systems)	X	X	X	X	X	X	X	X	X			X	X
	WYNN (Freedom Scientific)	X	X	X		X	X		X	X			X	X
	Read & Write Gold (TextHelp)	X	X	X		X	X	X	X				X	X
Voice recognition software	Microsoft XP Speech Recognition (Microsoft)	X	X	X		X	X	X	X		X	X	X	X
	Dragon Naturally Speaking Preferred (Nuance Communications)	X	X	X		X	X	X	X		X	X	X	X
	ViaVoice (Nuance Communications)	X	X	X		X	X	X	X		X	X	X	X

II

Instruction and Intervention

6

Academic Adaptations for Students with AAC Needs

Gloria Soto

Special education legislation has gradually specified that the general education curriculum should be the primary *content* of the education of students with disabilities and the instructional activities used to implement it are the primary *context* for these students to receive instruction. The need to develop appropriate adaptations has intensified as students who rely on augmentative and alternative communication (AAC) are provided access to general curriculum activities. Educators and related services professionals must be able to identify and develop the most appropriate instructional adaptations to support the participation of these students in the general curriculum goals and activities. It can be a daunting task. This chapter discusses current issues and effective practices central to the development of adaptations for students with AAC needs. The chapter begins with a discussion on the access to the general curriculum mandate and then moves to development of adaptations to support the participation of these students in the general curriculum.

ACCESS TO THE GENERAL CURRICULUM: WHAT DOES IT MEAN?

The Individuals with Disabilities Education Act Amendments (IDEA) of 1997 (PL 105-17) introduced important changes in the provision of special education services for students with disabilities. One of the most significant changes concerns the requirement that students with disabilities receive *access* to the general curriculum. Specifically, the amendments require that students with disabilities be involved in and make progress in the general curriculum to the maximum extent appropriate (Wehmeyer, Lattin, Lapp-Rincker, & Agran, 2003). The requirement to maximize students' involvement in the general curriculum means that students receiving special education services have the right to participate in the same instructional activities, with the same materials, and in the same progress-monitoring activities used with typically developing students. These mandates were explicitly articulated partly because special education had often been misunderstood as a parallel curriculum and students with disabilities had, for the most part, been omitted from the general education curriculum (Turnbull, Turnbull, Wehmeyer, & Park, 2003).

Spooner and Browder (2006) noted that access to the general curriculum is not synonymous with inclusion. According to IDEA 1997, special education is specially designed instruction to support the child's participation in the general curriculum, regardless of the setting where the student is being educated. Although general education settings may be easier and more likely to provide access to the general curriculum, inclusion is neither a prerequisite nor synonymous with general curriculum access (Wehmeyer et al., 2003). The focus of the access to the general curriculum mandate is not on *where* students are to be educated but on *what* is the content of the students' educational program. Students in all types of education settings must have access to their state's general curriculum (Spooner & Browder, 2006).

IDEA 1997 and the No Child Left Behind (NCLB) Act of 2001 (PL 107-110) further stipulated that states include students with disabilities in large-scale state assessments and specified that those assessments be linked to academic content standards, with accommodations when needed (see Chapter 1 for an extensive discussion of educational assessment). By requiring that all students be included in large-scale assessments and specifying that those assessments be linked to academic content standards, current policy implies the need to align instruction with academic content standards and teach language arts, mathematics, and science to all children regardless of the extent of their disabilities and the setting where they are being educated (Browder, Spooner, Wakeman, Trela, & Baker, 2006).

States are allowed to design alternate performance assessments for students with the most significant disabilities who are significantly below grade level and cannot participate in the statewide assessment system. These assessments are linked directly to the state's general content standards and reflect the portions of the content standards from kindergarten through high school that are accessible to students with the most significant cognitive disabilities (Browder et al., 2004). In addition to being aligned with academic domains, alternate achievement standards must also address the functional needs of these students (Browder et al., 2004; Browder, Wakeman, & Flowers, 2006). Yet, the expectation for all students is to have access to the academic content for their assigned grade level. For example, an 11-year-old student with disabilities who is in fifth grade will be exposed to the history and literature typically taught for this grade level but with simplified content and outcomes that differ from grade-level attainment. For instance, the student might use picture symbols to indicate the main character, the setting, and the sequence of events of a story that is read to him.

WHAT IS THE GENERAL CURRICULUM?

The general curriculum is often referred to as the state's academic content standards or the content to be learned by typically developing students at each specific grade level (Browder, Spooner, et al., 2006; Spooner & Browder, 2006; Wehmeyer, Lattin, & Agran, 2001). Content standards identify the knowledge, skills, and understanding that students should demonstrate in academic areas (Turnbull et al., 2003). Because there is no national curriculum, each state determines priorities for student learning and has its own standards (Browder, Spooner, et al., 2006). Thus, it is critical that clinicians and special educators become familiar with their own state standards and grade-level curriculum. These can typically be found on each state's educational agency web site.

The general curriculum is organized across academic domains, typically language arts, mathematics, science, social science, and so forth. Some states also include a life skills curriculum. Within each academic domain, the general curriculum includes the scope and sequence of skills students are to meet within and across grade levels. The general curriculum also includes the instructional materials used by teachers to work on the content standards, such as textbooks and worksheets adopted by the school system, as well as the activities used to monitor student progress, such as large-scale assessments to determine whether students are making progress in achieving state standards.

Although current policy involves the need for assessment of academic standards linked to grade-level content, it does not prevent the inclusion of instruction in functional skills that students with disabilities need (Browder, Wakeman, et al., 2006). Although most people in the special education community welcome the mandate for access to the general curriculum and the increase in expectations for students with disabilities, many warn that an emphasis on academic content alone runs counter to the ultimate intent of IDEA 1997, which is to prepare individuals with disabilities to live productive and independent adult lives to the maximum extent possible (Ford, Davern, & Schnorr, 2001; Hunt, Quirk, Ryndak, Halvorsen, & Schwartz, 2007; Turnbull et al., 2003). Academic outcomes are important, and measuring them is necessary, but not sufficient, to achieve the global outcome of quality of life for students with disabilities and their families. The unique needs of each individual requires educators to also address quality-of-life domains such as social-emotional adjustment, independence and responsibility, physical health, and communication (Hunt et al., 2007). For instance, for students with AAC needs, the curriculum needs to include both the general education curriculum as set forth by each state as well as additional curricular domains addressing their specific needs. In addition to the academic curriculum, students with AAC needs will require a specialized and intensive curriculum in other areas such as operational, strategic, linguistic, and social competence; functional life skills; and vocational and community-based instruction.

HOW CAN STUDENTS WITH DISABILITIES PARTICIPATE IN THE GENERAL CURRICULUM?

Involving students with disabilities in the general curriculum requires changes at multiple levels in the way special education instruction has been traditionally delivered. In fact, Wehmeyer and Agran (2006) have suggested changes at the district, school, and classroom level in a comprehensive reform. Districtwide, comprehensive reform efforts are necessary to ensure that content areas important to students with disabilities (e.g., functional or life skills) are well integrated into mandated areas such as reading, science, and mathematics. At the school level, administrators and faculty need to articulate a shared vision and a process to ensure that children with diverse abilities are successful and participate in the general curriculum to the maximum extent possible. This may include schoolwide implementation of positive behavior supports, disability awareness, flexible groupings, community-building activities, curriculum mapping, and Universal Design for Learning (UDL; Browder, Spooner, et al., 2006; Browder et al., 2007).

Universally designed classrooms respond to and accommodate the needs of all learners by addressing the barriers that can prevent student learning. Typically, educators and clinicians use a UDL plan for adaptations at three levels: representation, expression, and engagement. *Representation* often refers to how information is presented to students (i.e., input). Teachers incorporate UDL principles when they present content to students in multiple formats such as oral statements, text, digital text, graphic symbols, visual organizers, online resources, video-based materials, highlighters, and peer or adult supports. *Expression* refers to the need for alternate methods for responding (i.e., output) to the instructional content, which typically requires speaking, writing, manipulating, or drawing. Teachers incorporate UDL principles when they allow students to respond to content using multiple modalities such as speech-generating devices, adapted keyboards, customized software, role play, simulations, presentations, and peer-assisted assignments. Third, *engagement* includes a variety of strategies to support students' participation in the learning process (Browder, Wakeman, et al., 2006; Wehmeyer & Agran, 2006). Teachers who implement UDL principles provide students with an array of options to remain engaged and motivated, such as giving students choices regarding learning activities and materials, using multiple work locations, varying the length of activities, varying feedback strategies, and using adapted vocabulary (Salend, 2008). The Center for Applied Special Technology web site includes resources and tools to support clinicians and educators in the implementation of UDL principles (see http://www.cast.org).

Differentiated instruction (DI) is another reform that can be incorporated at the classroom level. DI is premised on the idea that *all* learners do not learn in the same way and refers to the practice of ensuring that each learner receives the methods and materials most suitable to his or her needs and abilities. Teachers who use DI incorporate the principles of UDL by using strategies that address students' strengths, interests, skills, and abilities in flexible learning environments (Hoover & Patton, 2004). During the course of a unit, a teacher who implements DI uses a wide range of instructional materials in a variety of formats and complexities to enable all students in his or her classroom to reach the objectives of the instructional unit (Broderick, Mehta-Parekh, & Reid, 2006). Teachers who use DI acknowledge and prepare for the range of aptitudes, needs, and interests that they find in their classrooms. The assumption underlying DI is that when a student (with or without disabilities) appears unengaged or unmotivated, it is likely that the student is unable to understand the nature of the task or finds the modality of the activity unattainable.

DI requires an analysis of the expectations of the instructional unit and the development of modifications. For instance, most classroom activities require communication skills such as participating in classroom conversations, following teacher directions, answering questions, and requesting clarifications, as well as understanding the teacher's explanations and descriptions. These expectations may be incompatible with the abilities and needs of students who use AAC. Adaptations will be necessary to ensure student participation. The following sections of the chapter describe specific tools, processes, and strategies for designing adaptations at the classroom and the instructional activity level to ensure participation and achievement in the general curriculum for students with AAC needs.

Due to the complex needs of students who rely on AAC, a comprehensive implementation of adaptations to ensure access to the general curriculum requires the collaboration of general educators, special educators, related services personnel, and family members. Indeed, many of this book's chapters identify a number of critical methods and strategies to support students' participation in curricular activities, such as communication strategies (Chapters 7 and 8), peer supports (Chapter 11), assistive technology (AT) integration (Chapter 12), and collaborative teaming (Chapter 13).

ADAPTATIONS TO PROMOTE THE PARTICIPATION OF STUDENTS WHO RELY ON AAC

The changes mandating the use of the general curriculum as the *content* and *context* for instruction and intervention for students with disabilities present the educational team with enormous opportunities and significant challenges. First, educators, clinicians, and families have a greater opportunity to reverse the trend of lowering standards for students with disabilities, which often reflects negative stereotypes of disability and biases against their participation in general education (Ford et al., 2001; Hoover & Patton, 2004; Turnbull et al., 2003). Instead of lowering standards or deriving parallel standards, educational teams are now challenged to do what is necessary to help students achieve proficiency within the state-mandated standards. Thus, educators must adapt specific instruction to ensure that all students are provided with opportunities to acquire content and skills associated with each standard. This requires a solid understanding of the curriculum and its components as well as methods and strategies to individualize instruction without resorting to a parallel curriculum, separate location, or special pull-aside activities (Ford et al., 2001; Hoover & Patton, 2004). There is an emerging body of literature in the special education field addressing evidence-based strategies to provide access to the general curriculum for students with a range of disabilities, many of whom use AAC (see, e.g., Browder, Spooner, et al., 2006; Orelove, Sobsey, & Silberman, 2004; Rief & Heimburge, 2006; Salend, 2008). AAC professionals can also draw from validated models used to design curricular adaptations for students with significant disabilities (e.g., Best, Heller, & Bigge, 2005; Giangreco & Doyle, 2000; Janney & Snell, 2004; Salend, 2008; Snell & Brown, 2005; Udvari-Solner, Causton-Theoharis, & York-Barr, 2004; Wehmeyer et al., 2001). Despite differences, all models use the general education activities as the referent (Wehmeyer & Agran, 2006; Wehmeyer et al., 2001).

Adaptations at the Classroom Level

The environmental conditions of the classroom affect students' ability to acquire information and demonstrate what they have learned (Wehmeyer & Agran, 2006). Adapting environmental conditions will be necessary for students with AAC needs to attend to and cope with the multiple demands that characterize classroom instruction. The type of adaptation will depend on the nature and extent of a student's disability. The most obvious adaptation is that of the physical environment to meet the mobility, sensory, and technology requirements of students with AAC needs. Environmental modifications range from the most obvious changes to facilitate accessibility, such as adding ramps to entryways, rearranging furniture to allow wheelchair maneuvering, and modifying transportation vehicles, to modifying conditions, such as lighting, noise level, visual and auditory input, and location of materials (Udvari-Solner et al., 2004). Elements of the environment need to be carefully engineered for students who experience sensory impairments and information processing and communication difficulties.

Classroom Layout   The literature supports the importance of physical space in creating positive learning environments. Research on classroom environments indicates that different environmental layouts seem to influence a child's learning (Mastropieri & Scruggs, 2006; Rief & Heimburge, 2006). *Classroom layout* refers to the spatial arrangement of the classroom (i.e., how and where students are seated in relation to the teacher and to one another, how classroom members move around the room, the overall sense of atmosphere and order). Existing research on classroom environments indicates that effective classrooms are organized to accommodate a variety of different activities, instructional groupings, and arrangements throughout the day. These may include group instruction, computer-assisted instruction, cross-age peer tutoring, instructional assistants, group instruction, and direct systematic instruction. Effective classrooms are those that minimize student distractions so that students are able to actively engage in classroom activities (Savage, 1999; Weinstein, 1992). Despite the role of classroom structure on student outcomes, there is very limited research specifically addressing how classroom layout may affect the engagement and communication opportunities available to and the learning outcomes of students with AAC needs (Hunt, Soto, Maier, Müller, & Goetz, 2002).

Creating Positive Learning Communities Through Cooperative Activities

Cooperative learning (CL) is defined as an instructional strategy in which a small heterogeneous group of students with equal status roles work together to achieve common learning goals (Jenkins, Antil, Wayne, & Vadasy, 2003; McMaster & Fuchs, 2002). CL activities provide many opportunities for peer communication as students help and support each other as they complete an instructional activity (Merritt & Culatta, 1998). By definition, *cooperative strategies* are interactive, language-based didactic structures that support the acquisition of conversational skills and social skills in general, both for children who use speech and children using AAC (Soto & von Tetzchner, 2003). During cooperation, students may provide or request information; recount past events; comment on or clarify some idea, event, or state of affair; resolve conflicts; and elaborate on others' ideas. As students acquire new competence in interacting with each other, they become partners within instructional exchanges with the opportunity to learn from and teach each other (Rogoff, Goodman, & Bartlett, 2001). A large body of literature documents the positive effects of CL on the academic achievement of students with learning disabilities (see McMaster & Fuchs, 2002, for a synthesis of empirical research), especially when CL is combined with other instructional supports such as computer-assisted instruction, reciprocal teaching, cross-age peer tutoring, instructional assistants, and direct instruction. The effects appear more robust in general education classrooms than in special education classrooms. Advocates of CL as an inclusive strategy argue that in general education classrooms, cooperative groups are more heterogeneous and hence provide more academic support to students with disabilities. The effects of CL on the academic achievement of students with significant disabilities are not well established. The majority of existing studies have highlighted social benefits such as increased classroom participation and interaction with peers (see Jenkins et al., 2003).

In an empirical study comparing the effects of different instructional groupings on the social acceptance of students with significant disabilities by their typically developing peers, Piercy, Wilton, and Townsend (2002) concluded that CL strategies resulted in higher indices of social acceptance than other types of groupings. In addition, the children in the CL group showed significant increases in positive social interaction with peers without disabilities. These findings were explained by the fact that in CL, the children had opportunities to learn about one another in multidimensional and dynamic ways. Cooperation afforded opportunities for the students with disabilities to reveal their areas of strength. They became individuals with likes, dislikes, fears, and joys, as opposed to stereotypical images.

Introduction of conversation books, peer buddy systems, and interactive activities has been found to be positively related to increases in communicative interaction between children who rely on AAC and their typically developing peers (see Chapter 11). Hunt and her colleagues (2002) reported that the number of reciprocal communicative interactions between students who used AAC and their typically developing peers in a general education classroom increased whenever CL activities were used. The authors were able to conclude that the use of CL activities with adaptations and support from peer partners promoted the students' active participation.

Peer support intervention is a strategy that seems to be more effective for students with significant disabilities than traditional CL (Carter & Kennedy, 2006). Peer support intervention uses one or more chronologically matched typically developing peers to provide academic and social support to a student with significant disabilities. In this type of approach, peers are trained to provide support by adapting instructional activities, communicating with and providing feedback to the student with disabilities, and, when appropriate, implementing positive behavior support strategies. When compared with other support strategies, it appears that peer support interventions contribute to improved academic performance, decreased levels of problem behavior, and increased levels of social interaction between students with and without disabilities (Carter & Kennedy, 2006; Spooner, Dymond, Smith, & Kennedy, 2006).

Adaptations at the Activity Level

At the activity level, the development of adaptations is determined by an analysis of the cognitive, sensory, motor, cultural, and linguistic demands of the instructional activity in contrast with the individual's needs and abilities. Students with AAC needs can participate in a wide range of general education activities when provided with appropriate curriculum adaptations and supports. Typically, students with AAC needs will require adaptations for the way in which the curriculum is delivered to them (i.e., presentation, input) and the way in which they are expected to engage in and respond to the curricular activity (i.e., response, output). Responding to the curriculum usually refers to the response demands, which may include writing, speaking, drawing, and manipulating.

Curriculum Presentation   Students with AAC needs may have physical, cognitive, and/or sensory impairments that can make access to instructional materials a challenge (Downing, 2005). Students with AAC needs require modified access to content materials that are consistent with their sensory and motor abilities and their learning preferences and needs. Adaptations in curriculum presentation modify the way the curriculum is conveyed or imparted (Wehmeyer et al., 2001). In the classroom, information is typically presented through written text or verbally. Yet, many students with AAC needs may not have the hearing or auditory comprehension to benefit from materials being spoken or read to them. For these students, alternative symbols such as pictures, photographs, objects, or parts of objects along with print can be used instead. They may also benefit from multiple means of representation that can be modified in size, shape, color, or format (e.g., from print to pictures; Browder, Spooner, et al., 2006). Some students may have additional visual impairments that affect their ability to process information presented to them through text or graphics. These students can benefit from digitized audio, books on tape, or text-reader programs. Modifications of the sensory characteristics of a learning environment are also necessary for students who have processing difficulties. These may include changes in lighting, background color, glare, noise level, or movement demands (see Blackstone, 1994, for in-depth information on the effects of vision problems on AAC system design). Using peer supports (e.g., peer buddies, peer tutors, cross-age peer tutors), personalized scaffolding, and options for repetition are ways to keep students engaged (Broderick et al., 2006).

Response   Written or oral responses are the typical ways that students engage with the curriculum. Adaptations will be required for students with AAC needs who have little or no functional speech and often have no functional handwriting. There are alternative ways to enable students to express their ideas and demonstrate their knowledge, such as providing additional time for task completion, allowing for alternatives to typical means of expression such as using a switch to select a picture, concept keyboards, word prediction programs, spell checkers, graphics and pictures, and augmentative communication devices.

In addition, it will be necessary to provide more than one opportunity per activity to demonstrate one's knowledge. Students with AAC needs will require multiple opportunities to engage with the curriculum and to practice assessment activities. Chapter 5 provides information on supportive equipment and software for students who are unable to gain access to and respond to curricular materials in conventional ways. It is also important for educators and clinicians to have a working knowledge regarding availability of appropriate technology, how to obtain equipment, and how to make effective use of technology within meaningful activities (Downing, 2006). The *Wisconsin Assistive Technology Initiative (WATI) AT Checklist* provides a simple yet effective way to identify the available range of low- to high-tech AT options that can be used to support student participation (see http://www.wati.org).

Adaptations at the Content Level

The adaptations described previously provide alternative ways for students with AAC needs to take in information or communicate their knowledge back to the teacher. The changes to the way the curriculum is presented to the student and the means the student uses to respond do not necessarily alter or lower the standards or expectations for a particular activity. When there is no difference in curricular expectation, one may say the student is participating in an *identical curriculum* to same-age peers, although adaptations are provided to ensure participation. These adaptations may include providing physical assistance, adapting materials, augmenting modalities, and providing different response requirements.

By contrast, a *modified curriculum* is when a student requires a substantial adaptation that results in a fundamental alteration to the content of the curriculum. In a modified curriculum lesson, the student with AAC needs participates in lessons targeting either modified grade-level standards or alternate achievement standards that are aligned to academic standards (Courtade-Little & Browder, 2005; see Chapter 1). Alternate achievement standards may reflect a narrower range of academic content (e.g., fewer objectives under a content standard) or learning less complex content at earlier grades that is considered a prerequisite to attaining grade-level proficiency (Karvonen, Wakeman, Flowers, & Browder, 2007). This shift to academic content represents a major challenge for professionals serving students with significant disabilities because they need to plan the curriculum, develop and adapt materials, and learn how to effectively teach academic skills to students with the most significant disabilities. Further complicating this shift is the lack of research-based strategies to teach general curriculum content to this population, a lack of understanding of the general curriculum among special education professionals, and the need to combine academic instruction with individual priorities represented in the student's individualized education program (IEP; Karvonen et al., 2007).

Educators need to consider both the content and demands of the curriculum and the needs and strengths of the student when making curriculum adaptations. Developing curriculum modifications for students with AAC needs requires a deliberate analysis of the cognitive, linguistic, sensory, and motor demands of the instructional activities at the content, presentation, and response levels. This analysis will assist the team in determining where the student is most likely to have difficulties and selecting appropriate adaptations. Deciding what modifications are necessary can be difficult and requires the collaboration of the entire educational team. The role of the speech-language pathologist (SLP) is critical in designing those adaptations.

Beginning the Process

Adapting the curriculum to the student's needs and abilities requires professionals to understand the cognitive, linguistic, sensory, and motor demands of the lesson. An activity analysis is helpful for identifying student difficulties and planning for intervention (Merrit & Culatta, 1998; Ukrainetz, 2006). There are a number of environmental observation forms that can be used toward this end (e.g., the *WATI Environmental Observation Form*; the *Team Planning Tool* in Gee, 2004; *the Discrepancy Analysis Tool* in Udvari-Solner et al., 2004). Yet, all forms require the team to engage in a process by which they compare the demands of the activity with the abilities of the student. Next, the steps of a process to follow when adapting an instructional activity are presented. The form in Figure 6.1 can be used to record this process.

1.   Provide a task analysis of the general education activity.

The use of task analysis enables the team to break down an activity into expected behavioral parts; that is, for each step of the activity, the team highlights what typically developing students are expected to do (Best et al., 2005; Wehmeyer & Agran, 2006).

2.   Identify the skill continuum.

Next, the team should identify the cognitive, linguistic, motor, and sensory skills that are required to perform each step of the task. The purpose is to find a mismatch between activity demands and student abilities and to isolate the factors contributing to that mismatch (Merritt & Culatta, 1998). Cognitive and language taxonomies are useful tools to classify the cognitive and linguistic demands of lessons. Bloom's taxonomy is perhaps the most widely known cognitive taxonomy (see University of Victoria, n.d.). The SLP is critical in helping educators understand the language demands of specific activities. Ukrainetz (2006) suggested using communicative competence lines to structure these demands into pragmatics, discourse structure, grammar, lexicon, word finding, self-regulation, and metalinguistics.

3.   Indicate the student's level of functioning on the skill continuum.

Once the skills have been identified, the team needs to indicate whether the target student possesses those skills. A plus sign (+) is used when the target student is able to perform a skill as would a typically developing student. A minus sign (–) is used when the target student is not able to perform the skill as would a typically developing student. The SLP is essential in helping educators understand the student's language skills.

4.   Determine the adaptations for presentation. (How will the student receive the information?)

Next, the team will have to determine necessary adaptations so the student can understand the lesson as presented to him or her. The SLP needs to assist the teacher to know how to adjust the language of instruction to the student's abilities and how to provide appropriate verbal and visual scaffolds during instruction. It may be that the student receives instructions through an FM system, through a graphic activity schedule outlining the steps of the tasks, or through a peer buddy.

5.   Determine the adaptations for response. (How will the student respond to the information?)

The team will have to identify the lesson response and performance requirements (e.g., handwriting, manipulating, drawing, speaking) and develop appropriate adaptations. It may be that the target student uses his or her AAC system to make choices or provide responses during the activity.

6.   Select an alternate objective if necessary.

If the team determines that the curricular expectations are in conflict with the student's abilities, despite the previous adaptations, then modifying the curricular content may be necessary. Curricular modifications change the content of what is being taught (Best et al., 2005) by relying on modified or alternate content standards (see Chapter 1).

Student: _____   Date: _____

Activity: _____   Team members involved: _____

Academic standard: _____

Objective: _____

Modified or alternate standard (if necessary): _____

Newly derived objective: _____

Task analysis Activity steps	Skill continuum	Student's performance in skill continuum	Adaptations for access	Adaptations for response
1.				
2.				
3.				
4.				
5.				
6.				
7.				
8.				
9.				
10.				

Figure 6.1. Form to record the adaptation of an instructional activity.

139

The process of designing useful adaptations is dynamic and collaborative. The educational team must be willing to be creative and work together to integrate the often complex array of technologies for learning, mobility, and participation that students with AAC needs bring to the classroom (Hunt et al., 2002; see Chapter 13 for specific strategies on collaborative teaming). It is important to remember that the provision of adaptations does not replace the need for systematic instruction. Most students will require direct instruction to learn the appropriate use of adaptations and to acquire the targeted skill. It is also important to remember the need for ongoing evaluation of student performance with and without adaptations. Adaptations must be modified, replaced, or eliminated based on changes in student abilities or task requirements (Udvari-Solner et al., 2004).

ROLE OF THE SPEECH-LANGUAGE PATHOLOGIST

IDEA 1997 also changed the professional roles of SLPs working in the schools. Most specifically, it challenged the manner SLPs plan and deliver services to children with communication impairments (Merritt & Culatta, 1998). According to IDEA 1997, the role of related services personnel is to support the child's access to the general curriculum. This means that the general curriculum serves as the context for 1) determining appropriate intervention needs and goals, 2) designing intervention activities, 3) selecting and modifying materials, and 4) monitoring progress (McCormick, Frome Loeb, & Schiefelbush, 2003).

In order to provide context-relevant services without jeopardizing the unique contributions they make to student learning and development, SLPs serving in educational teams need to be sensitive not only to the communication needs of the individual who relies on AAC but also to the specific classroom context within which the student will be using his or her communication system (Whitmire, 2000, 2002). The classroom is the environment that presents the most significant language and interaction demands as well as opportunities for students with AAC needs. Providing integrated language services for students with AAC needs requires SLPs and educators to rethink intervention approaches and commit to a collaborative course of action (Merritt & Culatta, 1998; Soto, Müller, Hunt, & Goetz, 2001). In addition, because intervention objectives should be related to state standards, the SLP needs to consider the ongoing activities of the classroom and target those language skills closely linked to academic and literacy success (Ukrainetz, 2006).

In addition to providing clinical services when needed, the SLP should also be able to maximize the student's social and academic participation in the classroom by collaborating to make curricular adaptations and facilitate social interaction with peers. The general curriculum and regular school activities become the context within which intervention targets are defined (Ehren, 2000; Whitmire, 2000). In order to support the classroom teacher, the SLP needs to have a working knowledge of state standards the teachers are working toward and an understanding of the language demands of that curriculum, because those will frame the intervention targets. The importance of understanding linguistic demands for determining intervention goals and strategies is stressed in the work of Merrit and Culatta (1998), Nelson (1998), and Ukrainetz (2006).

The increasing pressure within special education to use grade-level achievement standards as intervention objectives has pushed some SLPs to engage in task assistance rather than in therapeutic intervention (Ukrainetz, 2006). Although task assistance allows a student to participate in specific classroom activities, it is important that SLPs target underlying skills required for a student to become a more independent learner. Ukrainetz (2006) urged SLPs not to lose their therapeutic focus and to target those language skills that can be remediated fairly quickly, will have a significant effect in the student's participation in classroom activities, can be used in functionally equivalent activities, and will provide solutions for additional long-term problems.

CONCLUSION

IDEA 1997 mandates increased participation of students with disabilities in the general curriculum. This is possible only with systematic efforts affecting all levels of the educational system, beginning with district-, school-, and classroom-level changes, and involving curriculum options (standard setting) and curricular design. This chapter presented strategies that cover all these areas and, in doing so, will hopefully help increase the participation of students with AAC needs in the general curriculum. Given the impetus of the mandate for access to the general curriculum, it is imperative that researchers in the field of AAC engage in efforts to evaluate the efficacy of the adaptations and strategies described previously. Most of the existing research focuses on the effects of adaptations on the social participation of students who rely on AAC. The effect of adaptations on student achievement in core academic areas should also be examined. Only by doing so can the goal of curriculum access be truly attained.

REFERENCES

Best, S.J., Heller, K.W., & Bigge, J.L. (2005). *Teaching individuals with physical or multiple disabilities* (5th ed.). Upper Saddle River, NJ: Pearson/Prentice Hall.

Blackstone, S.W. (1994). The ABCs of vision and AAC. *Augmentative Communication News, 7*(5). Available online at http://www. augcominc.com/articles/7_5_2.html

Broderick, A., Mehta-Parekh, H., & Reid, D.K. (2006). Differentiating instruction for disabled students in inclusive classrooms. *Theory into Practice, 44,* 194–202.

Browder, D.M., Flowers, C., Ahlgrim-Delzell, L., Karvonen, M., Spooner, F., & Algozzine, R. (2004). The alignment of alternate assessment content with academic and functional curricula. *Journal of Special Education, 37,* 211–223.

Browder, D.M., Spooner, F., Wakeman, S.Y., Trela, K., & Baker, J. (2006). Aligning instruction with academic content standards: Finding the link. *Research and Practice for Persons with Severe Disabilities, 31,* 309–321.

Browder, D.M., Wakeman, S.Y., & Flowers, C. (2006). Assessment of progress in the general curriculum for students with disabilities. *Theory into Practice, 45,* 249–259.

Browder, D.M., Wakeman, S.Y., Flowers, C., Rickelman, R.J., Pugalee, D., & Karvonen, M. (2007). Creating access to the general curriculum with links to grade-level content for students with significant cognitive disabilities: An explication of the concept. *Journal of Special Education, 41,* 2–16.

Carter, E.W., & Kennedy, C.H. (2006). Promoting access to the general curriculum using peer support strategies. *Research and Practice for Persons with Severe Disabilities, 31,* 284–292.

Courtade-Little, G., & Browder, D.M. (2005). *Aligning IEPs to academic standards for students with moderate and severe disabilities.* Verona, WI: Attainment Company.

Downing, J. (2005). *Teaching communication skills to students with severe disabilities* (2nd ed.). Baltimore: Paul H. Brookes Publishing Co.

Downing, J. (2006). Building literacy for students at the presymbolic and early symbolic levels. In D.M. Browder & F. Spooner (Eds.), *Teaching language arts, math, and science to students with significant cognitive disabilities* (pp. 39–62). Baltimore: Paul H. Brookes Publishing Co.

Ehren, B.J. (2000). Maintaining a therapeutic focus and sharing responsibility for student success: Keys to in-classroom speech-language services. *Language, Speech, and Hearing Services in the Schools, 31,* 219–229.

Ford, A., Davern, L., & Schnorr, R. (2001). Learners with significant disabilities: Curricular relevance in an era of standards-based reform. *Remedial and Special Education, 22,* 214–222.

Gee, K. (2004). Developing curriculum and instruction. In F.P. Orelove, D. Sobsey, & R.K. Silberman (Eds.), *Educating children with multiple disabilities: A collaborative approach* (4th ed., pp. 67–151). Baltimore: Paul H. Brookes Publishing Co.

Giangreco, M.F., & Doyle, M.B. (2000). Curricular and instructional considerations for teaching students with disabilities in general education classrooms. In S. Wade (Ed.), *Inclusive education: A casebook of readings for prospective and practicing teachers* (pp. 51–69). Mahwah, NJ: Lawrence Erlbaum Associates.

Hoover, J.J., & Patton, J.R. (2004). Differentiating standards-based education for students with diverse needs. *Remedial and Special Education, 25,* 74–78.

Hunt, P., Quirk, C., Ryndak, D., Halvorsen, A., & Schwartz, I. (2007). *Meaningful student outcomes in an era of standards-based reform.* Paper presented at the Annual Convention of TASH, Seattle.

Hunt, P., Soto, G., Maier, J., Müller, E., & Goetz, L. (2002). Collaborative teaming to support students with AAC needs in general education classrooms. *Augmentative and Alternative Communication, 18,* 20–35.

Individuals with Disabilities Education Act Amendments (IDEA) of 1997, PL105-17, 20 U.S.C. §§ 1400 *et seq.*

Janney, R., & Snell, M.E. (2004). *Teachers' guides to inclusive practices: Modifying schoolwork* (2nd ed.). Baltimore: Paul H. Brookes Publishing Co.

Jenkins, J.R., Antil, L.R., Wayne, S.K., & Vadasy, P. (2003). How cooperative learning works for special education and remedial students. *Exceptional Children, 69,* 279–292.

Karvonen, M., Wakeman, S.Y., Flowers, C., & Browder, D. (2007). Measuring the enacted curriculum for students with significant cognitive disabilities. *Assessment for Effective Intervention, 33,* 29–38.

Mastropieri, M., & Scruggs, T. (2006). *The inclusive classroom: Strategies for effective instruction* (3rd ed.). Upper Saddle River, NJ: Prentice Hall.

McCormick, L., Frome Loeb, D., & Schiefelbush, R.L. (2003). *Supporting children with communication difficulties in inclusive settings: School-based language intervention.* Boston: Pearson Education.

McMaster, K.N., & Fuchs, D. (2002). Effects of cooperative learning on the academic achievement of students with learning disabilities: An update of Tateyama-Sniezek's review. *Learning Disabilities Research & Practice, 17,* 107–117.

Merritt, D.D., & Culatta, B. (1998). *Language intervention in the classroom.* San Diego: Singular.

Nelson, N.W. (1998). *Childhood language disorders in context: Infancy through adolescence* (2nd ed.). Boston: Allyn & Bacon.

No Child Left Behind Act of 2001, PL 107-110, 115 Stat. 1425, 20 U.S.C. §§ 6301 *et seq.*

Orelove, F.P., Sobsey, D., & Silberman, R.K. (2004). *Educating children with multiple disabilities: A collaborative approach* (4th ed.). Baltimore: Paul H. Brookes Publishing Co.

Piercy, M., Wilton, K., & Townsend, M. (2002). Promoting the social acceptance of young children with moderate-severe intellectual disabilities using cooperative learning techniques. *American Journal of Mental Retardation, 107,* 352–360.

Rief, S.F., & Heimburge, J.A. (2006). *How to reach and teach all children in the inclusive classroom: Practical strategies, lessons, and activities* (2nd ed.). San Francisco: Jossey-Bass.

Rogoff, B., Goodman, C., & Bartlett, L. (2001). *Learning together: Children and adults in a school community.* New York: Oxford University Press.

Salend, S.J. (2008). *Creating inclusive classrooms: Effective and reflective practices.* Upper Saddle River, NJ: Merrill/Prentice Hall.

Savage, T.V. (1999). *Teaching self-control through management and discipline.* Boston: Allyn & Bacon.

Snell, M., & Brown, F. (2005). *Instruction of students with severe disabilities* (6th ed.). Upper Saddle River, NJ: Prentice Hall.

Soto, G., Müller, E., Hunt, P., & Goetz, L. (2001). Professional skills for serving students who use AAC in general education classrooms: A team perspective. *Language, Speech, and Hearing Services in the Schools, 32,* 51–56.

Soto, G., & von Tetzchner, S. (2003). Supporting the development of alternative communication through culturally significant activities in shared educational settings. In S. von Tetzchner & N. Grove (Eds.), *Augmentative and alternative communication: Developmental issues* (pp. 287–299). London: Whurr.

Spooner, F., & Browder, D.M. (2006). Why teach the general curriculum? In D.M. Browder & F. Spooner (Eds.), *Teaching language arts, math, and science to students with significant cognitive disabilities* (pp. 1–14). Baltimore: Paul H. Brookes Publishing Co.

Spooner, F., Dymond, S.K., Smith, A., & Kennedy, C.H. (2006). What we know and need to know about accessing the general curriculum for students with significant cognitive disabilities. *Research and Practice for Persons with Severe Disabilities, 31,* 277–283.

Turnbull, H.R., Turnbull, A.P., Wehmeyer, M.L., & Park, J. (2003). A quality of life framework for special education outcomes. *Remedial and Special Education, 24,* 67–74.

Udvari-Solner, A., Causton-Theoharis, J., & York-Barr, J. (2004). Developing adaptations to promote participation in inclusive environments. In F.P. Orelove, D. Sobsey, & R.K. Silberman (Eds.), *Educating children with multiple disabilities: A collaborative approach* (pp. 151–193). Baltimore: Paul H. Brookes Publishing Co.

Ukrainetz, T.A. (2006). *Contextualized language intervention: Scaffolding pre-K–12 literacy achievement.* Eau Claire, WI: Thinking Publications.

University of Victoria. (n.d.). *Bloom's taxonomy.* Available online at http://www.coun.uvic.ca/learning/exams/blooms-taxonomy.html

Wehmeyer, M.L., & Agran, M. (2006). Promoting access to the general curriculum for students with significant cognitive disabilities. In D.M. Browder & F. Spooner (Eds.), *Teaching language arts, math, and science to students with significant cognitive disabilities* (pp. 15–38). Baltimore: Paul H. Brookes Publishing Co.

Wehmeyer, M.L., Lattin, D.L., & Agran, M. (2001). Achieving access to the general curriculum for students with mental retardation: A curriculum decision-making model. *Education and Training in Mental Retardation and Developmental Disabilities, 36,* 327–342.

Wehmeyer, M.L., Lattin, D.L., Lapp-Rincker, G., & Agran, M. (2003). Access to the general curriculum of middle school students with mental retardation: An observational study. *Remedial and Special Education, 24,* 262–272.

Weinstein, C. (1992). *Designing the instructional environment: Focus on seating.* Retrieved September 18, 2007, from http://eric.ed.gov

Whitmire, K. (2000). Action: School services. *Language, Speech, and Hearing Services in Schools, 31,* 194–199.

Whitmire, K. (2002). The evolution of school-based speech-language services: A half century of change and a new century of practice. *Communication Disorders Quarterly, 23,* 68–76.

7

Addressing the Communication Demands of the Classroom for Beginning Communicators and Early Language Users

Jennifer Kent-Walsh and Cathy Binger

ffective participation in classroom contexts requires many types of communication (Beukelman & Mirenda, 2005; Downing, 2005b). Students routinely are required to participate in speaking, listening, reading, writing, and social tasks within the context of an educational curriculum. These activities can be particularly challenging for beginning communicators and early language users given the underlying language requirements of these activities (Sturm & Clendon, 2004).

Reichle, Beukelman, and Light (2002) defined *beginning communicators* as individuals who have an expressive vocabulary of fewer than 50 words or symbols. Some of these individuals may not yet be symbolic communicators, and they may be learning to use aided or unaided symbols to represent basic communicative function messages (Beukelman & Mirenda, 2005). *Early language users* also include students who are beginning to combine symbols into very brief messages. A wide range of profiles is represented within these groups, including young students in the early school years and much older students who have larger gaps between their chronological ages and language skill levels. These students may be in elementary, middle, or high school within general or special education classrooms.

Across the age, ability, and school placement continuum, effective augmentative and alternative communication (AAC) systems are critical tools for students with complex communication needs (Beukelman & Mirenda, 2005). It is important to implement these AAC tools as early as possible (Romski, Sevcik, & Forrest, 2001). Even when early interventions have not been implemented, it is still imperative for "educators" (e.g., educational assistants, speech-language pathologists [SLPs], teachers, other support staff) to introduce AAC interventions as they attempt to help beginning communicators and early language users meet the communication demands of the classroom (e.g., Downing, 2005a, 2005b). Otherwise, these students end up having very different educational experiences from their typically developing peers.

KEY ISSUES: FACTORS AFFECTING
CLASSROOM SUCCESS FOR STUDENTS WITH AAC NEEDS

There are a number of key factors that may affect classroom success for students with AAC needs. These factors can be largely divided into two categories: internal factors and external factors. Internal factors include variables such as an individual's communication, language, cognitive, and motor abilities. External factors include environmental or communication partner factors such as the

---

Note: The authors made equal contributions to the writing of this chapter.

provision of AAC tools, available communication opportunities, engineered contexts, and targeted curricula. The interplay between these two types of factors sets the stage for students' language learning and communication (see Chapters 2 and 8 for more information on these issues). In addition, Downing (2005b) discussed how students with a complex array of internal factors, particularly students with severe communication disorders, can be integrated successfully into classrooms that contain their own complex mixtures of external factors (e.g., classmates with a wide variety of profiles; teachers with varying bases of knowledge, skills, and expertise; various classroom settings that place a range of demands on students).

Internal Factors

Educators should consider what communication capabilities a student brings to the classroom when they contemplate how to address the communication demands of the classroom for beginning communicators and early language users. Research indicates that children who use AAC often 1) are passive communicators, 2) initiate few interactions, 3) respond infrequently, 4) produce a limited number of communicative functions, and 5) use restricted linguistic forms (e.g., Kent-Walsh & McNaughton, 2005; Light, Collier, & Parnes, 1985). It is important for educators to determine if these characteristics are relevant to the student in question and how the characteristics may relate to individual characteristics unique to specific disabilities. For example, a student with an autism spectrum disorder (ASD) may exhibit different manifestations of the previous interaction patterns as a result of the tendency to learn communicative functions sequentially as opposed to simultaneously. Similarly, students with other disabilities (e.g., developmental delay, cognitive impairments, multiple disabilities, cerebral palsy, suspected childhood apraxia of speech) will have additional communication characteristics that must be considered as educators monitor their interaction patterns.

External Factors

In addition to initial internal factors that are relevant to facilitating language acquisition for beginning communicators, there are a number of external factors that educators must consider in order to create educational contexts in which communication opportunities exist. The following categories may be relevant to students who use AAC and their educators: 1) general practice barriers, 2) communication partner characteristics, 3) curriculum considerations, and 4) environmental variables.

General Practice Barriers   There are a number of general practice issues that may be specifically relevant to students who use AAC. For example, children with complex communication needs often have multiple demands placed on their time throughout the school day, including necessary time for speech, AAC, physical therapy, and other highly specific interventions. Similarly, in many instances, the professionals involved in these interventions face unique time barriers of their own related to high caseloads and collaborative teaming activities (American Speech-Language-Hearing Association [ASHA], 2004; Soto, Müller, Hunt, & Goetz, 2001).

Some additional barriers that educators may encounter include working with professionals and family members who subscribe to myths relating to how AAC should only be used as last resort (Romski & Sevcik, 2005) and working with students who have not received early or ongoing AAC interventions (McSheehan, Sonnenmeier, Jorgensen, & Turner, 2006). Furthermore, many educators have not received training or had experience in providing AAC services (Kent-Walsh & Light, 2003; Koul & Lloyd, 1994). Therefore, as much as they may want to provide appropriate and relevant interventions for their students, they understandably may struggle to do so.

Communication Partner Characteristics   Both educators and other communication partners (e.g., parents, peers) may engage in interaction patterns that do not facilitate the language development of students who use AAC. These patterns include partners taking the majority of conversational turns, providing few opportunities for communication, asking predominantly yes-no questions, failing to acknowledge students' communicative attempts, interrupting individuals using AAC, and focusing on the technology instead of the individual (e.g., Blackstone, 1999; Houghton, Bronicki, & Guess, 1987; Kent-Walsh & McNaughton, 2005; Light et al., 1985; Sigafoos, 1999). In educational contexts, such partner interaction tendencies can affect how students using AAC are able to engage with the curriculum and their peers, thus jeopardizing their academic progress.

Curriculum Considerations   It is also noteworthy that educators may or may not work in a context in which a particular curriculum with a language basis or emphasis is implemented (Spooner & Browder, 2006). Typically, each state or province adopts particular achievement standards for each grade level and then individual school districts choose their preferred instructional/curricula materials. For example, some curricula used by a school district may provide helpful guidance to educators by targeting student skills within more traditional categories such as language, literacy, mathematics, science, social, creative expression, and self-esteem (e.g., High/Scope K–12, California Department of Education Alternate Performance Assessment Blueprints) or by targeting student skills within a more creative or holistic framework (e.g., Montessori). Although such curricula typically do not specifically speak to the needs of students who use AAC, they do guide educators with respect to academic goals and instructional techniques. Educators can then incorporate relevant target skills and techniques, such as those covered later in this chapter, within an existing framework. The reality, however, is that not all educators are provided with such a structural framework via mandated curricula. In such cases, educators may need acute guidance because AAC goals need to be infused within the curricular option in which the student is participating. Table 7.1 contains a suggested framework for making decisions about adapting materials and instruction effectively and also provides suggestions for various types of adaptations specifically for beginning communicators and early language users. Furthermore, Figures 7.1, 7.2, and 7.3 provide case examples for adapting the curriculum for students with various communication profiles.

Environmental Variables   A range of factors relating to how classrooms are engineered also must be considered by educators attempting to facilitate students' communication in educational settings. Providing students with access to necessary tools and supports in the classroom setting becomes central in this type of discussion. For example, students with complex communication needs must have appropriate access to their AAC systems and other supports for early language and literacy activities. Without this type of access, it is exceptionally difficult for these students to fully participate in classroom activities and to achieve relevant academic goals (Downing, 2005a, 2005b; Sturm & Clendon, 2004; Sturm et al., 2006). Chapter 6 provides practical strategies for addressing these types of concerns.

APPLICATION

Upon consideration of the range of internal and external factors discussed previously, educators must identify relevant target skills, intervention techniques, partner interventions, service-delivery coordination approaches, and methods for tracking student progress. Frameworks for consideration in each of these areas are presented next.

Communication Skills

All states have alternate standards for communication and language arts for students who have significant disabilities. These alternate standards allow educators to address the skills that are minimally required. A variety of communication skills must be targeted to help students achieve competency in the classroom. For students with AAC needs, skills that assist in contributing to social competency (i.e., initiating, maintaining, and terminating interactions) and linguistic competency

Table 7.1. Nine suggested material/instructional adaptation steps for beginning communicators and early language users

Step	General description	Specific action options
1. Create a plan for adapting materials.	Adapting materials is just one part of an overall plan for students using augmentative and alternative communication (AAC). To be effective, adaptations will require sustained development and support. Decisions must be made within the framework of a larger curricular or unit context.	Identify the mandated curriculum or choose one yourself. Involve your administrator and curriculum or program coordinator as you develop your plan. Identify exactly who (e.g., paraprofessionals, school volunteers, speech-language pathologist [SLP], teacher) will be responsible for making, implementing, supporting, and evaluating the adaptations throughout the year because you will need help. Strive to make adaptations that can benefit an entire class or several classes or students to facilitate long-term maintenance.
2. Identify the demands that the student is not meeting.	Observe how the students using AAC perform when they are given tasks requiring the use of typical instructional materials.	For identified difficulties, determine at which of the following levels the difficulties are occurring: • *Level 1:* Acquiring or getting the important content from oral or printed instruction • *Level 2:* Storing or remembering information presented in materials to allow information to be used at a later date • *Level 3:* Expressing information or demonstrating competence on performance measures
3. Develop goals for teaching strategies and making adaptations.	Determine how identified difficulties will be addressed. Some difficulties can be handled by adaptations, whereas other problems may signal the need for intensive instruction in skills with the use of specified techniques, as described previously in this chapter.	Within the context of the students' instructional goals and individualized education programs (IEPs), approach adaptations as short-term solutions within the context of a long-term plan for teaching skills and strategies that will promote the students' independence as learners and, ultimately, reduce the need for the adaptations.
4. Determine the need for content adaptations versus format adaptations.	Consider content adaptation only when the students' IEPs note that the curriculum is inappropriate for them in order to maintain compliance with current local and state education standards. In cases in which the curriculum is considered appropriate for the students, focus adaptations on format, not on content, because content adaptations can affect the fulfillment of curriculum standards. Format adaptations should be used to enhance or compensate for mismatches between the presentation or design of the materials and the skills and strategies of the students without altering critical concepts or instructional goals.	Suggested content adaptations[a] • *Size adaptations:* Adjust the number of items students are expected to learn or complete. • *Time adaptations:* Adjust the amount of time allowed for learning, completing tasks, or testing. • *Level of support adaptations:* Adjust the amount of personal assistance or technology use. • *Input adaptations:* Adjust how instruction is delivered. • *Output adaptations:* Adjust how the students are expected to demonstrate learning or mastery of critical content. • *Difficulty adaptations:* Adjust the skill level, problem type, or rules about how the students approach the activity. • *Participation adaptations:* Adjust how the students are involved in the activity.

5. Identify the features of the materials that need to be adapted.

Determine how the design of materials may be creating problems for students using AAC within the following categories:

- *Abstractness:* Content appears too conceptual, hypothetical, or impractical.
- *Organization:* Organization is not clear or is poorly structured.
- *Relevance:* Information does not appear to have any relationship to students or their lives.
- *Interest:* Information or presentation of the information is boring.
- *Skills:* Information is written at a level that assumes and requires skills beyond those possessed by students.
- *Strategies:* Information is presented in ways that assume that students strategically know how to approach tasks effectively and efficiently.
- *Background:* Students lack the experiences and concepts to make new information meaningful.
- *Complexity:* Information or tasks have too many parts or layers.
- *Quantity:* There is too much difficult or complex information to remember.
- *Activities:* Instructional activities do not lead to understanding or mastery.
- *Outcomes:* Information does not cue students how to think about or study information to meet intended outcomes.
- *Responses:* Material does not provide options for students to demonstrate competence in different ways.

Suggested design adaptations

- *Abstractness:* Provide concrete examples, analogies, interpretations, or experiences.
- *Organization:* Use graphic organizers and cues to focus attention.
- *Relevance:* Present rationales and tie information to experiences.
- *Interest:* Present information and assignments that build on student attention, participation, strengths, and interests.
- *Skills:* Present information to build on students' skills and provide explicit skill instruction.
- *Strategies:* Provide explicit learning strategy instruction, and use cues to guide students in task completion.
- *Background:* Provide background experiences.
- *Complexity:* "Chunk" information, steps, and tasks.
- *Quantity:* Explicitly teach memory strategies.
- *Activities:* Provide scaffolded learning experiences that include additional or alternative instructional activities, sequences, or practice experiences.
- *Outcomes:* Inform students about performance expectations.
- *Responses:* Provide varied opportunities for students to demonstrate their knowledge.

6. Determine adaptations that will allow the students to meet the demand.

Determine if format adaptations should involve

- Altering existing materials
- Mediating existing materials
- Selecting alternate materials

Suggested format approaches

- *Altering existing materials:* Rewrite, reorganize, add to, or recast information in alternate ways so that students can gain access to regular curriculum materials independently.
- *Mediating existing materials:* Provide additional instructional support, guidance, and direction to students in using existing materials. Alter instruction to mediate the barriers presented by the design of the materials. Directly lead the students to respond to and interact with existing materials in different ways.
- *Selecting alternate materials:* Select or develop a new set of curriculum materials and assistive technologies that are more sensitive to student needs.

(continued)

Table 7.1. *(continued)*

Step	General description	Specific action options
7. Inform parents and students about the adaptation.	Directly inform parents and students about adaptations, how they will be implemented, and how they relate to earlier experiences or adaptations.	Inform parents of any role that they might play in terms of helping the students use the adaptation in school or at home.
		Develop simple policies and implementation sheets to keep parents informed about how they might become involved.
		Discuss adaptations and make key content decisions at IEP meetings and parent–teacher conferences.
8. Implement, evaluate, and adjust the adaptation.	Use adaptations consistently/systematically.	Provide necessary instruction on strategies that will gradually increase student independence.
	Evaluate effectiveness of adaptations and make adjustments to ensure desired outcomes are achieved across time.	
9. Fade the adaptation when possible.	Fade or change adaptations and assistive technologies as students' skills/needs change.	Teach students how adaptations are implemented, how to advocate use of accommodations, and about their legal rights to accommodations and assistive technologies related to their disabilities.

Note: This table is adapted from the "Adapting Language Arts, Social Studies, and Science for the Inclusive Classroom" page of the *Teacher Vision* web site (http://www.teachervision.fen.com/educational-research/teaching-methods/8538.html).

[a]Based on Cole, S., Horvath, B., Chapman, C., Deschenes, C., Ebeling, D., & Sprague, J. (2000). *Adapting curriculum and instruction in inclusive classrooms* (2nd ed.). Port Chester, NY: National Professional Resources.

(i.e., understanding and using the symbols and grammatical rules of languages used at home and at school) may be appropriate targets for classroom intervention. In addition, many children may require assistance with attaining operational competency—that is, the technical skills to operate their AAC systems. A wide variety of skills that fall into these categories have been studied and can be adapted for use in classroom settings.

Social Competency Skills

Beginning communicators may require specific instruction to develop a range of social skills. An overview of critical early social skills is provided next.

Rejecting, Accepting, Requesting, and Choice Making

Some beginning communicators may need to be taught how to accept preferred items and reject nonpreferred items (Sigafoos, Drasgow, O'Reilly, & Tait, 2004; Sigafoos & Mirenda, 2002; Sigafoos & Roberts-Pennell, 1999). Some students may not demonstrate rejection or acceptance at all, some may demonstrate these behaviors inconsistently, and some may demonstrate socially inappropriate variations of these behaviors (e.g., rejecting by throwing objects). Many beginning communicators who do demonstrate acceptance and rejection in some manner may have more difficulties with the next steps, which include requesting and making basic choices. Requesting items (e.g., objects, activities) and making basic choices (e.g., choosing between at least two different items) share an important component with acceptance and rejection—the student must demonstrate his or her preferences (Beukelman & Mirenda, 2005). Learning to accept and reject individual items are typically prerequisite skills for learning to make choices and requests. Once a student learns to accept or reject a single object or activity, then he or she may then be ready to move on to ask for a particular item or make a choice between two or more options. Sigafoos and Mirenda (2002) proposed a continuum of formats for requesting, ranging from an *elicited offered choice* (e.g., the educator initiates the interaction and offers two or more explicit choices, such as offering a choice between coloring a picture blue or red) to a *user-initiated request*, in which the student initiates a request independently.

There are many different types of requests. Some students may need to learn to request social interaction in a socially appropriate manner. For example, Johnston, Nelson, Evans, and Palazolo (2003) taught three children with ASD to request entrance into a play activity by using a graphic symbol representing, CAN I PLAY? Another common classroom occurrence is for a student to want to continue with a preferred activity (e.g., being pushed on a swing). Gee, Graham, Goetz, Oshima, and Yoshioka (1991) taught three elementary-age students to request the continuation of routine activities (e.g., assistance with food preparation and consumption) by activating their AAC devices (a buzzer or voice output with the message COME HERE, PLEASE). Other communicative requests that students who are beginning communicators and early language users may need to learn include requesting objects, requesting more (e.g., MORE JUICE), requesting an alternative (e.g., milk instead of juice), and requesting action or assistance (e.g., help with opening a heavy door; Sigafoos & Mirenda, 2002).

Turn Taking

Improving turn-taking skills is another social skill with which many beginning communicators and early language users require assistance (e.g., Hunt, Alwell, & Goetz, 1991; Kent-Walsh, 2003). Many students who use AAC have demonstrated notoriously low turn-taking ratios with their partners, in both one-to-one and group settings (e.g., Houghton et al., 1987; Kent-Walsh, 2003). Part of the reason that beginning communicators and early language users tend to take so few turns has to do with the dynamic interplay of internal and external factors; that is, many students fail to take turns due, in part, to their inherent challenges with communication, but research has shown that when the communication partners make a few, simple changes to the ways in which they communicate with these students, the students make rapid and significant gains in the number of turns that they take (Kent-Walsh, 2003). Figure 7.4 provides a detailed example of one method for teaching turn taking.

Student name: _Bridget_

Other characteristics: _Passive communicator, developmental delays_

Primary disability: _Cerebral palsy_

Communication modes: _Dynamic display augmentative and alternative communication (AAC) device (DynaVox V), gaze, gestures, and vocalizations_

School placement: _Inclusive first-grade classroom_

Primary educators/communication partners: _Classroom teacher, educational assistant, exceptional education teacher, peers, speech-language pathologist (SLP)_

Targeted skill	Curriculum context	Targeted activity	Assistive technologies	Vocabulary selection and organization	Intervention techniques[a]	Potential tools for tracking student progress
Increasing communicative turn taking	Language arts	Reading storybooks	DynaVox V adapted storybooks	Select vocabulary from pack-aged curriculum and relevant vocabulary in storybook Develop theme-based communication displays for each story-book with Fitzgerald Key lay-out (see Figure 7.5 for example)	Least-to-most prompting hierarchy: natural cue (e.g., reading the story) + aided AAC model → open-ended question + aided AAC model → answer question + aided AAC model; natural consequences (nonverbal and verbal) Note: This is the "RAA" hierarchy in Figure 7.4.	Percent correct, rate, Goal Attainment Scaling (GAS), EasyTally, elec-tronic language sample
Increasing multisymbol message production	Science	Assembling an ant farm	DynaVox V	Select vocabulary from pack-aged curriculum and analyze the activity Develop theme-based communication displays for ant farm activity with Fitzgerald Key lay-out (see Figure 7.5 for example)	Least-to-most prompting hierarchy: natural cue (e.g., comment about ant farm) → expectant delay → point toward device → two-symbol aided AAC model, followed by expansion, extension, or imitation	Percent correct, rate, GAS, EasyTally, elec-tronic language sample
Furthering concept development (colors, verbs)	Art	Coloring and assembling cardboard cut-out char-acters (dress-up activity)	DynaVox V Adapted glue Pencil grips	Develop theme-based communication displays for character dress-up activity with Fitzgerald Key layout (see Figure 7.5 for example)	Aided AAC modeling, binary choices, and open-ended questions, followed by natu-ral consequences (verbal)	Rate, GAS

Figure 7.1. Example of adapting the curriculum for Bridget, a student with cerebral palsy. (Key: [a]The intervention techniques specified in this column are suggested for teaching this specific skill in this specific context. Other intervention techniques may be appropriate for use in this and other contexts. Additional evidence-based examples similar to this case include Binger, Kent-Walsh, Berens, Del Campo, & Rivera, 2008; Binger & Light, 2007; and Kent-Walsh, 2003.)

Student name: _John_   Primary disability: _Autism_

Other characteristics: _Beginning to use single symbols, challenging behaviors (throwing, yelling)_

Communication modes: _Picture Exchange Communication System (PECS), gestures, and vocalizations_

School placement: _Middle school self-contained classroom_

Primary educators/communication partners: _Classroom teacher, educational assistant, peers, speech-language pathologist (SLP)_

Targeted skill	Curriculum context	Targeted activity	Assistive technologies	Vocabulary selection and organization	Intervention techniques[a]	Potential tools for tracking student progress
Reject undesired objects (currently throws undesired items)	Lunch	Selecting lunch items	Big Mack	Program NO, THANK YOU into Big Mack	Most-to-least prompting hierarchy: physical guidance → direct verbal prompt → point toward augmentative and alternative communication (AAC) device → expectant cue → natural cue	Percent correct, rate, Goal Attainment Scaling (GAS)
Request action or assistance	Science	Assembling shoebox solar system	Big Mack	Program I NEED HELP, PLEASE into Big Mack	High-probability request or most-to-least prompting hierarchy: physical guidance → direct verbal prompt → point toward AAC device → expectant cue → natural cue	Rate, GAS
Transition across activities (currently yells and throws self on floor)	Class change	Moving from classroom to any other room	Picture symbols, visual schedule	Create visual schedule containing various locations / Select appropriate picture symbols	Preferred item as distractor, followed by natural consequences (nonverbal and verbal)	Percent correct, GAS

Figure 7.2. Example of adapting the curriculum for John, a student with autism. (Key: [a]The intervention techniques specified in this column are suggested for teaching this specific skill in this specific context. Other intervention techniques may be appropriate for use in this and other contexts. Additional evidence-based examples similar to this case include Bopp, Brown, & Mirenda, 2004.)

Student name: *Violet*

Primary disability: *Down syndrome, significant cognitive impairment*

Other characteristics: *Severe motor-speech impairment (apraxia), generally compliant*

Communication modes: *Static display multilevel aided augmentative and alternative communication (AAC) device (Tech/Speak), manual signs, gaze, gestures, and vocalizations*

School placement: *High school self-contained classroom*

Primary educators/communication partners: *Classroom teacher, educational assistant, peers, speech-language pathologist (SLP)*

Targeted skill	Curriculum context	Targeted activity	Assistive technologies	Vocabulary selection and organization	Intervention techniques[a]	Potential tools for tracking student progress
Make choices	Family and consumer sciences	Cook in small group (with one or two peers)	Tech/Speak	Select vocabulary from cooking lesson plan Develop theme-based communication displays for each cooking activity	Aided and unaided AAC models (from peers and educators), binary choice, and open-ended questions (e.g., "What do you need next?"), followed by natural consequences (nonverbal and verbal)	Percent correct, Goal Attainment Scaling (GAS)
Share information	Social studies	Current/recent events (Hurricane Katrina)	Tech/Speak	Select vocabulary from lesson plan Theme-based communication display containing hurricane vocabulary	Open-ended questions, point toward AAC device, followed by natural consequences (verbal)	Rate, GAS
Improve receptive vocabulary	Art	Photography	Tech/Speak, visual supports for key concepts	Select vocabulary from lesson plan Theme-based communication display containing photography vocabulary	Aided and unaided AAC models (from peers and educators) and open-ended questions, followed by natural consequences (nonverbal and verbal)	Percent correct, GAS

Figure 7.3.   Example of adapting the curriculum for Violet, a student with Down syndrome. (Key: [a]The intervention techniques specified in this column are suggested for teaching this specific skill in this specific context. Other intervention techniques may be appropriate for use in this and other contexts. Additional evidence-based examples similar to this case include Downing, 2005a.)

Intervention technique	Description		Interactive storybook reading example
1. Pretest and commitment to instructional program	Educators • Take pretraining measurements of communication partners' spontaneous use of the targeted technique(s) or prompting hierarchy and the communication of the students who use augmentative and alternative communication (AAC) in the typical school context (e.g., classroom) • Introduce the technique(s) or hierarchy and the training protocol to communication partners • Discuss communication partners' pretraining strengths and weaknesses in implementing the targeted technique(s) or hierarchy • Obtain a formal participation commitment to the instructional program from the communication partners	Introductory session Individual instructional session lasting approximately 90 minutes	Speech-language pathologist (SLP) • Took pretraining videos of the educational assistants reading with the students using AAC during library time at school • Explained that the purpose of the instructional program was to teach the educational assistants how to implement a cueing hierarchy in order to increase the communicative turn taking of their students using AAC • Briefly described the hierarchy and its component techniques (aided AAC system modeling, expectant delay, open-ended question asking, and increased responsivity to communicative attempts) and the instructional protocol • Reviewed and signed instructional contract with the educational assistants.
2. Hierarchy description	Educators • Describe the targeted techniques and method for remembering the hierarchy steps • Discuss the effect of implementing the targeted technique(s) or hierarchy on the students using AAC with the communication partners	Introductory session (continued)	SLP • Showed four videotapes of herself during interactive storybook reading sessions with unfamiliar students using AAC: two without use of the hierarchy and two tapes with use of the hierarchy • Guided a discussion about 1) the differences noted in student communicative participation in the "without hierarchy" and "with hierarchy" tapes (e.g., increased communicative participation by students), 2) the implications of these differences (e.g., increased opportunities for students to develop language and emergent literacy skills), and 3) the potential benefits of implementing the hierarchy with the students (e.g., increased student involvement in classroom activities) • Described in detail all of the techniques involved in the hierarchy

(continued)

Figure 7.4. Eight suggested steps for communication partner instruction. (Sources: Kent-Walsh, 2003; Kent-Walsh & McNaughton, 2005.)

Figure 7.4. *(continued)*

Intervention technique	Description		Interactive storybook reading example
3. Hierarchy demonstration	Educators • Model use of the targeted technique(s) or hierarchy and explain all the steps	Introductory session (continued)	The SLP provided the following demonstrations during role plays with the educational assistants: • Implementation of the individual techniques • Sequential use of each of the techniques • Talk-aloud statements during the role play to illustrate the thought process involved (e.g., "I'm looking at you and waiting for you to say something. I'm counting to 8 seconds. You still haven't said anything, so now I'm going to ask you an open-ended question.")
4. Verbal practice of hierarchy steps	Communication partners practice naming and describing all steps required to implement the technique(s) or hierarchy	Introductory session (continued)	With the use of a visual aid, the SLP • Reviewed a pneumonic to help the educational assistants remember how to correctly implement the techniques within the prompting hierarchy: "RAA" (R = read, A = ask, A = answer) • Used rote verbal rehearsal to learn to "read, ask, and answer" and discussed how each step in RAA was combined with AAC modeling and followed by an expectant delay
5. Controlled practice and feedback	Communication partners practice implementing the technique(s) or hierarchy in a controlled environment with gradual fading of educator prompting and feedback	Practice session One individual instructional session lasting approximately 45 minutes each	SLP • Demonstrated use of the RAA hierarchy again during a role play • Switched roles with the educational assistants, thus allowing them the opportunity to practice implementing the targeted hierarchy • Asked the educational assistants to add the next sequential step in the hierarchy until they were able to sequentially implement all of the targeted steps

6. Advanced practice and feedback	Communication partners practice implementing the technique(s) or hierarchy in multiple situations within the natural classroom environment with gradual fading of educator prompting and feedback	Practice session One individual instructional session lasting approximately 45 minutes each	Educational assistants • Practiced implementing the hierarchy with the student using AAC with gradually faded feedback from the SLP • Asked questions if they were unsure of how to proceed • Were given feedback on the accuracy of their implementation of the hierarchy after each page they read with the students
7. Posttest and commitment to long-term hierarchy use	Educators • Document and review communication partners' mastery of the technique(s) or hierarchy and check performance against the pretraining measurements • Elicit feedback on the effect of the communication partners' implementation of the technique(s) or hierarchy • Assist communication partners in generating action plans for maintenance and generalization of the technique(s) or hierarchy	Instructional follow-up session One individual instructional session lasting approximately 30 minutes	SLP and educational assistants • Watched randomly selected 5-minute pre- and postinstructional video segments • Discussed 1) the educational assistants' communication, 2) the effects of the training on the communication of the students using AAC, 3) the overall effect of the instructional program, and 4) the importance of maintaining use of the targeted interaction hierarchy
8. Generalization of targeted hierarchy use	Communication partners practice implementing the technique(s) or hierarchy across a wide range of settings and plan for long-term implementation	Instructional follow-up session (continued)	SLP and educational assistants • Discussed options for generalized use of the hierarchy during novel classroom activities (e.g., circle time, craft activities, classroom games) • Developed action plans for adaptations of the hierarchy in such novel activities

Commenting/Nonobligatory Turn Taking   Making comments (also known as taking nonobligatory turns) that are relevant to school life is one specific type of turn that is important in the classroom setting. It is important to note that nonobligatory turns are not required turns (i.e., they are not in response to direct questions). Instead, these turns place the student in a position to be an active, spontaneous communicator. Davis and colleagues (Davis, Reichle, & Southard, 1998) taught two teenagers (one with Down syndrome and one with cerebral palsy) to use their AAC devices to take nonobligatory turns following comments made by a communication partner (e.g., I'D LIKE TO GO SHOPPING.). Prior to intervention, these two students failed to respond to these types of comments, even though they were highly likely to respond to direct questions. Both teenagers took significantly more nonobligatory turns following intervention. Light and Binger (1998) provided examples of general, flexible comments/nonobligatory turns that may be preprogrammed onto a student's device (e.g., THAT'S GREAT! NO WAY! UH OH. YEAH!) and used in a variety of situations. Having access to such flexible vocabulary can assist a student with increasing classroom participation with both teachers and peers across a wide variety of activities and create improved social competence by increasing the turn-taking symmetry between students who use AAC and their communication partners.

Using an Introductory Strategy   An *introductory strategy* (Light & Binger, 1998), which is a message that is written on or programmed into the student's AAC device that can be used with new communication partners, is another type of nonobligatory turn. These messages typically include information on how the person communicates (e.g., I USE THIS COMPUTER TO TALK TO PEOPLE.) and how to cope with communication breakdowns (e.g., IF YOU DON'T UNDERSTAND ME, PLEASE ASK ME TO REPEAT MYSELF.). Sometimes, a student will also need to state his or her name, but this is not socially appropriate for all situations (e.g., placing an order in a restaurant).

Asking Partner-Focused Questions   In the same series of studies, Light, Binger, and colleagues (Light & Binger, 1998; Light, Binger, Agate, & Ramsey, 1999) taught a wide variety of individuals who used AAC to ask partner-focused questions. These types of questions are similar to comments/nonobligatory turns in that they place the student using AAC in a very active communication role and, indeed, as an initiator of communication. To ask a partner-focused question, the student simply asks a peer or educator (e.g., teacher, SLP, paraprofessional, other adult) a question that is about the peer or educator and not about the student him- or herself. For example, a high school student might ask another high school student, "What's up?" or "What are you doing this weekend?" Typically, these messages are preprogrammed onto a student's AAC device to maximize communicative efficiency.

Building Peer Relationships   Building friendships is one of the cornerstones of growing up, and finding ways to support such relationships must be included in educational plans for beginning communicators and early language users (see Chapter 11). Building peer relationships is one of the themes across many of the previous social skills. A student with AAC needs can request an object from a peer, make choices within an activity in which other students are making similar choices, take more turns when conversing with a peer, and make comments and ask partner-focused questions with peers—and that student may use AAC to accomplish each of these tasks. In a research review of inclusive educational programs, Hunt and Goetz (1997) concluded that "students with severe disabilities realize acceptance, interactions, and friendships in inclusive settings" and that "parents report acceptance and belonging as a major positive inclusion outcome" (p. 26). Hunt and colleagues (Hunt, Soto, Maier, & Doering, 2003; Hunt, Soto, Maier, Liboiron, & Bae, 2004; Hunt, Soto, Maier, Müller, & Goetz, 2002) have conducted a number of investigations examining the effect of a collaborative teaming approach to service provision with students with disabilities, many of whom were beginning communicators and early language users. One component of the educational program used in each study was to build social skills. For example, the inclusion support teacher made a photo conversation book for one student to assist the student with building and maintaining peer relationships (Hunt et al., 2003). These researchers have shown that by using a collaborative teaming approach to intervention and setting goals that are geared toward improving social relationships, students who are beginning communicators and early language users can participate with peers at similar levels to other students in the classroom (Hunt et al., 2003; Hunt et al., 2004).

Decreasing Challenging Behaviors   Although some of the social skills discussed may not directly relate to curricular items, it is clear that many of these skills are precursors to making achievements within the curriculum (e.g., a child who cannot make choices cannot accurately select materials for a science project). Working on these skills also may have a direct effect on reducing challenging behaviors for many children. Sigafoos, Arthur-Kelly, and Butterfield (2006) discussed a wide variety of communication-based replacements for challenging behaviors, all of which may be accomplished by using aided or unaided AAC. For example, if a student tends to reject unwanted items by throwing the items, then he or she might be taught to use a spoken approximation of "no," shake his or her head to indicate "no," point to a graphic symbol that represents NO, or select a symbol on a voice output device that says NO, THANK YOU. Thus, the student learns to improve his or her social skills while simultaneously decreasing challenging behaviors.

Linguistic Competency Skills

Beginning communicators and early language users are, by definition, at the early stages of language learning, and it is critically important to support their early language development.

Language Comprehension   Improving language comprehension is one major area that often does not receive adequate attention. Children must be able to understand spoken language to function within most classrooms, and building that comprehension must be an explicit focus for some children—some beginning communicators may exhibit little to no comprehension of spoken words. Sevcik and Romski (2002) pointed out that beginning communicators face not only the task of learning to comprehend spoken language, just as children without disabilities do, but they also must learn to comprehend the AAC symbols that the child is expected to use. Frequently, graphic symbols (e.g., photographs, line drawings) are used to support language comprehension. One common example is a visual schedule, which "is an intervention that depicts the sequence of activities, steps, or rules that apply to specific individuals or routines" (Bopp, Brown, & Mirenda, 2004, p. 14). Visual schedules are often used with students who have autism or other developmental disabilities and help these students to understand what it is they are supposed to do either within a classroom activity or across different activities.

Receptive Vocabulary   Building receptive vocabulary skills is one part of supporting overall language development, including language comprehension. Here, the educator teaches the student the meaning of specific vocabulary words. Educators may provide instruction to promote comprehension of spoken words, AAC symbols, or both. For example, Drager and colleagues (2006) taught two children with autism to improve both their spoken and graphic symbol receptive vocabulary within typical classroom activities; that is, the students improved their ability to identify the correct object when they were directed to "Show me [verbal label for object]" or "Show me [point to graphic symbol of object]."

Expressive Vocabulary   Building receptive vocabulary goes hand in hand with building expressive vocabulary; indeed, the same vocabulary items may be targeted receptively and expressively using the same or similar intervention techniques (Drager et al., 2006). As early language users begin to use language expressively, they must begin to build their expressive vocabulary skills. Often, increases in expressive vocabulary occur while targeting other skills. For example, to increase turn taking during story reading, Kent-Walsh (2003) created communication pages within voice output devices that were specific to each storybook, such as a communication page that included the vocabulary CLIFFORD, EMILY ELIZABETH, BIG, RED, and DOG and other graphic symbols relevant to the book

Clifford the Big Red Dog (Bridwell, 1998). In many cases, the children did not have access to and did not use these specific graphic symbols prior to the onset of the investigation. By increasing their turn-taking skills, these students necessarily increased their expressive vocabulary. This is true for many other skills discussed previously, including requesting, commenting/nonobligatory turns, using an introductory strategy, and asking partner-focused questions. In all cases, the student will likely be using new vocabulary words when using his or her new skills.

Sometimes, it may be important to set specific goals for increasing particular types of vocabulary words. For example, if an early language user relies heavily on nouns, it is important to teach the student to begin using other types of word classes, such as verbs and adjectives. Students who only have access to and who are only taught to use object or noun symbols will not have the vocabulary necessary to achieve the next step in linguistic development, which is learning to combine symbols.

Multisymbol Messages   Finally, educators can teach early language users who comprehend and use a number of words and/or AAC symbols to begin to combine symbols, just as a child who speaks and who is using single-word utterances begins to use brief sentences. Binger and colleagues have taught a number of children to begin using symbol combinations during storybook reading and other activities (Binger, Kent-Walsh, Berens, Del Campo, & Rivera, 2008; Binger & Light, 2007).

Operational Skills   Many beginning communicators and early language users also need to learn operational skills to gain access to their AAC systems because each AAC component places an array of motor, visual, auditory, and cognitive demands on a student. In addition, teachers, SLPs, and other support staff must take responsibility for many operational demands, such as programming the AAC device. Some operational requirements are often embedded within social goals. For example, in a study conducted by Gee and colleagues (1991), three students had to learn the operational skills of activating and holding down switches for a set period of time to activate their AAC devices (i.e., either call buttons or a simple message that said, COME HERE, PLEASE) in order to gain the attention of their communication partners. For each of these students, learning to operate the device was not a separate objective. They learned to use single-switch devices within a communicative context. This approach is preferable, whenever possible, as the student learns from the very beginning that using AAC results in desirable communicative outcomes. At times, however, students may need to learn operational skills separately from their social and linguistic goals. For example, scanning is a complicated process that involves many steps, and many students require explicit instruction to learn to use this selection technique (Treviranus & Roberts, 2002). When the student is first learning to scan, it may be useful to provide decontextualized instruction so that the student can give his or her full attention to this cognitively demanding task. As soon as the student begins to scan functionally, however, it is important to provide instruction in the classroom so that the student learns to scan functionally in response to the natural cues and natural consequences in his or her typical communication environment.

In addition, beginning communicators and early language users require the assistance of others to manage other aspects of operational competency, including the selection, representation, and organization of vocabulary. For example, the educational team must determine how to best represent vocabulary for beginning communicators and early language users. They must decide if the student's aided AAC symbols will take the form of real objects, partial objects, miniature objects, remnants, photographs, line drawings, or some combination of these symbol types (see Chapter 14 for additional information). In addition, they must determine when symbols will represent single concepts (e.g., HUG) versus whole messages (e.g., CAN I HAVE A HUG, PLEASE?). In some cases, it may be appropriate to consider using symbols that represent multiple concepts (e.g., Semantic Compaction and Unity software on devices such as the Vanguard from Prentke Romich Co.). In addition, the team must decide the best method for organizing vocabulary within an aided AAC device. For example, symbols may be organized by using a taxonomic organization (i.e., using semantic categories such as a people page, places page, insects page, mammals page), Fitzgerald Keys (i.e., organizing vocabulary from left-to-right following typical syntactic patterns, such as agents on the left, actions in the middle, and objects on the right), or visual scene displays. Frequently, combinations of these approaches can be used. For example, a taxonomic organization can be used for various classroom activities, such as having a series of pages that all relate to science activities (e.g., for a unit on insects, there may be one page for spiders, another for caterpillars, and another for ants), and then certain pages can be organized using a Fitzgerald Key (e.g., a page for building an ant farm; see Figure 7.5).

A variety of potential social, linguistic, and operational skills may be appropriate for a given student, and the team must prioritize the targeted skills. Of course, curricular priorities will help determine which skills to target within particular circumstances. For example, if students are completing a science unit on insects and are building ant farms, then the student using AAC can improve his or her requesting skills by taking nonobligatory turns and making comments about the ants inside the ant farm (e.g., DID YOU SEE THAT? WOW!).

Intervention Techniques

A wide variety of intervention techniques have been used successfully to teach students the skills discussed previously.

Social and Linguistic Competency Techniques   Figure 7.6 contains a description and an example of each technique, in addition to indicating which techniques may be helpful for teaching a variety of social and linguistic skills. The first section of Figure 7.6 lists techniques that create opportunities for communication and provide students with the time and opportunities required for communication to take place. Educators and other communication partners fail to provide communication opportunities for students who use AAC when the classroom environment is highly structured. One of the first steps to providing communication opportunities is for educators to become aware of and take advantage of natural cues that occur in the classroom. For example, simply walking into the classroom in the morning can be a natural cue to say, "Good morning." An

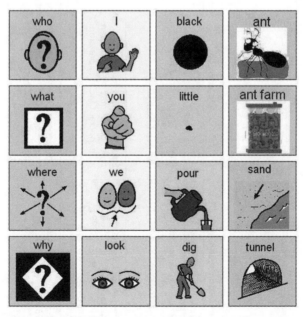

Figure 7.5. Sample communication board for an ant farm activity organized using a Fitzgerald Key. Color coded for ease of recognition. The Picture Communication Symbols © 1981–2008 by Mayer-Johnson LLC. All Rights Reserved Worldwide. Used with permission.

Social and linguistic skills

Intervention technique	Description	Example	Accept/reject	Ask partner-focused questions	Comment	Improve listening comprehension	Improve receptive vocabulary	Increase expressive vocabulary	Make choices	Produce multisymbol messages	Request	Respond contingently	Transition across activities	Take communicative turns	Use partner-focused questions
Create opportunities for communication															
Blocked response/interrupted behavior chain (Goetz, Gee, & Sailor, 1985)	Student is prevented from completing an activity or a necessary item is removed from view.	Students are making an ant farm in science class. Educator gives student the ant farm but no sand.	X		X					X	X	X		X	
Expectant delay/time delay (e.g., Gee, Graham, Goetz, Oshima, & Yoshioka, 1991; Light, Binger, Agate, & Ramsey, 1999)	Educator pauses for an extended time; pause may be accompanied by an expectant facial expression.	Educator gives student the ant farm and waits 15 seconds.	X	X	X	X	X	X	X	X	X	X		X	X
Natural cue (Light & Binger, 1998)	Educator provides student with any type of opportunity to communicate that would occur naturally.	Educator hands student the ant farm and pauses. *or* Educator approaches student and pauses.	X	X	X	X	X	X	X	X	X	X	X	X	X
Open-ended/*wh-* question (Kent-Walsh, 2003)	Educator asks open-ended question to prompt a communicative response.	Educator hands student the ant farm and asks, "What goes in the ant farm?"			X	X	X	X	X	X	X	X	X	X	X
Guide communicative behaviors															

Technique	Description	Example									
Aided, unaided, or multimodal AAC model (Binger & Light, 2007)	Educator provides a model using AAC; the partner may model the behavior that is expected from the student.	Educator says, "Here's the sand. Sand."	X	X	X	X	X	X	X	X	X
Binary choice (Sigafoos & Mirenda, 2002)	Educator offers student a choice between two items/activities.	Educator gives student an empty ant farm and says, "Do you want sand or rocks?" (while holding up a bag of sand and a bag of rocks).			X	X	X	X	X	X	X
Direct verbal prompt	Educator provides student with direct verbal instruction; may be highly directive or general prompt.	Educator says, "Tell me, 'sand'" (highly directive). *or* Educator says, "Your turn" (general prompt).	X	X	X	X	X	X	X	X	X
High-probability request (Davis, Reichle, & Southard, 1998, 2000)	Educator provides three to five antecedent requests that the student is highly likely to complete immediately before targeted low-probability request.	Educator says, "Give me five" (student complies), "Touch your nose" (student complies), and "Point to your shirt" (student complies; all high-probability requests). Educator says, "Pour in the sand" (a low-probability request).				X	X	X	X	X	
Physical guidance (Sigafoos, 1999; Sigafoos, Drasgow, O'Reilly, & Tait, 2004)	Educator assists student with creating a manual sign or directs hand toward AAC device.	Educator says, "Sand or rocks?" (offers binary choice between sand and rocks). Student has no response. Educator directs student's hand toward the sand.	X	X	X	X	X	X	X	X	X
Point toward student or AAC device (Light & Binger, 1998)	Educator points toward the student (if using unaided AAC) or the AAC device; may be highly directive or a general point.	Educator provides general point toward aided AAC device. *or* Educator points directly toward AAC symbol for SAND	X	X	X	X	X	X	X	X	X
Preferred item as distractor (Davis et al., 2000)	Educator presents preferred item immediately before low-probability (target) request.	Educator hands student a Superman action figure and says, "Walk to the ant farm."		X			X		X		X

Figure 7.6. Intervention techniques to teach selected social and linguistic skills to beginning communicators and early language users. [a]Expansions, extensions, and imitations are other examples of natural consequences that are verbal.

(continued)

Figure 7.6 *(continued)*

Intervention technique	Description	Example	Accept/reject	Ask partner-focused questions	Comment	Improve listening comprehension	Improve receptive vocabulary	Increase expressive vocabulary	Make choices	Produce multisymbol messages	Request	Respond contingently	Transition across activities	Take communicative turns	Use partner-focused questions
Responding to/reinforcing communicative behaviors															
Expansion (verbal)	Educator repeats student's message and adds new information.	Student says, "SAND ANT FARM." Educator says, "Yes, you put sand in your ant farm."	X		X			X	X	X	X	X		X	X
Extension (verbal)	Educator adds new information and changes meaning of student's message.	Student says, "SAND ART FARM." Educator says, "Yes, and ants go in the ant farm, too."			X			X	X	X	X	X		X	
Imitation (verbal)	Educator imitates student's message to reinforce the message.	Student says, "SAND ART FARM." Educator says, "Sand ant farm."	X		X				X	X	X	X		X	
Natural consequences (nonverbal)	Educator provides nonverbal, contingent response to student's communicative attempt.	Student says, "SAND." Educator gives the student the sand.	X	X		X	X	X	X	X	X	X	X	X	X
Natural consequences (verbal)	Educator provides verbal, contingent response to student's communicative attempt.	Student uses preprogrammed message to say "THIS IS FUN." Educator says, "Yes, I think building an ant farm is fun, too."[a]	X	X	X	X	X	X	X	X	X	X	X	X	X

effective next step for many students is for the educator (or peer) to provide an expectant delay—that is, an extended pause that is sometimes accompanied by an expectant facial expression (Light & Binger, 1998). Expectant delays provide the student with a silent cue that it is his or her turn to communicate, and they also provide the student with time to process the natural cue and to formulate his or her own message. This processing time may be essential for many beginning communicators and early language users. Blocked responses or interrupted behavior chains may be provided in conjunction with expectant delays. Here, the educator prevents the student from completing an activity and waits for the student to communicate (Goetz, Gee, & Sailor, 1985). For example, if the student is completing an art project, then the educator may hand the student some paper but no markers; the educator then waits to see what the student will do. Asking open-ended or *wh*-questions (i.e., who, what, where, when, why) can also create communication opportunities. During storybook reading activities, Kent-Walsh (2003) taught educational assistants to ask questions such as, "What is Clifford doing?" to prompt students to take their conversational turns. These types of questions are important because they prompt higher content turns than yes-no questions (e.g., "Is Clifford eating ice cream?") and provide opportunities for students to expand their expressive vocabulary.

The items listed in the second set of techniques in Figure 7.6 are used to guide the student toward explicit communicative behaviors. Some of these techniques are highly directive and designed to elicit quite explicit communicative turns, including providing a binary choice ("Do you want the car or the truck?" while pointing to the symbols for CAR and TRUCK), providing a direct verbal prompt ("Point to TRUCK"), and physically guiding the student's hand toward a particular AAC symbol (guide the student's hand to the TRUCK symbol). When using a preferred item as a distractor (Davis, Reichle, & Southard, 2000), the educator provides the student with a motivating, distracting item before making a request that the student might prefer not to perform (e.g., handing the student a favorite action figure before the educator selects LET'S GO TO THE BATHROOM on the child's AAC device). A high-probability request is a highly structured cue in which the educator provides three to five antecedent requests that the student is very likely to perform, followed by a request that the student typically prefers not to complete (Davis et al., 2000). For example, the educator might say, "Give me five," "Point to your eye," and "Snap your fingers" (all high-probability requests), followed by "Tell me, LET'S GO TO THE BATHROOM" (a low-probability request). With both preferred item distractors and high-probability requests, the educator typically expects a very specific response from the child (e.g., walking to the bathroom), and a positive event (or events) precedes the low-probability event. Pointing toward the child to indicate that it is his or her turn or pointing toward the AAC device/symbols is a less-directive prompt that provides the child with more communicative choices. Here, the student can select his or her own message to convey. Finally, providing AAC models—that is, the educator using the communication modes that the student is expected to use (e.g., gesturing, signing, selecting graphic symbols)—is a semi-directive technique that can be a very effective teaching technique (Binger & Light, 2007). These models are semi-directive in that the student may or may not choose to imitate the AAC model that the educator provides; direct prompts are not necessarily part of the model. In many cases, students may select novel messages following an aided AAC model (Binger, Berens, Kent-Walsh, & Taylor, 2008). The idea is simply to provide models of how the student could choose to communicate. AAC models can be provided in conjunction with other types of cues. For example, in the preferred item as a distractor example, the educator used an AAC model when selecting LET'S GO TO THE BATHROOM on the student's AAC device. Infusing the classroom with AAC models is critical. Educators cannot expect a student to learn to use an alternate communication mode if the student rarely sees others using that communication mode, just as one would not expect a child to learn to talk if the child never sees and hears other people talking.

The third section of Figure 7.6 provides a variety of ways for educators to respond to the student once the student has demonstrated the targeted skill. For example, once a child who is learning to reject provides a socially appropriate method for rejecting an item (e.g., wrinkling his or her nose to indicate that he or she does not want to look at a book about spiders), the educator can provide the nonverbal natural consequence of removing the item (e.g., the book about spiders) and/or a verbal natural consequence by saying, "Oh, you don't want that." In another example of a child with more advanced skills, a child might ask a partner-focused question that is preprogrammed onto her device (e.g., WHAT'S UP?), and the educator provides a verbal natural consequence (e.g., "Not much. What's up with you?"). Expansions, extensions, and imitations are all responses that an educator can use to respond to the student and simultaneously assist the student with building his or her language skills. For example, if an early language user is requesting items for an art activity and says CRAYON on the AAC device, then the educator can imitate and confirm the student's selection by selecting CRAYON, or the educator can provide an expansion by saying, "Blue crayon." If the student says BLUE CRAYON, then the educator may provide an extension—that is, add new information that changes the meaning slightly—by saying, "You're going to draw with your crayon," while selecting DRAW CRAYON on the student's AAC device.

In many cases, it is appropriate to combine multiple intervention techniques within prompting/cueing hierarchies. For example, Light, Binger, and colleagues (Light & Binger, 1998; Light et al., 1999) used a least-to-most cueing hierarchy to teach students (as well as adults) who used AAC to take appropriate communicative turns, ask partner-focused questions, and use an introductory strategy. The components of the least-to-most prompting hierarchy used in these investigations included a natural cue, an expectant delay, a general point toward the AAC device, and an aided AAC model. In some cases, it may be necessary to add an additional final step that includes physical guidance. For example, to teach a student to ask partner-focused questions, the educator might enter the room and say, "Good morning, Tommy" (natural cue), provide Tommy with a 15-second pause accompanied by an expectant facial expression (expectant delay), point toward Tommy's AAC device (point toward device), and then select the message HI, HOW ARE YOU? on Tommy's AAC device (aided AAC model). If Tommy did not select the message, then the educator could add a final step of guiding Tommy's hand to the correct symbol on his device. Each successive step in this hierarchy, as in all least-to-most prompting hierarchies, is more directive. One benefit of this approach is that the student is only presented with the amount of prompting that he or she needs to be successful, thus preventing prompt dependency. For a more detailed example of another least-to-most prompting hierarchy, see Figure 7.4.

In some cases, educators may need to use a most-to-least prompting hierarchy. One circumstance in which this type of hierarchy is appropriate is when students exhibit challenging behaviors. For example, if Tommy demonstrates rejection by throwing things, then a prompting hierarchy that is the reverse of the one presented previously might be appropriate for teaching Tommy to express rejection in a more socially appropriate manner. That is, as soon as Tommy is presented with a known, undesirable object, the educator immediately guides his hand toward a simple voice output device that says, NO, I DON'T WANT THAT (physical guidance). Slowly, the educator fades the physical prompt until the educator just points toward the device. Eventually, this prompt is faded too, until the educator merely presents the undesirable object while providing an expectant delay until the point that Tommy selects the message as soon as the object is presented (i.e., at the natural cue level). See Figures 7.1, 7.2, and 7.3 for further applications of social and linguistic intervention techniques.

Operational Competency Techniques   Operational competency instruction must be as basic as possible for beginning communicators and early language users. There is no inherent value in learning operational skills. Learning to hit a switch, for example, only has value when hitting the switch results in a desired curricular, communicative, or social success. The time and effort spent on developing operational competencies will vary widely across beginning communicators and early language users depending, in great part, on the presence and severity of their physical impairments.

With unaided AAC, operational competency will involve learning to produce clear, meaningful gestures and manual signs. Aided AAC operational competencies may range from very basic to quite complex. If using low-tech aided AAC, such as a communication book, the student may require instruction in securing the book at appropriate times and in locating the correct page of his or her communication book for a given activity (e.g., finding the ant farm page). If using a very simple, one-hit voice output device, then the only operational competency expected of the student may be for him or her to learn to press down on the switch to activate the message. Students using higher-level devices will obviously require higher levels of operational competency with their devices, which may include instruction in selecting from a variety of symbols, requesting that a new overlay be placed on the device (for devices that have static displays), or navigating across various pages on a device that has a dynamic display. Some students with severe motor impairments may need to learn to scan, which may require very explicit instruction for early language users.

Whenever possible, it is desirable to teach students to use unaided and aided AAC systems within communicative contexts. As such, many students do not require isolated instruction in the use of their AAC systems, and the intervention techniques described in the previous section will suffice for teaching such students to use their AAC systems. For students who do require explicit operational instruction, such as students who gain access to their aided AAC devices via scanning, the student's motor control (Treviranus & Roberts, 2002) and cognitive capabilities (Rowland & Schweigert, 2002) must be taken into consideration. For example, Treviranus and Roberts outlined three phases of learning to use automatic scanning. In the first phase, the student spends time learning to understand the scanning pattern, learning the movement needed to activate the switch, becoming familiar with the timing of making a selection, determining how to correct errors, and learning the keyboard layout. In phase two, the student learns to integrate the skills from phase one in a more fluid manner. During this phase, errors decrease and scanning speed and task endurance might increase. For these two phases, instruction should take place in a decontextualized setting to minimize distractions for the student. In the final phase, the student can pay more attention to message formulation. As scanning becomes more automatic, the student can allocate more resources toward what he or she wishes to say. Once the student achieves this level of operational competency, it is important to provide instruction within natural contexts in the classroom to ensure that he or she is using messages for truly functional communicative purposes.

Educators and other team members are typically responsible for other operational demands of the AAC system for beginning communicators and early language users, including symbol representation, vocabulary selection, and vocabulary organization. Some of the techniques that may be used to make these determinations can be based on the student's language development level. For example, with respect to symbol representation, if Maria is building her single-word vocabulary and is expected to learn to begin to combine symbols, she must have access to single-meaning symbols so that she can learn to combine them. For building an ant farm, some of this single-symbol vocabulary might include the following: I, WE, NEED, POUR, BLACK, SIX, ANT FARM, SAND, LEGS. A wide variety of two to three symbol messages can be created from these symbols (e.g., I POUR SAND, BLACK ANT, SIX LEGS). Preprogrammed messages are also appropriate for many students. Maria, for example, could use the message DID YOU SEE THAT? to direct her peers' attention toward a new tunnel that appeared in the ant farm. Often, then, a combination of single-meaning symbols and whole messages is the best option for supporting both language development needs and immediate communication needs.

As evidenced in the previous example, one primary technique for choosing appropriate vocabulary for a student is to examine and document the vocabulary that is used within each classroom context. This information can be gathered by investigating classroom materials (e.g., items needed to build an ant farm, books about ants and other insects that students will be reading) and by documenting the vocabulary used by peers in the classroom by taking an environmental inventory. To conduct an environmental inventory, educators observe peers in the classroom and document the vocabulary that the peers use within various classroom settings (typically developing peers who rely on speech to communicate). Educators can then decide which of these vocabulary items would be useful to include within the student's AAC system. Communication diaries may also be used to determine appropriate vocabulary—educators keep a running record of vocabulary that the student might need within various activities. For younger children, vocabulary checklists, such as the MacArthur Communicative Development Inventories (CDI; Fenson et al., 1993) or the Language Development Survey (Rescorla, 1989), can be used for ideas for relevant vocabulary as well. Finally, aided AAC modeling, which is typically discussed as a method for building linguistic and social skills (see Figure 7.6 for a description), is also a powerful and efficient tool for vocabulary selection. Here, the educator uses AAC when communicating with the student. These models are typically designed to be at or just above the student's current communicative level. When using AAC in this manner, the educator rapidly discovers which vocabulary items or messages are missing within the student's AAC system. For example, if Maria's educator is using Maria's voice output device during the ant farm activity, then the educator may realize that key symbols, such as DIG and TUNNEL, are missing on the device.

Finally, the team must decide how to organize the student's vocabulary. Many beginning communicators may initially experience the most success with using single symbols. For example, the Picture Exchange Communication System (PECS; Bondy & Frost, 1994) is an intervention approach that makes use of single-concept graphic symbols. Visual scene displays, also known as integrated scenes, offer other options that may benefit beginning communicators and early language users (Beukelman & Mirenda, 2005). The student uses a photograph or drawn picture that depicts an entire scene (e.g., students engaged in an ant farm activity), and the student selects items within that scene to communicate (e.g., pointing to an ant inside the ant farm). These scenes may be in hard copy communication board format or may be programmed within an electronic device. A major benefit of visual scene displays is that all vocabulary appears within a meaningful context, which may assist with comprehension for some beginning communicators and early language users (Drager, Light, Speltz, Fallon, & Jeffries, 2003). For students who can manage having vocabulary organized within more traditional grid formats, vocabulary may be organized taxonomically (e.g., insects page versus mammals page) by using a Fitzgerald Key (see Figure 7.5) or by a combination of these two approaches. Overall, then, many operational requirements need to be considered when creating AAC solutions for beginning communicators and early language users in order to optimize the students' chances for success with using AAC. See Chapter 12 for further information on teaching operational competencies.

Framework for Teaching Partners How to Facilitate Communication in the Classroom

Although the previously described intervention techniques can be helpful to educators as they are attempting to facilitate their students' communication development, not all educators will be sufficiently familiar with the individual techniques to start working on specific skills with their students independently. It is critical that all involved educators be taught to use appropriate intervention techniques and prompting hierarchies because the communication needs of students using AAC cannot be addressed adequately by one single educator in a classroom. Too often, when a team member attempts to provide other educators with instruction on using intervention techniques, the instruction takes place in a quick and informal manner. One common scenario would be an SLP providing the classroom teacher and educational assistant with very brief instructions on how to use an AAC device within a particular activity. Frequently, the result is that the SLP is frustrated when the classroom teacher and educational assistant fail to follow through on the recommendations, and the classroom teacher and educational assistant are frustrated because they feel inadequately prepared to follow through on the SLP's instructions. In the end, the students suffer far too often as their AAC devices sit either unused or underutilized. To alleviate this common classroom dilemma, this section provides guidance for educators to teach other educators, parents, and peers how to implement the intervention techniques addressed in this chapter.

Figure 7.4 details a communication partner instructional protocol and includes descriptions of the eight-component evidence-based instructional steps described by Kent-Walsh and McNaughton (2005). Figure 7.4 also incorporates a detailed example of how these instructional steps could be used to teach partners to use an evidence-based least-to-most prompting hierarchy to target increased communicative turn taking. The child in the example uses AAC in an interactive storybook reading context, as described by Kent-Walsh (2003). The prompting hierarchy described in the example includes the following instructional techniques described in the previous section: aided AAC modeling, expectant delay, open-ended question asking, and increased responsivity to communicative attempts (increased responsivity includes all of the items in the Responding to/Reinforcing Communicative Behaviors section in Figure 7.6). For information on other approaches for teaching communication partners how to support communication within the classroom, readers are directed to the works of Giangreco and colleagues (Giangreco, Broer, Stephen, & Edelman, 1999, 2001; Giangreco, Edelman, & Broer, 2001a, 2001b) and Jorgensen and colleagues (Jorgensen, McSheehan, & Sonnenmeier, 2007; McSheehan et al., 2006; Sonnenmeier, McSheehan, & Jorgensen, 2005).

Coordinating Services and Tracking Student Progress

There are a number of tools available that can assist educators in coordinating the student's educational program. For example, Choosing Outcomes and Accommodations for Children (COACH; Giangreco, Cloninger, & Iverson, 1998) is a program that helps educators identify long-term visions and goals for students. A related option is the Vermont Interdependent Services Team Approach (VISTA; Giangreco, 1996), a collaborative team approach that is designed to help educators determine which services are needed to support students' educational programs and who will provide the necessary services. This program encourages not only educators but also peers (i.e., using natural supports) to assist students with meeting their goals. A similar program called the Unified Plan of Support helps teams determine what supports a student needs to meet his or her goals and who is responsible for assisting with each goal (e.g., Hunt et al., 2003; Hunt et al., 2004; Hunt et al., 2002). These processes can be helpful in determining specific educational targets, which is often challenging with students who have so many educational needs.

Once educators have identified appropriate communication skills to target with their students, key intervention techniques, suitable classroom activities, relevant communication partner interventions, and a method for coordinating student services, they must then consider how they will monitor and track their students' progress. This section offers several examples of tracking options. At the most basic level, simple calculations can offer educators options for tracking progress across time. Frequently, progress attained on individual skills is documented in an individualized education program (IEP) as a percentage correct. For example, one objective for Troy, a child with severe intellectual and physical disabilities, is to request continuation of a desired activity at least 70% of the time. To calculate percent correct, the educator must keep track of each opportunity the student has to complete the desired skill. In many cases, it is impractical or impossible to track all opportunities. Therefore, tracking the rate of progress may be helpful in such cases. For example, Consuelo is a beginning communicator who tends to be very passive, and one of her objectives is to increase her rate of communicative turn taking during social activities. Instead of attempting to calculate percent correct, a clear way to track her progress is to keep track of how many times she attempts to communicate within a given time frame (e.g., take at least 5 communicative turns within a 20-minute small-group activity).

Another option is Goal Attainment Scaling (GAS), which "is a simple and precise method for evaluating individual progress toward unique goals" (Schlosser, 2002, p. 485) that is conducive for tracking progress with everyday interventions and allows for consensus-based goal setting. This approach has been suggested as a particularly appropriate way to track progress on individual skills for students who use AAC (Schlosser, 2002). GAS does not look at just one outcome measure that the student either achieves or fails to achieve (e.g., the student will take at least 5 turns within 20 minutes). Instead, five possible outcomes are determined for each goal. Typically, the expected outcome receives a weighting of 0, the two "above expectations" levels of +1 and +2, and the two "below expectations" levels of –1 and –2. In this manner, the student's level of achievement, even if that level falls above or below the expected outcome, can be tracked and charted.

Table 7.2 contains an example of GAS for a student named Consuelo. Goal 1 for Consuelo is to increase her turn-taking skills, and the expected outcome might be for her to take at least 4–6 turns during a 20-minute small-group activity. If she attains this level of achievement, then she would receive a rating of 0, which is the expected outcome. If she fails to meet the criterion but still occasionally takes turns, then she receives a rating of –1, and if she fails to take any turns, then she receives a rating of –2. If Consuelo exceeds expectations by taking at least 7–8 turns, then she receives a rating of +1 and a rating of +2 if she takes at least 9 turns within a 20-minute small-group activity. More important, GAS is also a way to measure progress across multiple goals. For

Table 7.2. Example of Goal Attainment Scaling for Consuelo

Goal attainment levels	Goal 1: Increase turn taking	Goal 2: Ask partner-focused questions	Goal 3: Respond contingently to questions
Best expected outcome (+2)	Takes at least 9 turns during 20-minute small-group activity	Asks at least two partner-focused questions to at least two different people when arriving in the classroom in the morning (no prompts)	Responds to at least 70% of open-ended questions posed by educator (no prompts)
More than expected outcome (+1)	Takes at least 7–8 turns during 20-minute small-group activity	Asks at least two partner-focused questions with one person when arriving in the classroom in the morning (no prompts)	Responds to at least 60% of open-ended questions posed by educator (no prompts)
Expected outcome (0)	Takes at least 4–6 turns during 20-minute small-group activity	Asks one partner-focused question to one person when arriving in the classroom in the morning (no prompts)	Responds to 50% of open-ended questions posed by educator (no prompts)
Less than expected outcome (–1)	Takes 1–3 turns during 20-minute small-group activity	Asks one partner-focused question to one person when arriving in the classroom in the morning (following expectant delay or point toward augmentative and alternative communication [AAC] device)	Responds to 50% of open-ended questions posed by educator (following expectant delay)
Worst expected outcome (–2)	Takes no turns during 20-minute small-group activity	Asks one partner-focused question to one person when arriving in the classroom in the morning (following aided AAC model)	Responds to fewer than 50% of open-ended questions posed by educator (following expectant delay or more intrusive prompt)

example, for the goals listed in Table 7.2, if Consuelo achieves a rating of 0 for Goal 1, a −1 for Goal 2, and a +1 for Goal 3, then her overall progress is at the 0 level (i.e., 0 + [−1] + 1 = 0). In other words, she met expectations for the overall level of expected progress, even though she did not meet expectations with one of her goals. This type of feedback can be both helpful and encouraging for educators and families.

There are also electronic methods for keeping track of student progress. The EasyTally of Performance, developed by the Augmentative and Alternative Communication–Rehabilitation Engineering Research Center (AAC-RERC), is a free software program that an educator can use to track progress for each skill being targeted for a given student. The educator can input data to track percent correct for each target, percent correct for each skill, number of opportunities to practice each target, and levels of cueing that the student required (Ball, 2007). In addition, some AAC devices now have the capability to track and print out all messages that are created on the device (i.e., an automatically created language sample). This feature comes, for example, with all Prentke Romich Company devices and also on the DynaVox IV and V models. Furthermore, the Universal Language Activity Monitor (U-LAM) is designed to enable other AAC devices, including older devices, to have this feature and is available for a free 60-day trial (AAC Institute, n.d.).

Caution is warranted, however, when enabling this feature on any AAC device. It is critical that the educator has permission from the student as well as the parents to collect data from an AAC device. Students, like everyone else, are entitled to have private conversations with others, and it is unethical to examine messages that were created outside of the immediate presence of the educator without explicit consent. Furthermore, there are particular concerns when working with minors who may not be able to provide true informed consent or assent, which will likely be the case with many early language users. In addition, unless the educator is present, it is not possible to determine precisely who authored a particular message on a device. This concern has implications not only for confidentiality but also for analysis. Educators must be confident that the data that they are analyzing were truly generated by the student. One method for controlling this issue is to only turn on the language monitoring feature when the educator is present. Also, as educators should be using aided AAC modeling throughout the school day, determining authorship of messages can be challenging (although some devices enable special codes for alternative users). Educators must keep all of these issues in mind if they choose to use this feature on devices.

Once transcripts are generated, one option for automatically analyzing the electronic data is to use the Performance Report Tool (PeRT), which provides 17 measures based on the electronically generated language samples (AAC Institute, 2007). This program can be used to analyze data created on Prentke Romich Company devices and the DynaVox DV4 and MT4 devices. It is important to remember, however, that students who use AAC are multimodal communicators. Beginning communicators and early language users typically use many modes to communicate, and an electronically generated language sample and analysis will not capture the full range of communication for these students. Some students, for example, will use multiple modes within one message, such as a student who signs MORE and then uses his or her device to add APPLE. The device, in this case, would only capture the word APPLE, even though the student generated a two-symbol message. When educators are fully aware of these issues, they can use these helpful tools responsibly to assist with the complex task of monitoring their students' progress.

CONCLUSION

Many children in school settings are beginning communicators or early language users. This chapter presented a framework for considering relevant skills, intervention techniques, partner training, and curricular contexts for these students. Irrespective of the specifics of an individual student's profile or the specific circumstances of a given classroom, there is consistent evidence for the types of skills that can be targeted and the manner in which these skills can be addressed by educators attempting to assist beginning communicators and early language users with communication development. With internal and external factors taken into consideration and appropriate AAC systems in place, educators can feel confident in their efforts to identify and target functional goals with their students in the classroom context and beyond. In this way, students receive critical preparation for demanding classrooms and have opportunities to meet challenging and relevant academic goals.

REFERENCES

AAC Institute. (2007). *Performance Report Tool* (PeRT). Retrieved from http://www.aacinstitute.org/Resources/ProductsandServices/PeRT/intro.html

AAC Institute. (n.d.). *Universal Activity Language Monitor* (U-LAM). Retrieved from http://www.aacinstitute.org/Resources/ProductsandServices/U-LAM/intro.html

American Speech-Language-Hearing Association. (2004, November). *Supply and demand for speech-language pathologist's resource list.* Retrieved from http://www.asha.org/NR/rdonlyres/9D2ECE6A-AC53-4968-A4973-4960AF4558CC4964D4974/4960/WorkforceUpdateSLP.pdf

Ball, L. (2007). *EasyTally of Performance.* Retrieved from http://aac.unl.edu/reference/EasyTally.doc

Beukelman, D.R., & Mirenda, P. (2005). *Augmentative and alternative communication: Supporting children and adults with complex communication needs* (3rd ed.). Baltimore: Paul H. Brookes Publishing Co.

Binger, C., Berens, J., Kent-Walsh, J., & Taylor, S. (2008). The impacts of aided AAC interventions on AAC use, speech, and symbolic gestures. *Seminars in Speech and Language, 29,* 146–154.

Binger, C., Kent-Walsh, J., Berens, J., Del Campo, S., & Rivera, D. (2008). Teaching Latino parents to support the multi-symbol message productions of their children who require AAC. *Augmentative and Alternative Communication, 24*(4).

Binger, C., & Light, J. (2007). The effect of aided AAC modeling on the expression of multi-symbol messages by preschoolers who use AAC. *Augmentative and Alternative Communication, 23,* 30–43.

Blackstone, S. (1999). Clinical news: Communication partners. *Augmentative Communication News, 12,* 1.

Bondy, A.S., & Frost, L.A. (1994). The Picture Exchange Communication System. *Focus on Autistic Behavior, 9*(3), 1–19.

Bopp, K., Brown, K., & Mirenda, P. (2004). Speech-language pathologists' roles in the delivery of positive behavior support for individuals with developmental disabilities. *American Journal of Speech-Language Pathology, 13,* 5–19.

Bridwell, N. (1998). *Clifford the big red dog.* Pueblo, CO: Scholastic.

Cole, S., Horvath, B., Chapman, C., Deschenes, C., Ebeling, D., & Sprague, J. (2000). *Adapting curriculum and instruction in inclusive classrooms* (2nd ed.). Port Chester, NY: National Professional Resources.

Davis, C.A., Reichle, J., & Southard, K. (1998). Teaching children with severe disabilities to utilize nonobligatory conversational opportunities: An application of high-probability requests. *Journal of The Association for Persons with Severe Handicaps, 23,* 57–68.

Davis, C.A., Reichle, J., & Southard, K. (2000). High-probability requests and a preferred item as a distractor: Increasing successful transitions in children with behavior problems. *Education & Treatment of Children, 23,* 423–440.

Downing, J. (2005a). Inclusive education for high school students with severe intellectual disabilities: Supporting communication. *Augmentative and Alternative Communication, 21,* 132–148.

Downing, J. (2005b). *Teaching communication skills to students with severe disabilities* (2nd ed.). Baltimore: Paul H. Brookes Publishing Co.

Drager, K., Light, J., Speltz, J., Fallon, K., & Jeffries, L. (2003). The performance of typically developing 2 1/2-year-olds on dynamic display AAC technologies with different system layouts and language organizations. *Journal of Speech, Language, and Hearing Research, 46,* 298–312.

Drager, K., Postal, V., Carrolus, L., Castellano, M., Gagliano, C., & Glynn, J. (2006). The effect of aided language modeling on symbol comprehension and production in two preschoolers with autism. *American Journal of Speech Language Pathology, 15,* 112–125.

Fenson, L., Dale, P., Reznick, S., Thal, D.J., Bates, E., Hartung, J., Pethick, S., & Reilly, J. (1993). *MacArthur Communicative Development Inventories.* San Diego: Singular Publishing Group.

Gee, K., Graham, N., Goetz, L., Oshima, G., & Yoshioka, K. (1991). Teaching students to request the continuation of routine activities by using time delay and decreasing physical assistance in the context of chain interruption. *Journal of The Association for Persons with Severe Handicaps, 16,* 154–167.

Giangreco, M. (1996). What do I do now? A teacher's guide to including students with disabilities. *Educational Leadership, 53,* 56–59.

Giangreco, M., Broer, S., Stephen, M., & Edelman, S. (1999). The tip of the iceberg: Determining whether paraprofessional support is needed for students with disabilities in general education settings. *Journal of The Association for Persons with Severe Handicaps, 24*(4), 281–291.

Giangreco, M., Broer, S., Stephen, M., & Edelman, S. (2001). Teacher engagement with students with disabilities: Differences between paraprofessional service delivery models. *Journal of The Association for Persons with Severe Handicaps, 26*(2), 75–86.

Giangreco, M.F., Cloninger, C.J., & Iverson, V.S. (1998). *Choosing Outcomes and Accommodations for Children (COACH): A guide to educational planning for students with disabilities* (2nd ed.). Baltimore: Paul H. Brookes Publishing Co.

Giangreco, M., Edelman, S., & Broer, S. (2001a). Paraprofessional support of students with disabilities: Literature from the past decade. *Exceptional Children, 68*(1), 45–63.

Giangreco, M., Edelman, S., & Broer, S. (2001b). Respect, appreciation, and acknowledgement of paraprofessionals who support students with disabilities. *Exceptional Children, 67*(4), 485–498.

Goetz, L., Gee, K., & Sailor, W. (1985). Using a behavior chain interruption strategy to teach communication skills to students with severe disabilities. *Journal of The Association for Persons with Severe Handicaps, 10,* 21–30.

Houghton, J., Bronicki, B., & Guess, D. (1987). Opportunities to express preferences and make choices among students with severe disabilities in classroom settings. *Journal of The Association for Persons with Severe Handicaps, 12,* 18–27.

Hunt, P., Alwell, M., & Goetz, L. (1991). Interacting with peers through conversation turntaking with a communication book adaptation. *Augmentative and Alternative Communication, 7*(2), 117–126.

Hunt, P., & Goetz, L. (1997). Research on inclusive educational programs, practices, and outcomes for students with severe disabilities. *Journal of Special Education, 31,* 3–35.

Hunt, P., Soto, G., Maier, J., & Doering, K. (2003). Collaborative teaming to support students at risk and students with severe disabilities in general education classrooms. *Exceptional Children, 69,* 315–332.

Hunt, P., Soto, G., Maier, J., Liboiron, N., & Bae, S. (2004). Collaborative teaming to support preschoolers with severe disabilities who are placed in general education early childhood programs. *Topics in Early Childhood Special Education, 24,* 123–142.

Hunt, P., Soto, G., Maier, J., Müller, E., & Goetz, L. (2002). Collaborative teaming to support students with augmentative and alternative communication needs in general education classrooms. *Augmentative and Alternative Communication, 18,* 20–35.

Johnston, S., Nelson, C., Evans, J., & Palazolo, K. (2003). The use of visual supports in teaching young children with autism spectrum disorder to initiate interactions. *Augmentative and Alternative Communication, 19,* 86–103.

Jorgensen, C.M., McSheehan, M., & Sonnenmeier, R.M. (2007). Presumed competence reflected in the educational programs of students with IDD before and after The Beyond Access professional development intervention. *Journal of Intellectual & Developmental Disability, 32,* 248–262.

Kent-Walsh, J. (2003). *The effects of an educational assistant instructional program on the communicative turns of students who use augmentative and alternative communication during book-reading activities.* Unpublished doctoral dissertation, Penn State University, University Park, PA.

Kent-Walsh, J., & Light, J. (2003). General education teachers' experiences with inclusion of students who use augmentative and alternative communication. *Augmentative and Alternative Communication, 19,* 104–124.

Kent-Walsh, J., & McNaughton, D. (2005). Communication partner instruction in AAC: Present practices and future directions. *Augmentative and Alternative Communication, 21,* 195–204.

Koul, R.K., & Lloyd, L.L. (1994). Survey of professional preparation in augmentative and alternative communication in speech-language pathology and special education programs. *American Journal of Speech-Language Pathology, 3,* 13–22.

Light, J.C., & Binger, C. (1998). *Building communicative competence with individuals who use augmentative and alternative communication.* Baltimore: Paul H. Brookes Publishing Co.

Light, J., Binger, C., Agate, T.L., & Ramsey, K.N. (1999). Teaching partner-focused questions to individuals who use augmentative and alternative communication to enhance their communicative competence. *Journal of Speech, Language, and Hearing Research, 42,* 241–255.

Light, J., Collier, B., & Parnes, P. (1985). Communicative interaction between young nonspeaking physically disabled children and their primary caregivers: Part I: Discourse patterns. *Augmentative and Alternative Communication, 1,* 74–83.

McSheehan, M., Sonnenmeier, R.M., Jorgensen, C.M., & Turner, K. (2006). Beyond communication access: Promoting learning of the general education curriculum by students with significant disabilities. *Topics in Language Disorders, 26,* 266–290.

Reichle, J., Beukelman, D.R., & Light, J.C. (Eds.). (2002). *Augmentative and alternative communication series: Exemplary practices for beginning communicators: Implications for AAC.* Baltimore: Paul H. Brookes Publishing Co.

Rescorla, L. (1989). The Language Development Survey: A screening tool for delayed language in toddlers. *Journal of Speech and Hearing Disorders, 54,* 587–599.

Romski, M.A., & Sevcik, R. (2005). Augmentative communication and early intervention: Myths and realities. *Infants and Young Children, 18,* 174–185.

Romski, M.A., Sevcik, R.A., & Forrest, S.C. (2001). Assistive technology and augmentative communication in inclusive early childhood programs. In M.J. Guralnick (Ed.), *Early childhood inclusion: Focus on change* (pp. 465–479). Baltimore: Paul H. Brookes Publishing Co.

Rowland, C., & Schweigert, P.D. (2002). Cognitive skills and AAC. In D.R. Beukelman & J. Reichle (Vol. Eds.) & J.C. Light, D.R. Beukelman, & J. Reichle (Series Eds.), *Augmentative and alternative communication series: Communicative competence for individuals who use AAC: From research to effective practice* (pp. 241–276). Baltimore: Paul H. Brookes Publishing Co.

Schlosser, R. (2002). Outcomes measurement in AAC. In D.R. Beukelman & J. Reichle (Vol. Eds.) & J.C. Light, D.R. Beukelman, & J. Reichle (Series Eds.), *Augmentative and alternative communication series: Communicative competence for individuals who use AAC: From research to effective practice* (pp. 479–513). Baltimore: Paul H. Brookes Publishing Co.

Sevcik, R.A., & Romski, M.A. (2002). The role of language comprehension in establishing early augmented conversations. In D.R. Beukelman & J. Reichle (Vol. Eds.) & J. Reichle, D.R. Beukelman, & J.C. Light (Series Eds.), *Augmentative and alternative communication series: Exemplary practices for beginning communicators: Implications for AAC* (pp. 453–474). Baltimore: Paul H. Brookes Publishing Co.

Sigafoos, J. (1999). Creating opportunities for augmentative and alternative communication: Strategies for involving people with developmental disabilities. *Augmentative and Alternative Communication, 15,* 183–190.

Sigafoos, J., Arthur-Kelly, M., & Butterfield, N. (2006). *Enhancing everyday communication for children with disabilities.* Baltimore: Paul H. Brookes Publishing Co.

Sigafoos, J., Drasgow, E., O'Reilly, M., & Tait, K. (2004). Tutorial: Teaching communicative rejecting to children with severe disabilities. *American Journal of Speech-Language Pathology, 13,* 31–42.

Sigafoos, J., & Mirenda, P. (2002). Strengthening communicative behaviors for gaining access to desired items and activities. In D.R. Beukelman & J. Reichle (Vol. Eds.) & J. Reichle, D.R. Beukelman, & J.C. Light (Series Eds.), *Augmentative and alternative communication series: Exemplary practices for beginning communicators: Implications for AAC* (pp. 123–156). Baltimore: Paul H. Brookes Publishing Co.

Sigafoos, J., & Roberts-Pennell, D. (1999). Wrong-item format: A promising intervention for teaching socially appropriate forms of rejecting to children with developmental disabilities. *Augmentative and Alternative Communication, 15,* 135–140.

Sonnenmeier, R.M., McSheehan, M., & Jorgensen, C.M. (2005). A case study of team supports for a student with autism's communication and engagement within the general educational curriculum: Preliminary report of the beyond access mode. *Augmentative and Alternative Communication, 21,* 101–115.

Soto, G., Müller, E., Hunt, P., & Goetz, L. (2001). Critical issues in the inclusion of students who use augmentative and alternative communication: An educational team perspective. *Augmentative and Alternative Communication, 17*(2), 62–72.

Spooner, F., & Browder, D.M. (2006). Why teach the general curriculum? In D.M. Browder & F. Spooner (Eds.), *Teaching language arts, math, and science to students with significant cognitive disabilities* (pp. 1–13). Baltimore: Paul H. Brookes Publishing Co.

Sturm, J., & Clendon, S.A. (2004). AAC, language, and literacy: Fostering the relationship. *Topics in Language Disorders, 24,* 76–91.

Sturm, J., Spadorcia, S.A., Cunningham, J.W., Cali, K.S., Staples, A., Erikson, K., et al. (2006). What happens to reading between first and third grade? Implications for students who use AAC. *Augmentative and Alternative Communication, 22,* 21–36.

Treviranus, J., & Roberts, V. (2002). Supporting competent motor control of the AAC system. In D.R. Beukelman & J. Reichle (Vol. Eds.) & J.C. Light, D.R. Beukelman, & J. Reichle (Series Eds.), *Augmentative and alternative communication series: Communicative competence for individuals who use AAC* (pp. 199–240). Baltimore: Paul H. Brookes Publishing Co.

8

Supporting More Advanced Linguistic Communicators in the Classroom

Carole Zangari and Gail Van Tatenhove

Proficiency in language and discourse is a critical skill for success in school (Corson, 1988). Children spend about 1,000 hours per year in school engaged in a range of language-rich activities, including listening to the teacher, asking and answering questions, collaborating with classmates, participating in discussions, reading literature, and writing text. Almost all activity within the general education classroom is linked to the assumption that children come to school with the knowledge of how to engage in extended discourse (McCabe & Rollins, 1994), with most learning occurring when teachers talk with students and students talk with each other.

Most typically developing students enter school having mastered the fundamentals of their native language and can use that language effectively in the classroom. At school entry, children generally have a basic understanding of what language is and "have an implicit command of the linguistic-communicative system for the everyday demands of comprehension and production" (Silliman & Wilkinson, 1991, p. 42). It is assumed that children coming to school have already learned to talk so that they can "talk to learn."

By definition, children with significant expressive communication impairments do not fit this student profile, though many do enter school with a great deal of linguistic knowledge (Lund & Light, 2003). In this chapter, the phrase *more advanced linguistic communicator* refers to a student with language production skills corresponding to 36 months of age and beyond. These students communicate in sentences and use morphological features, such as regular plurals (e.g., *shoes*), present progressive verb tenses (e.g., *going, seeing, eating*), irregular verb tenses (e.g., *fell, ate*), prepositions (e.g., *in, on*), possessives (e.g., *daddy's*), early conjunctions (e.g., *but, and),* and question words (e.g., *who, what, where*). Students with more advanced language skills have made two transitions: 1) from illocutionary to locutionary communication and 2) from a focus on semantics to a focus on syntax (Paul, 1997). These students may or may not be sufficiently competent with their augmentative and alternative communication (AAC) systems to participate actively and fully within the classroom. In most cases, they are not yet using literate language[1]. Even children without communication difficulties have limitations in semantics, grammatical concepts, and morphology at this level. Students with AAC needs will undoubtedly experience even greater limitations. Thus, it is important to acknowledge that although these students have a good start in language acquisition, they are not functioning at the level of their peers. There is still much that these students need to learn to use language successfully within the classroom.

The road to literate language can be bumpy. Many students who use AAC must develop skills in their native language while simultaneously learning their AAC tools and strategies (Kovach &

---

[1]Westby (1985) described literate language as the use of language "to monitor and reflect on experience, and reason about, plan, and predict experiences" (p. 181). See Paul (2007) for a discussion of the relationship between oral and literate language.

Kenyon, 2003; Williams, 2005). These dual priorities—further development of language and of AAC-related skills—make well-planned, clearly defined goals and objectives essential for the educational achievement of these students. This chapter discusses three areas significant to the development of more advanced language in students who use AAC. It begins by delineating some of the critical characteristics of AAC systems for this population and then presents priority roles for speech-language pathologists (SLPs) and educators. The chapter concludes with a discussion of language intervention related to vocabulary, grammar, and narrative language.

CRITICAL CHARACTERISTICS OF AAC SYSTEMS

Students with more advanced language skills may or may not enter the classroom with an effective AAC system in place. The team of people supporting them will be challenged to develop a system that facilitates language development while meeting the educational demands of the classroom. It is beyond the scope of this chapter to discuss all the possible variations of AAC systems that could be designed; rather, critical characteristics of AAC systems are discussed as they relate to the more advanced linguistic communicator in the classroom.

AAC Systems Must Include Multiple Modalities

It is a misconception to think of AAC as synonymous with technology. Rather, AAC represents a broad range of strategies and technologies. To meet the educational demands of the classroom, advanced linguistic communicators must tap into their full repertoire of multimodal communication strategies (Foreman & Crews, 1998; Iacono, Mirenda, & Beukelman, 1993). In addition to unaided strategies, such as natural speech, signs, and gestures, students with more advanced language abilities generally require both sophisticated AAC technology and low-tech communication aids.

_____   Jeremiah, a kindergartner with significant apraxia of speech, is an example of a student whose AAC system is emerging to meet his language needs. He uses his natural speech and gestures across contexts and supplements his messages with a high-tech speech-generating device (SGD). His teacher recently introduced the use of an alphabet card to provide him with a quick way of responding to the many classroom activities that involve discussions of letters and letter names. The team recognized the need for a more comprehensive AAC tool to serve as a back-up for the SGD and is in the process of creating a portable communication book for this purpose. _____

AAC Systems Must Be Linguistically Based

The second critical component is that the AAC system be linguistically based. Linguistically based systems are those that provide sufficient language power to support the student with more advanced language in the classroom. A linguistically based system must have sufficient and appropriate vocabulary along with morphological variations of root words. Although many other strategies might be used to meet a short-term communication need (e.g., a topical/activity-based picture display on the planets), students with more advanced language require personal communication systems that allow them to manipulate word forms and express novel messages. These personal, linguistically based systems often include both SGDs and manual (i.e., nonelectronic or no-tech) communication aids.

There are more than 100 commercially available SGDs on the market, each with a variety of features. While some of these are linguistically based, others are not. Some devices are simple, single message devices, while other, more sophisticated, devices have the potential to hold thousands of prestored words, phrases, and sentences. Some devices include features, such as the ability to play MP3 files, accessibility to cell phone technology, and built-in digital cameras. While many of these features make for interesting applications with the SGD, the key feature of a linguistically based SGD is how it provides and manages language for both oral and written language output. Other device features may be desirable and provide extra benefits, but a device that cannot adequately support language in the classroom cannot adequately support the student in the classroom.

Prior to the invention of SGDs, language was provided to students needing aided AAC systems through nonelectronic (manual) communication boards and books. In many places throughout the world, manual communication tools continue to be the primary means of aided communication. They are typically custom designed and built for individual students (Vanderheiden & Grilley, 1976; Vicker, 1974).

One of the main challenges of making manual boards and books for students with more advanced language involves "real estate," or ways in which messages are situated on the aid. The intent of the nonelectronic tool is to give the preliterate student sufficient vocabulary and morphology to develop and express language. For students who use wheelchairs, there is a limited amount of real estate available on the laptray. For ambulatory students, there is a limited amount of real estate a student can carry. If a student who uses a wheelchair has a laptray that measures 20 inches wide and 10 inches deep, the tray can hold a picture display with approximately 200 one-inch pictures. Two hundred pictures/words is a good start but provides access to significantly less words than those used by a typically developing student.

The challenge is daunting. How can the preliterate student have access to more words with a limited amount of space? To expand the real estate available other designs evolved, including multiple simultaneous displays and multiple sequential displays (Vanderheiden & Grilley, 1976; Vicker, 1974). Both designs provide access to key vocabulary needed for the use of generative language in spontaneous conversation. Multiple *sequential* displays do this by arranging vocabulary on different pages, levels, or screens. In this approach, students may have to navigate through several pages or screens to construct a single sentence. This type of display is used frequently by students of different ages. Porter and her colleagues have demonstrated the use of multiple sequential displays with children who access messages through partner-assisted scanning (Porter, 2000; Porter, Kirkland, & Dunne, 1998). Multiple *simultaneous* displays provide continuous access to a set of key words and provide additional options in selected categories of words. For example, a communication board might have a fixed set of pronouns in one area and a set of descriptors on miniature pages (a set of strips attached to the board) that the student can page through. Figure 8.1 depicts examples of both types of communication tools.

Some linguistically based communication aids use combinational strategies to increase the total number of concepts that can be represented within the confines of a restricted space. In this approach, symbols representing concepts such as *opposite*, *same as*, or *sounds like* are added to the display. When used in combination with existing words, students have access to a broader range of concepts they can express. Landon, for example, is able to use these strategies to convey additional ideas. In his communication book, *big* + /same as/ could be used to express words such as *large* or *huge*, and *yell* + /opposite of/ could represent *whisper*. Although this approach does not give students the full control they would have with an unlimited vocabulary set, it does offer preliterate students an opportunity to express a wider variety of concepts than would otherwise be available to them. Linguistically based communication aids should also include the alphabet, whenever possible, both to take advantage of and to further develop literacy skills.

Manual communication boards and books are neither outdated nor obsolete. They remain a valuable option in the range of AAC options useful for students with more advanced language skills. These tools can be used for language instruction, for removing operational issues from the language learning process, and as a back-up system to any SGD.

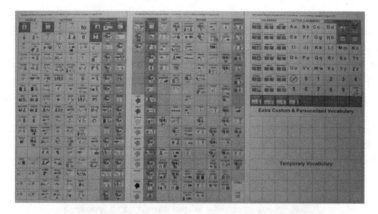

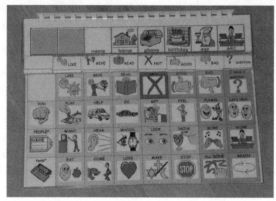

Figure 8.1.   Examples of linguistically based communication tools.

AAC Systems Must Feature Core Vocabulary

Core vocabulary refers to high-frequency, multipurpose, commonly occurring words from a range of word classes that are a central part of an individual's AAC system. These high-frequency words include approximately 78% of what adults and children actually say and are drawn from a core of fewer than 400 words (Beukelman, Jones, & Rowan, 1989). These reusable, common words are consistent across clinical populations, activities, places, topics, and demographic groups, including individuals using AAC systems (Marvin, Beukelman, & Bilyeu, 1994; Stuart, Beukelman, & King, 1997).

Core vocabulary is the central element of linguistically based AAC systems. Linguistically based SGDs have the potential to be programmed with a robust set of 300–400 high-frequency words that can help students become literate language users. A robust set of reusable, common words should be drawn from all word classes, including pronouns (e.g., *I, me, you, him*), verbs (e.g., *go, want, put, get, let*), helping verbs (e.g., *is, can, could, will, was, did),* adjectives (e.g., *good, bad, more*), adverbs (e.g., *again, now, here, there*), prepositions, (e.g., *in, on, with, of, for*), determiners (e.g., *this, that*), conjunctions (e.g., *and, or, because*), interjections (e.g., *yes, no, please, sorry*), questions words (e.g., *who, when, where*) and finally nouns (e.g., *idea, way, thing, stuff).* (See http://aac.unl.edu/VLN1.html for a partial listing of robust core vocabulary.)

Becoming a fluent user of core vocabulary is a top priority for students who use AAC and are on the path to literate language. Because they are used so frequently, core vocabulary words should be situated on the SGD in a place that allows for quick and easy access. Instruction geared toward mastering conversation with core words should figure prominently in the individualized education program (IEP), with sufficient opportunities for initial teaching, building automaticity, and generalizing skills across activities and environments.

AAC Systems Must Provide Access to Morphological Variations

A linguistically based AAC tool includes grammatical markers (Sutton, Gallagher, Morford, & Shahnaz, 2000). Students with advanced language skills need communication tools that will allow them to communicate in a precise and grammatically correct fashion. Although precision and grammar do not always have the highest priority in an interactive exchange, students with more advanced language skills need opportunities to further develop and practice these skills. Their AAC systems must allow them to pluralize, vary verb tenses, create comparative and superlative adjectives, and delineate possession, among other things. Table 8.1 lists 14 of the most critical morphemes that should be available to students with more advanced language in order for them to become linguistically proficient. Although typically developing children generally master use of these morphemes by age 5, children who use linguistically based AAC tools may not use them correctly until later in childhood, especially if access to an appropriate SGD has been limited (Brown, 1973).

To develop literate language, students using SGDs must have early and consistent access to morphological variations that permit productions of mature, grammatically correct forms. For example, a low-tech SGD might simply have the student add an -ed ending to a word to make it past tense. In English, however, many of the most frequently used verbs are irregular in the past tense (e.g., tell/told, go/went, eat/ate, say/said). Having access to a strategy of simply attaching an -ed is an improvement over systems without past tense options but remains quite limiting and may prevent these children from speaking in a grammatically correct fashion. One would assume that this approach would hinder further language development, but it is also likely to influence how these students are perceived by themselves and others. Given a choice between speaking incorrectly (e.g., "I knowed the answer." "He getted a new car.") and not speaking at all, some students will choose the latter. While experimentation with correct morphological forms is a common language learning experience, we generally do not want to limit students who use AAC and require them to communicate this way in the classroom. Experimentation with morphological forms is a natural part of language acquisition, and students who use AAC should have the freedom to engage in verbal play. However, students must also be given tools that allow them to experiment with the grammatically correct form and not be forced to communicate telegraphically, imprecisely, or incorrectly.

Table 8.1. Critical morphemes for inclusion in linguistically based AAC systems

Morpheme	Examples
Present progressive	Jared writing
Preposition in	Computer in classroom
Preposition on	Tia on swing
Regular plural -s	Books, legs, glasses
Irregular past	Went, said, came, told
Possessive 's	Teacher's desk; Jared's girlfriend
Uncontractible copula (i.e., to be as a main verb)	(Who's absent?) She is.
Articles	Write the date, add a picture.
Regular past -ed	Needed, worked, believed
Regular third person -s	Gives, knows, helps
Irregular third person	Has, does
Uncontractible auxiliary	(Who is going?) We are. (Who copied it?) She did.
Contractible copula	Jared's tall. They're always late.
Contractible auxiliary	Emma's not happy. She'll be fine.

Source: Brown (1973).

AAC Systems Must Have the Potential for Growth and Expansion

Linguistically based systems provide the architecture for language growth in that they can be systematically expanded to include additional linguistic forms and structures. This is very important for students with more advanced language, particularly in vocabulary acquisition and the development of narrative language skills. Teams who are supporting these students should consider how the AAC system accommodates the addition of new core vocabulary and new morphological forms. Teams should also evaluate the ways in which the student's AAC system accommodates infrequently used vocabulary that may only be used temporarily, such as content words from a science lesson or place names associated with an upcoming field trip.

Much of this relates to vocabulary organization. Teams should carefully consider how words are stored on each component of a student's AAC system. Because literacy skills are developed over several years, language is generally represented on AAC tools using pictures accompanied by the written gloss (meaning). There are currently three picture-based strategies for organizing and retrieving vocabulary in high-tech SGDs. Each offers advantages and has limitations that affect students who use AAC in the classroom.

Multiple Levels, Screens, or Pages   One approach for organizing vocabulary employs multiple pages, screens, or levels using pictures that have a one-to-one correspondence to each word, phrase, or sentence in the AAC tool. Students must learn and memorize the meaning of each picture, which may be easier for some word classes (e.g., object nouns, action verbs) than for abstract concepts that are more difficult to depict (e.g., *with, some, for, can*). The picture symbols are most often arranged in grid format (although the use of visual scene displays is becoming more common). This approach is frequently used and is the traditional way for developing manual communication boards and pages for communication books/wallets (see discussion on multiple sequential and multiple simultaneous displays). It is also used on many SGDs with static displays and dynamic screens. How students compose their messages depends on the way in which vocabulary is organized on the various pages. In general, students using this type of communication aid must navigate between pages, levels, or screens. Because this approach requires a one-to-one correspondence between vocabulary entries (referents) and pictures (symbols), it can result in a large number of individual pictures across multiple pages, screens, or levels.

Semantic Encoding   A second approach used in SGDs is semantic encoding, which draws on the multiple meanings inherent in pictures (e.g., apple makes a person think of *apple, food, eat, red, hungry*). These multiple meaning pictures are displayed in traditional grids of pictures and combined into short sequences (i.e., 1–3 pictures) to communicate individual words, phrases, or sentences. This approach is designed to reduce the number of pictures within the system by using each picture in multiple ways. Students using this approach must learn a system of associations so that they can retrieve words through their picture sequences. Semantic encoding, like the multiple page approach, also has roots in the development of manual communication boards, particularly manual boards that systematically used word-altering strategies.

Visual Screen Displays   A third, relatively new approach is through visual screen displays (VSDs). VSDs use a highly contextualized visual scene, such as a photograph of the child in the family kitchen sitting at the table, with messages embedded under different elements of the photograph. This approach portrays generic and/or personalized contexts with a variable number of words, phrases, or sentences embedded in "hotspots" on each page or screen. To communicate a word or idea not embedded in that screen requires navigating to different scenes to locate the required word and select the hotspot. Research on this type of approach is optimistic in terms of the initial learning of vocabulary (Light et. al., 2004), but the approach is too new to determine its long-range application for providing a child with a linguistically based system, as defined in this chapter.

Summary   Each of these architectural approaches manages vocabulary and morphology growth in a different manner, and decisions regarding which approach to utilize should be made following a comprehensive evaluation with the input of important stakeholders. Teams should carefully consider how each component of the student's multi-modal AAC system supports the development of literate language and accommodates growth and expansion.

PRIORITY ROLES FOR
SPEECH-LANGUAGE PATHOLOGISTS AND EDUCATORS

Helping students with AAC needs achieve their academic and communicative potential is a daunting responsibility. This section discusses six priority roles for educators and SLPs who support these students that align with Paul's (2007) practitioner guidelines for changing language behavior through facilitation, maintenance, and induction.

- *Priority 1:* Provide students with immediate access to an AAC system with which they can effectively formulate novel utterances, participate in academic and social interactions, and express their needs and desires.

Students with AAC needs who have more advanced linguistic skills must be given quick access to tools and strategies that allow them to use their language skills to participate, learn, and develop and maintain social relationships. An AAC system with multiple components should be developed so that the student can bid for conversational turns, share unique and spontaneous thoughts, and communicate highly predictable utterances in a timely fashion. This system must allow the student to demonstrate what he or she is learning so that instruction can be appropriately tailored to meet his or her needs.

_____   Tia's initial AAC system in the third grade emphasized her ability to express concepts despite the relative lack of specific academic terms. While she could not use it to say *Pluto*, she could say *small, most far away, not one anymore, 8 not 9,* and *big mistake.* This gave her teacher considerable insight into what Tia really understood about the status of Pluto. In actuality, Tia demonstrated more of what she knew using these imprecise descriptions than would have been the case if someone had programmed in the exact name of this planetlike body into her SGD.   _____

- *Priority 2:* Develop and implement a long-range AAC plan for systematically developing the student's AAC system beginning in preschool and continuing through elementary, middle, and high school. The AAC system must contain the critical characteristics described in the introduction (e.g., linguistically based, multimodal) to optimize the student's chance of developing literate language.

Long-range planning is an essential element of a well-developed AAC system. The plan should essentially explain how the student's initial AAC system will develop into a complex and sophisticated system that leads to a coordinated progression of language and literacy skills.

_____   At a later stage, Tia's AAC system became more precise and allowed her to use the comparative and superlative forms (e.g., *smaller, farthest*). In some cases, curriculum-specific fringe vocabulary was added (e.g., *perimeter, civil rights, friction*), but the emphasis remained on expanding core vocabulary to include a richer pool of Tier 2 words (Beck, McKeown, & Kucan, 2002). Words from vocabulary lessons, such as *especially, base,* and *productive,* were added to her expressive communication tools to allow Tia to experiment with these words and use them in face-to-face interaction and writing. Adding words that had multiple meanings allowed Tia to use language creatively. Having a larger pool of words helped Tia's vocabulary mature and gave depth and richness to her language.   _____

- *Priority 3:* Develop and implement a long-range plan for building literate language.

In addition to a long-range plan for the AAC system, practitioners must develop an intervention plan that is theoretically sound and builds an expressive language base of standard core vocabulary, personalized core vocabulary, and fringe vocabulary (Smith, 2006). The long-range plan should describe a systematic approach for language intervention that expands the student's skills in morphology, syntax, and discourse. It should build semantics, narrative skills (both personal narratives and fictional stories), and promote development of meta-linguistic skills. Finally, it should be jointly implemented by the SLP and educator in a model that best matches the student's learning profile.

_____ In Tia's case, vocabulary development (semantics) and the use of more complex phrases and sentences were high priorities. The teacher modeled correct syntax and grammar but did not correct Tia's errors in those areas during interactions where lexical richness was a high priority. For example, when asked to recall the definition of *orphans* during a read-aloud segment, the teacher accepted Tia's response, "They doesn't parents," and replied with a recast ("Tia's right. They don't have parents.") that reinforced her efforts at learning new words. By recognizing what Tia did well (shared the correct content) and then modeling the grammatically correct form, the teacher provided both encouragement and instruction. _____

- *Priority 4:* Build a classroom communication environment that prioritizes linguistic expression.

Students with AAC needs require classrooms geared for frequent student–student and student–teacher interactions that maximize opportunities for further language development. The environment must require the student to communicate at his or her current language level and extend the student's learning of new language skills. It must maximize active learning opportunities and meaningful participation and allow the student to use the communication tool and strategy best suited to the context. Adults in the environment should regularly model use of the AAC system (unless the student is completely competent with it). They must use appropriate language facilitation strategies throughout the school day as language learning occurs not just during curricular lessons but in every academic and social encounter.

_____ Adults in Tia's classroom often modeled the use of her SGD as they conversed. Because Tia was a fairly competent device user, the teacher generally required Tia's help to find the specific word she wanted. For example, the teacher might model use of the SGD during conferences about writing and use a think-aloud approach to subtly solicit Tia's assistance (e.g., "Okay, I have *say* but I really want to say *tell*. I wonder if there is a power strip that can help me."). The teacher knew that Tia would most likely rush to show her how to retrieve the desired word. This co-construction of messages equalized the skill differential and maximized Tia's motivation to work hard at verbal expression. _____

- *Priority 5:* Interact with the student in a way which conveys high expectations for the student, models the AAC system, and elicits language at the student's highest level.

It is essential that others in the school set high standards for communicative interaction by consistently expecting and supporting high-level linguistic expression. Adults must gear the interaction so that the student routinely uses utterances appropriate in modality, content, and form for the context at hand.

_____ In Tia's classroom environment, adults made comments peppered with new vocabulary and asked questions that required responses rich in content. They were flexible in allowing students to participate with a single word (signed, spoken, or using AAC) in selected instances but more typically expected phrases and sentences. For example, in shared writing Tia might contribute descriptors such as *good* or *pretty*. As she did with all students, the teacher encouraged Tia to "put tired words to bed" and substitute more precise and vivid language. _____

- *Priority 6:* Train communication partners to use appropriate language elicitation strategies and encourage more advanced linguistic production whenever they communicate with the student.

To achieve their academic potential and become literate linguistic communicators, students with AAC needs require the support of a great many people. Teachers and SLPs must work together to identify ways of eliciting language that is effective in the classroom and develop and implement a plan to train other teachers, aides, therapists, peers, and family members. This may mean helping those individuals gain awareness of what language the student can and should be using in different situations. These stakeholders can also be taught specific language facilitation strategies, such as aided AAC modeling and cloze procedures (Binger & Light, 2007; Blockberger & Johnson, 2003).

INSTRUCTION AND INTERVENTION ISSUES AND STRATEGIES

There is limited published research on how students with AAC needs develop more advanced language skills. Students with AAC needs have different ability levels and styles of language learning (Iacono, 1992; Martinsen & von Tetzchner, 1996). There is evidence that many of these children have reduced comprehension and expression due, at least in part, to limited experiences with linguistically based AAC systems (Berninger & Gans, 1986; Redmond & Johnston, 2001; Sutton & Gallagher, 1993; Udwin & Yule, 1987, 1990). Like other children with communicative challenges, most of these students will need explicit instruction (Goldstein, 2006). This may be particularly true for students who use AAC systems in which the output modalities (e.g., SGDs) differ from the linguistic input they receive (Nelson, 1992). Explicit instruction is efficacious (Rosenshine & Stevens, 1986; Ellis & Worthington, 1994; Tarver, 1996) and may be helpful in addressing challenges that are unique to AAC (Bruno & Trembath, 2006; Sutton, Soto, & Blockberger, 2002). This section of the chapter addresses some of the key issues and strategies that can aid interventionists in planning and implementing instruction that moves the student toward language proficiency.

Many of the language intervention techniques used for speaking students can also be useful for helping students who use AAC gain more mature skills in grammar and vocabulary. Indirect methods, such as modeling the target behavior, are well suited to classroom use. For example, teachers who know their students need to learn to use verbs in the future tense may pepper their own speech with these constructions providing opportunities for incidental learning (e.g., "Art is after lunch with Mrs. McAllister. We *will be going* every Thursday"). Other techniques are used to elicit new word meanings or forms and provide opportunities for practice. These include obligatory adult utterances, such as mands (demands, commands; e.g., "You need to tell your partner if you don't understand"), direct questions, and cloze (i.e., fill-in-the-blank) sentences.

Direct questions can be used for various purposes and can be constructed to elicit many different target behaviors. They can be very effective at helping students formulate ideas (e.g., "How do you think Birdie felt after the storm?") and assess comprehension (e.g., "What part of paragraph one tells us that this happened a long time ago?"). They can also be used to help students elaborate on an initial response (e.g., "Can you tell us more about that?") and identify alternative responses (e.g., "Do you need me? You can say, 'I need some help, please' or ask, 'Can you look at this?'"). Contingent queries are another questioning strategy that can be used to elicit more detailed or specific information (e.g., Student: "Sticker book." SLP: "What about it?" Student: "Take it home." SLP: "Oh, you want to borrow the sticker book and take it home?"). While effective, direct questioning and mands have some significant drawbacks. One limitation is that they cast students in the role of respondent rather than building their capacity for initiating interaction. They also tend to elicit shorter, simpler sentences than less directive approaches. Well-formed comments and declarative statements can often do double duty, eliciting the target word/structure while building the student's ability to communicate under nonobligatory conditions.

_____   Rather than asking Tia specific questions (e.g., "How did Madison feel?"), the SLP routinely used comments to elicit responses (e.g., "I wonder how Madison was feeling when they started without her"). In cases where Tia failed to respond, the teacher could then follow-up with a more directive prompt, either in the form of a question (e.g., "How do you think she felt?") or a declarative sentence (e.g., "I'd like to hear what you think about how she felt." "Tia, we haven't heard from you in awhile"). By using direct questions and mands sparingly, the teacher allowed Tia to become a more proactive user of her language skills.   _____

Another effective intervention technique is to construct sentences with pauses or blank spaces that serve to cue the student to add words that complete the utterance. Also known as cloze or fill-in-the-blank sentences, this technique helps students to understand that a communicative response is expected without being highly directive. Environmental arrangements, such as purposefully providing a wrong answer or feigning misunderstanding, are also effective in eliciting certain linguistic behaviors (Cleave & Fey, 1997). A teacher, for example, might create opportunities for the students to use negative forms like *no, not,* and *don't* by labeling the states incorrectly on a map she is drawing on the board. The reader is referred to Paul (2007) for a more extensive discussion of these and other language teaching techniques.

Vocabulary Instruction

It is estimated that children learn an average of 3,000 new word meanings each year from kindergarten through Grade 12, though the semantic development of students in middle and high school is not well understood (Botting & Adams, 2005; Graves, 1986). Each year, only 300–400 of those new words are taught through direct instruction in the classroom (Stahl, 1991). Students who use AAC need and benefit from explicit instruction in semantics and morphology. Although a portion may need planned intervention to expand their receptive vocabularies, all students with AAC needs require instruction to increase the number of words they use at some point during their school years. All students with AAC needs should have systematic instruction to improve word knowledge and usage; however, there is no existing research that compares various approaches to semantic instruction with this population (Wilkinson & Albert, 2001).

There are two main areas to be considered in designing a program of appropriate vocabulary instruction: expanding the words students *know* and expanding the words they *use*. Indirect strategies, such as listening to adults read aloud and engaging in independent reading, can be part of an effective vocabulary-building program. Direct vocabulary instruction is also needed and may include things such as providing definitions, discerning meanings from contextual cues, and engaging in language experience activities. Many students who use AAC may require more intense vocabulary instruction due to limitations in their background knowledge; however, other elements of robust vocabulary instruction will likely be the same as (or very similar to) instruction for students without disabilities.

Instructional practices in vocabulary development have been criticized for lacking intensity and for overreliance on context (e.g., Beck, McKeown, & McCaslin, 1983; Johnson, 2001) among other things. A systematic approach to teaching new words has been advocated by Beck, McKeown, and Kucan (2002), who categorize vocabulary into three tiers for the purpose of planning instruction. Tier 1 vocabulary are those high-frequency words that form the basis of core vocabulary in many AAC systems (e.g., *happy, she, with, girl*). These words are assumed to be background knowledge in general education programs and are not typically targeted for instruction. Tier 2 words are used fairly often by mature language users and have applicability across a variety of contexts (e.g., *effort, convince, ridiculous*). Tier 2 words make good targets for intervention because of their capacity for frequent use in academic and social situations. Words in Tier 3 are used with much less frequency and are limited to more specific knowledge domains (e.g., *radius, barometer, simile*). Beck and her colleagues have noted that while these types of words are frequently part of content-area instruction, the teaching of vocabulary at the Tier 2 level is likely to provide students with longer-lasting, more functional gains in their word usage patterns. Beck and her colleagues suggest that explicit vocabulary instruction of Tier 2 words can be used to teach 400 words each academic year.

Explicit instruction includes providing a clear explanation of the word meaning using words the students already understand (i.e., student-friendly definitions) and having the students say the word using their natural speech or an AAC modality. Students can then be assisted to look up words in a dictionary or glossary and relate the denotation to their own understanding of the word. Illustrating the word through multiple examples is another important step in vocabulary teaching (e.g., "Let's think about things that are *mandatory*. Taking the math test was not a choice. We *had* to take it. Taking the test was *mandatory*. Can anyone else think of something they *had* to do—something *mandatory*?"). Using graphic organizers can be useful for students who are visual learners (see Figure 8.2 for an example). Comprehension checks can be used to determine how well the students are grasping the semantic concept (e.g., "Give me a thumbs-up for the ones that are *mandatory*. Going swimming. Voting. Coming to school.") and identify concepts that need further instruction.

Vocabulary instruction should help students relate new words to background knowledge and deepen their understanding of word meanings (Carr & Wixon, 1986) and should be conducted in engaging, interactive activities (Stahl, 1999, 2004). It should promote integration of new words with existing knowledge; provide sufficient practice and repetition; and support use in typical reading, writing, listening, and speaking tasks (Nagy, 1988). Nelson and Van Meter (2005) described several strategies for vocabulary development useful for affecting word usage patterns in conversational and written language. Vocabulary instruction can focus on teaching specific words and/or techniques for new word learning. In both situations, students benefit from frequent opportunities for learning and practice. Using a variety of activities ensures that students have multiple exposures to the new words they are learning. Because ample practice with new words is so essential, effective vocabulary programs generally include planned opportunities for students to encounter newly learned words in several different contexts.

_____   Juliana, a fourth grader who is rapidly becoming proficient in her use of a high-tech SGD, attended a language and literacy camp for students who use AAC. Her camp included different activities designed to enhance new word learning and embed word learning in meaningful contexts throughout the day. New words were introduced during the Morning Meeting, with each camper choosing a word he or she wishes to learn and practice. Definitions were provided, and discussions were held to help the children link the new word to concepts with which they were already familiar. Campers sometimes acted out things related to their words.

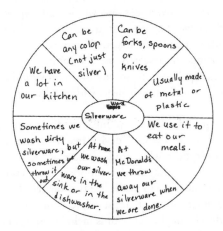

Figure 8.2.   Example of a graphic organizer used in vocabulary instruction.

On some days, they got word stickers that were placed around the room to remind people to use the new words. Campers had fun keeping score and making tally marks to keep track of how many times each new word was used. Later in the day, they engaged in more in-depth activities, such as the creation of semantic webs to intensify their understanding of the new word. _____

     Semantic webs are a type of graphic organizer or diagram used to teach new words or concepts. Also known as *semantic maps* or *concept maps*, they are often completed as part of an interactive activity and are very useful in demonstrating associations and relationships between words (Hyerle, 1996). Although these diagrams are easily customized to meet the specific needs of students, semantic webs for new vocabulary may include things like the definition, part of speech, associated attributes, and examples (see Figure 8.2).

     There are several other research-supported strategies that have been used to teach new vocabulary to students with language difficulties (Stahl, 1999). Activities that teach synonyms and antonyms, for example, establish a link between known words and new words. They give students an opportunity to consider the important attributes of the new word and relate those back to words they already know. Similarly, providing examples and nonexamples requires students to evaluate a word's attributes. This is particularly useful when the examples are highly individualized (e.g., "Mr. Gupta's hard algebra tests and pop quizzes made him *infamous*"), providing added relevance to the word meaning. Having students explain the examples provides insight into their understanding of the word and further reinforces the new concept. Sorting activities are also good for vocabulary teaching. Students can sort new words based on predefined characteristics, (e.g., noun/verb/adjective; prefix/suffix) or create their own categories ("guess my sorting pattern"). Some words can be analyzed and broken down into smaller segments that give clues to their meaning (e.g., *bio*graphy, use*less*). Finally, students can use their own words to explain the new word meaning, paraphrase the definition, or create sentences that demonstrate their understanding of the new word.

     See Table 8.2 for a list of additional language intervention strategies used for vocabulary instruction and the teaching of grammatical skills. Specific practices to be avoided in semantic instruction include using dictionary definitions to provide meaning, requiring students to copy definitions, teaching words in isolation or failing to relate them to students' experiences, using rote memorization, and making instruction tedious (Nelson & Van Meter, 2005). Instead, vocabulary instruction should be engaging, multifaceted, and relevant. New word learning should be integrated across the curriculum so that there are frequent opportunities for practice and repetition.

     Another challenge for interventionists involves expanding the words that are used by students with AAC needs so that their expressive vocabularies grow along with their knowledge of new words. Students are likely to overuse some words and neglect other words that they know. This is much like the challenge that many students without disabilities face in their writing: they use a small set of words so frequently that their communication can be overly simplistic, repetitive, and dull. In the absence of research on overcoming this barrier in students with AAC needs, it is reasonable to extrapolate from studies on improving the variety in the writing of children with learning disabilities as well as their peers without disabilities (e.g., Beck et al., 2002; Gersten & Baker, 2001).

     Lexical (or semantic) diversity refers to the number of different words used in a given language sample. Limitations in the student's AAC device frequently cause him or her to communicate with a restricted set of words. Even when students have access to a device with a larger pool of words, their experiences with that device (and appropriate instruction) are extremely limited. Thus, they may not yet have the proficiency to utilize the rich variety of words available to them. To enhance linguistic performance, interventionists must create frequent opportunities to model and elicit new words. Strategies used to highlight new words include displaying them on bulletin boards and badges.

Table 8.2.   Strategies for vocabulary and grammar instruction

Instructional strategy	Description
Joint book reading (Bedrosian, 1997; Bellon & Ogletree, 2000; Crowe, Norris, & Hoffman, 2004; Davie & Kemp, 2002; Koppenhaver et al., 2001; Liboiron & Soto, 2006; Soto & Dukhovny, 2008; Wood & Hood, 2004) and book discussions (Harmon, 1998)	These strategies provide an instructional context for learning new words and grammatical structures. Books are selected based on the opportunities they provide for the student to practice target language patterns. Adults read interactively with students, breaking from the text to interject carefully planned language that activates background knowledge, relates known concepts to the new information, provides models and examples of the target, poses relevant questions, elicits the target skill, and provides instructive feedback. Shared book reading approaches vary in terms of their discourse structure, with some approaches being highly naturalistic and others quite scripted.
Modeling via expansions, extensions, recast sentences, buildups and breakdowns, and aided language stimulation (Binger, 2008; Binger & Light, 2007; Bradshaw, Hoffman, & Norris, 1998; Cleave & Fey, 1997; Romski & Sevcik, 2003)	This strategy provides a model of the target skill (i.e., new word, linguistic pattern, or structure; e.g., target structure = if/then: "If we watch High School Musical, then we won't have time to go to the library."). Expansions and extensions both add additional information. Expansions add grammatical markers and detail that make the sentence more adultlike. Extensions explain the new concept by providing additional information (e.g., target word = superb: "Hannah Montana is superb. She is really good in that movie. She's excellent!"). Recasts focus attention on the target word/structure by elaborating and rephrasing the student's utterance (e.g., target word = superb; Student: "Hannah Montana good." Adult recast: "Yes, isn't Hannah Montana superb?"). Buildups highlight the target by adding new information around the target word/structure (e.g., target structure = after: "We have to read Chapter 4. After the bell. We have to read it after the bell.") Breakdowns separate longer utterances into chunks in order to focus attention on the target structure (e.g., target structure = after: "We have to read Chapter 4 after the bell. We have to read it. After the bell"). Aided language stimulation involves adults modeling the use of AAC tools, such as the student's speech-generating device or a poster-sized version of a communication board.
Semantic feature analysis (SFA: Crais, 1990; Rider, Wright, Marshall, & Page, 2008)	This strategy expands knowledge of vocabulary already in the student's repertoire through the use of a grid. Curriculum or other new words appear on one axis, and relevant attributes appear along the other axis. Students are helped to complete the grid. New words, attributes, and grids are added as needed.
Visual or concept mapping; Semantic webbing (Elshout-Mohr & van Daalen-Kapteijns, 1987)	This strategy teaches new words or enhances understanding of known words through the use of a graphic organizer (see Figure 8.2).
Scripts (Olswang & Bain, 1991)	This strategy embeds new words and patterns in a predictable routine to highlight a specific linguistic concept and provide opportunities for practice. Existing routines can be modified to teach the new skill or new routines can be created specifically for this purpose. Once established, the routine can be violated to elicit the target language behavior (e.g., target form = regular past tense; Routine: students read the teacher's daily message explaining what the class will do that day. The routine is violated by having the student read that message as if the activities were already completed).

Grammar and Morphosyntax

Children who use AAC lag behind their peers in the acquisition of morphological markers and syntactic forms (Blockberger & Johnston, 2003). At times, grammatical errors made by students who use AAC reflect an individual preference for message speed and efficiency over grammatical precision. For example, a student who is capable of using grammatically correct utterances (e.g., "May I please finish my assignment later?") may choose to truncate the message (e.g., "Finish later, please?") to conserve time and effort. Students with AAC needs, however, often have real difficulty acquiring adultlike grammatical skills. This may be because their expressive communication tools (i.e., SGDs and no-tech communication aids, such as boards and books) are limited in the number of words or word fragments that can be displayed at any one time. In many cases, linguistic performance is hindered by AAC systems that fail to provide full access to important grammatical elements, such as bound morphemes that indicate plural or possessive word forms. Secondly, there is a significant discrepancy between the input modality (i.e., the speech they hear) and their output modalities using their AAC systems. Learning abstract constructions is especially challenging since the morphological endings necessary to produce grammatically correct sentences are difficult to depict. Students who depend on these devices must learn to use graphic symbols, generally pictures, to represent abstract constructs and conventions. Grammatical instruction is likely to be highly variable because while some students with AAC needs already have an intact underlying language system onto which AAC can be mapped, many others do not.

There is very little research in the area of grammatical and morphological intervention for children who use AAC (Binger, 2008; Binger & Light, 2008; Bruno & Trembath, 2006). In her research teaching bound morphemes to children who used semantic compaction, Binger (2008) used story reading to explore the effect of modeling and recasting in a multiple baseline single subject design study. She found that while all children learned all three of the bound morphemes, they did not retain their knowledge of the first bound morpheme they were taught. Researchers have called for additional investigations of treatment efficacy and have suggested that, in the interim, it may be prudent to employ strategies that have been efficacious for students with language impairments. Paul (2007) provided a comprehensive review of language intervention strategies. Table 8.2 includes several strategies, which have been effectively used to improve morphology in students with language difficulties.

The development of advanced syntactic forms is another area where students who use AAC may require explicit instruction. Two areas that may be especially beneficial for these students are 1) the elaboration of noun and verb phrases and 2) the use of varied sentence forms. Paul (2007) discussed a variety of strategies useful in addressing these linguistic targets through systematic instruction. In this way, students who use relatively simple sentence structures, such as noun + verb + object, can become more sophisticated language users.

_____   Graciela, a fifth grader, learned to use elaborated noun phrases to make her sentences more vivid and interesting. When prompted, she was able to modify relatively simplistic sentences (e.g., "She was nice") by using more specific terms and adding descriptive elements (e.g., "My old teacher was really super nice"). Graciela also expanded the range of sentence types in her expressive repertoire when her SLP targeted advanced forms such as interrogatives with embedded phrases (e.g., "Why is he going to be gone for so long?" "Do you know if she is coming back to camp?"). _____

Fey (2008) outlined five principles of grammatical intervention that have specific relevance to AAC (see Table 8.3) that are based on earlier works relating to students with specific language impairment (Fey, Long, & Finestack, 2003). Strategies used to improve grammar include modeling (Binger & Light, 2007; Blockberger & Johnson, 2003), explanations of specific rules (Sutton & Gallagher, 1993), expectant delay (Alpert & Kaiser, 1992), elicitation questions (Fey, Cleave, Long, & Hughes, 1993), imitation (Camarata & Nelson, 1992), cloze procedures and judgment tasks (Blockberger & Johnson, 2003), and corrective feedback (Lund & Light, 2003). Binger and Light (2008) reviewed 31 studies that investigated grammar intervention with individuals of all ages who use AAC as well as some typically developing individuals who used AAC for research purposes. They noted a paucity of research in grammar instruction for this population. Although research in teaching grammatical skills to children with AAC needs is quite limited, there are a number of promising strategies that have strong empirical support with other clinical populations. A good example is the use of recasts, in which an adult responds to a child's communicative attempt by reformulating it. Recasts

Table 8.3.   Principles of grammar instruction that have high relevance to children who use AAC

Principle	Implication
Principle 1: The basic goal of all grammar interventions should be to help children improve in the use of grammar so they become better communicators in conversation, narration, exposition, and other textual genres in written and oral modalities.	Students should receive grammar intervention in meaningful, functional contexts. Interventions in nonfunctional contexts must have an explicit plan to build generalization to daily living.
Principle 2: The specific goals of grammatical intervention should be based on the child's functional readiness and need for the targeted forms.	Grammatical intervention goals must be based on thorough assessment of the student's receptive and expressive language abilities rather than on a general curriculum or developmental sequence.
Principle 3: The social, physical, and linguistic contexts of intervention should be manipulated to provide opportunities for adult models of and for student (mis-) use of specific grammatical targets.	The student's AAC system must allow for expression of the grammar skills targeted for instruction. The student needs to be exposed to a high rate of targeted constructions in the spoken and AAC modalities. Frequent opportunities for learning and practice of targeted grammar skills must be provided in situations where there are high levels of motivation or need for those skills.
Principle 4: Immature child utterances should be systematically contrasted with more grammatically complete adult forms, using sentence recasts.	Adults should use sentence recasts to provide students with grammatically correct and complete models of the target constructions on a regular and frequent basis. When possible, these should be modeled using appropriate AAC modalities.
Principle 5: Telegraphic models should be avoided and replaced by grammatical models in well-formed phrases and sentences.	Adults should communicate in well-formed sentences, and model them using the AAC system, when possible.

Sources: Fey (2008); Fey, Long, & Finestack (2003).

must be the first response following the child's utterance and should copy at least one content word from the student's original message (Fey et al., 2003). They make reference to the same event and share meaning with the original message; they reformulate the original message to provide a grammatically correct and complete model of the target construction.

For both grammatical and morphological skills to develop, students need exposure to a variety of adult forms. Researchers, such as Fey (1986), have argued for the provision of adult forms as opposed to the use of telegraphic speech (or, by extension, AAC input) for a number of reasons. First, telegraphic models may make language learning more difficult in that they reduce students' exposure to more advanced morphosyntactic forms and lessen their opportunities for incidental learning. In addition, they diminish morphosyntactic and prosodic cues to sentence, phrase, and word meaning. Poster-sized communication boards, such as the example in Figure 8.3, can be used to model target language constructions in the classroom.

Narrative Intervention

It comes as no surprise that students who use AAC and have difficulty with language complexity, grammar, and lexical diversity will also have difficulty formulating narratives. Narratives produced by students who use AAC tend to be shorter and less complete, with pronounced problems in clarity and cohesion (Bedrosian, Lasker, Speidel, & Politsch, 2003; Grove & Tucker, 2003; Soto & Hartmann, 2006; Soto, Yu, & Henneberry, 2007; Soto, Yu, & Kelso, 2008; Waller et al., 2001). Language difficulties, such as the absence of elaborated noun phrases and conjoining clauses, often punctuate the narratives of students who use AAC. These students' narratives often lack key story constituents, such as characters and settings. They are also, in many cases, less independent in the formation of narratives. Soto and Hartmann (2006) noted that the four students in their study relied

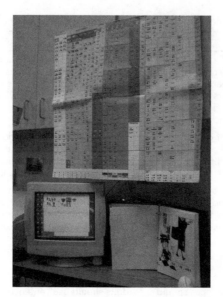

Figure 8.3. Example of a communication board that can be enlarged and used by teachers and adults to model target language skills in the classroom.

heavily on their communication partners to co-construct stories in a variety of narrative elicitation tasks. Given the depth and breadth of their difficulties with narrative production, it is likely that students who use AAC will need supportive intervention over and above what is offered as a regular part of the curriculum.

Many of the researchers who have examined storytelling in students who use AAC recommend a multifaceted approach to narrative intervention that includes a comprehensive assessment of narrative abilities. A thorough assessment of the student's narrative skills using a comprehensive tool such as the Narrative Assessment Profile (Bliss, McCabe, & Miranda, 1998)[2] can identify student strengths and limitations, yielding information that is essential for the development of an instructional plan. Frequent opportunities to hear and produce a variety of narratives are needed and should be provided in an environment that scaffolds the student's language abilities. For students who use AAC, this often means that they co-construct stories. Students may need partner support to compose narratives that have clear main ideas and supporting details and to order that information in a cohesive fashion.

Soto and her colleagues found that visual supports, such as story maps and templates with sentence starters, were useful in helping students create more meaningful narratives (Soto & Hartmann, 2006; Soto et al., 2007; Soto et al., 2008). In their studies, students typically engaged in narrative intervention tasks, such as story reading and retelling, recounting personal stories, and telling fictional narratives, 3–5 times per week. Students were provided with strategic messages (e.g., "What I want to say is the noun of ____" "What I want to say is similar to ____") that allowed them to convey concepts not available via their SGDs. During the intervention, contingent queries and verbal redirection were used to help the students clarify ambiguous messages. Their work suggests that through the provision of focused treatment and opportunities to be supported in the development of narratives, students who use AAC can greatly improve their storytelling skills, use more complete sentences, expand their expressive vocabularies, and formulate more complex utterances. In addition, they observed a trend toward greater independence: student narratives were more comprehensible without partner scaffolding (Soto et al., 2008).

---

[2]See Chapter 3 for additional information on the Narrative Assessment Profile and other narrative assessment tools.

An important consideration in narrative intervention relates to genre. Although personal narratives appear to be the most common form of storytelling in daily conversation (Preece, 1987), most approaches to narrative assessment and intervention focus on fictional narratives (Cannizzaro & Coelho, 2002; Finestack, Fey, Sokol, Ambrose, & Swanson, 2006; Gillam, McFadden, & van Kleeck, 1995; Hayward & Schneider, 2000; Swanson, Fey, Mills, & Hood, 2005). Explicit instruction in both forms is important as they have distinct forms and elements (McCabe & Bliss, 2003; McCabe, Bliss, Barra, & Bennett, 2008), and the two genres may follow different developmental paths (Bourg, Bauer, & van den Broek, 1997). Research by Peterson and McCabe (1983), for example, indicates that the ability to include precipitating events and resolutions appears in personal narratives prior to being demonstrated in fictional narratives. It is important to recognize, however, that narratives differ in their topography. Intervention plans, support materials (e.g., graphic story maps), and assessment procedures must take these differences into account.

_____   Tia's narratives frequently went into a portfolio so that her teacher could assess student progress. While evaluation of personal narratives employed a high point analysis, assessment of Tia's fictional narratives focused on story grammar elements. This allowed the team to see how she was progressing in both genres over a period of months. _____

Instruction in different types of narrative language is valuable because each genre makes a unique contribution to our lives. Competence in telling personal stories, for example, enriches our social interactions at home, in school, and in the community. On the other hand, the ability to create or retell fictional stories promotes success in literacy and academics. Thus, narrative intervention for students who use AAC can be viewed as a long-term process, with interventionists providing instruction on multiple genres.

What comprises good narrative intervention for students who use AAC? Research on the effectiveness of instructional strategies with students who have AAC needs is in the early stages, but is yielding interesting and potentially useful results. However, if we broaden our consideration to include narrative instruction for students with other types of language difficulties (e.g., Cannizzaro & Coelho, 2002; Davies, Shanks, & Davies, 2004; Hayward & Schneider, 2000; Swanson et al., 2005), a number of empirically supported guidelines emerge.

1. All students who use AAC and have more advanced linguistic skills (as defined previously) should receive explicit narrative instruction by knowledgeable interventionists. In most cases, the student will need individualized narrative intervention that complements curricular instruction.

2. Narrative instruction should be eclectic, multifaceted, and include frequent opportunities for structured learning and supported practice. It should be planned and implemented with input from important stakeholders on the IEP team.

3. Narrative intervention should encompass multiple genres and address both structural and cohesive elements. The instructional plan should be tailored to the type of narrative that is the focus of that particular lesson.

4. Partner support is a critical aspect of effective narrative intervention. Partners must become proficient in using open-ended queries, verbal redirection, encouragement, and other forms of scaffolding, gradually fading those supports as the student's skills increase.

5. Additional supports, such as graphic story maps, may be needed for students who have limited vocabulary on their AAC devices and those who are still learning to be proficient with their SGDs.

6. AAC tools, such as SGDs and communication books, should be configured to include vocabulary and messages that support narrative development.

CONCLUSION

Students who use AAC and are more advanced linguistic communicators will, in most cases, need the ongoing support of educators and SLPs to develop literate language and use it effectively. Teams must face the challenge of ensuring that these students always have access to well-functioning AAC systems that fully support generative language. Together with the student and family, professionals must continually evaluate the student's AAC system and make refinements that will allow further development of linguistic competence. Students who use AAC will vary in their need for language intervention, and, at times, may need intensive support to build more sophisticated language skills. As these students mature and move into new environments, their communication partners will need training on how best to support language through AAC. Like their peers without communication difficulties, students who use AAC have the potential to continue to develop their vocabulary, grammar, narrative, and other language skills beyond their formal schooling. Working together, teams can support these students and help them to achieve their goals and potential in academic settings and on into their adult years.

REFERENCES

Alpert, C.L., & Kaiser, A.P. (1992). Training parents as milieu language teachers. *Journal of Early Intervention, 16,* 31–52.

Beck, I.L., McKeown, M.G., & Kucan, L. (2002). *Bringing words to life: Robust vocabulary development.* New York: Guilford Press.

Beck, I.L., McKeown, M.G., & McCaslin, E. (1983). All contexts are not created equal. *Elementary School Journal, 83,* 177–181.

Bedrosian, J. (1997). Language acquisition in young AAC system users: Issues and directions for future research. *Augmentative and Alternative Communication, 13*(3), 179–185.

Bedrosian, J., Lasker, J., Speidel, K., & Politsch, A. (2003). Enhancing the written narrative skills of an AAC student with autism: Evidence-based issues. *Topics in Language Disorders, 24,* 305–324.

Bellon, M.L., & Ogletree, B.T. (2000). Repeated storybook reading as an instructional method. *Intervention School Clinic, 2,* 75–81.

Berninger, V., & Gans, B. (1986). Language profiles in nonspeaking individuals of normal intelligence with severe cerebral palsy. *Augmentative and Alternative Communication, 2,* 45–50.

Beukelman, D., Jones, R., & Rowan, M. (1989). Frequency of word usage by nondisabled peers in integrated preschool classrooms. *Augmentative and Alternative Communication, 5,* 243–248.

Binger, C. (2008). Bound morpheme intervention for children who use AAC. *Perspectives on AAC, 17,* 60–66.

Binger, C., & Light, J. (2007). The effect of aided AAC modeling on the expression of multisymbol messages by preschoolers who use AAC. *Augmentative and Alternative Communication, 23,* 30–43.

Binger, C., & Light, J. (2008). The morphology and syntax of individuals who use AAC: Research review and implications for effective practice. *Augmentative and Alternative Communication, 24*(2), 123–138.

Bliss, L.S., McCabe, A., & Miranda, A.E. (1998). Narrative assessment profile: Discourse analysis for school-age children. *Journal of Communication Disorders, 31,* 347–362.

Blockberger, S., & Johnson, J.R. (2003). Grammatical morphology acquisition by children with complex communication needs. *Augmentative and Alternative Communication, 19,* 207–221.

Botting, N., & Adams, C. (2005). Semantic and inferencing abilities in children with communication disorders. *International Journal of Language and Communication Disorders, 40,* 49–66.

Bourg, T., Bauer, P.J., & van den Broek, P.W. (1997). Building the bridges: The development of event comprehension and representation. In P.W. van den Broek, P.J. Bauer, & T. Bourg (Eds.), *Developmental spans in event comprehension and representation: Bridging fictional and actual events* (pp. 385–408). Mahwah, NJ: Lawrence Erlbaum Associates.

Bradshaw, M., Hoffman, P., & Norris, J. (1998). Efficacy of expansions and cloze procedures in the development of interpretations by preschool children exhibiting delayed language development. *Language, Speech, and Hearing Services in the Schools, 29,* 85–95.

Brown, R. (1973). *A first language: The early stages.* London: George Allen & Unwin.

Bruno, J., & Trembath, D. (2006). Use of aided language stimulation to improve syntactic performance during a weeklong intervention program. *Augmentative and Alternative Communication, 22*(4), 300–313.

Camarata, S., & Nelson, K. (1992). Treatment efficacy as a function of target selection in the remediation of child language disorders. *Clinical Linguistics and Phonetics, 20,* 563–571.

Cannizzaro, M.S., & Coelho, C.A. (2002). Treatment of story grammar following traumatic brain injury: A pilot study. *Brain Injury, 16,* 1065–1073.

Carr, E., & Wixon, K.K. (1986). Guidelines for evaluating vocabulary instruction. *Journal of Reading, 29,* 588–595.

Cleave, P., & Fey, M. (1997). Two approaches to the facilitation of grammar in children with language impairments: Rationale and description. *American Journal of Speech Language Pathology, 6,* 23–32.

Corson, D. (1988). *Oral language across the curriculum.* Clevedon, England: Multilingual Matters.

Crais, E. (1990). World knowledge to word knowledge. *Topics in Language Disorders, 10*(3), 45–62.

Crowe, L., Norris, J.A., & Hoffman, P.R. (2004). Training caregivers to facilitate communicative participation of preschool children with language impairment during storybook reading. *Journal of Communicative Disorders, 37,* 177–196.

Davie, J., & Kemp, C. (2002). A comparison of the expressive language opportunities provided by shared book reading and facilitated play for young children with mild to moderate intellectual disabilities. *Educational Psychologist, 22,* 445–460.

Davies, P., Shanks, B., & Davies, K. (2004). Improving narrative skills in young children with delayed language development. *Educational Review, 56,* 271–286.

Ellis, E.S., & Worthington, L.A. (1994). *Research synthesis on effective teaching principles and the design of quality tools for educators* (Technical Report No. 5). Eugene: University of Oregon, National Center to Improve the Tools of Educators.

Elshout-Mohr, M., & Van Daalen-Kapteijns, M. (1987). Cognitive processes in learning word meanings. In M.G. McKeown & M.E. Curtis (Eds.), *The nature of vocabulary acquisition* (pp. 53–72). Hillsdale, NJ: Lawrence Erlbaum Associates.

Fey, M.E. (1986). *Language intervention with young children.* Austin, TX: PRO-ED.

Fey, M. (2008, June). Thoughts on grammar intervention in AAC. *Perspectives on AAC, 17,* 43–49.

Fey, M.E., Cleave, P.L., Long, S.H., & Hughes, D.L. (1993). Two approaches to the facilitation of grammar in children with language impairment: An experimental evaluation. *Journal of Speech, Language, and Hearing Research, 36,* 141–157.

Fey, M.E., Long, S.H., & Finestack, L. (2003). Ten principles of grammar facilitation for children with specific language impairments. *American Journal of Speech Language Pathology, 12*(1), 3–15.

Finestack, L.H., Fey, M.E., Sokol, S.B., Ambrose, S., & Swanson, L.A. (2006). Fostering narrative and grammatical skills with "syntax stories." In A. van Kleeck (Ed.), *Sharing books and stories to promote language and literacy* (pp. 319–346). San Diego: Plural.

Foreman, P., & Crews, G. (1998). Using augmentative and alternative communication with infants and young children with Down syndrome. *Down Syndrome Research and Practice, 5,* 16–25.

Gersten, R., & Baker, S. (2001). Teaching expressive writing to students with learning disabilities: A meta-analysis. *Elementary School Journal, 101*(3), 251–272.

Gillam, R., McFadden, T.U., & van Kleeck, A. (1995). Improving narrative abilities: Whole language and language skills approaches. In S.F. Warren & M.E. Fey (Series Eds.) & M.E. Fey & J. Windsor (Vol. Eds.), *Communication and language intervention series: Vol. 5. Language intervention: Preschool through the elementary years* (pp. 145–182). Baltimore: Paul H. Brookes Publishing Co.

Goldstein, H. (2006). Language intervention considerations for children with mental retardation and developmental disabilities. *Perspectives on Language Learning and Education, 13*(3), 21–26.

Graves, M.F. (1986). Vocabulary Learning and Instruction. In E.Z. Rothkopf & L.C. Ehri (Eds.), *Review of research in education* (Vol. 13, pp. 49–89). Washington, DC: American Educational Research Association.

Grove, N., & Tucker, S. (2003). Narratives in manual sign by children with intellectual impairments. In S. von Tetzchner, & N. Grove (Eds.), *Augmentative and alternative communication: Developmental issues* (pp. 229–255). London, UK: Whurr Publishers.

Harmon, J.M. (1998). Vocabulary teaching and learning in a seventh-grade literature-based classroom. *Journal of Adolescent and Adult Literacy, 41*(7), 518–529.

Hayward, D., & Schneider, P. (2000). Effectiveness of teaching story grammar knowledge to pre-school children with language impairment. An exploratory study. *Child Language Teaching and Therapy, 16,* 255–284.

Hyerle, D. (1996). *Visual tools for constructing knowledge.* Alexandria, VA: ASCD.

Iacono, T. (1992). Individual language learning styles. *Augmentative and Alternative Communication, 8*(1), 33–40.

Iacono, T., Mirenda, P., & Beukelman, D. (1993). Comparison of unimodal and multimodal AAC techniques for children with intellectual disabilities. *Augmentative and Alternative Communication, 9,* 83–93.

Johnson, D.D. (2001). *Vocabulary in the elementary and middle school.* Boston: Allyn & Bacon.

Koppenhaver, D.A., Erickson, K.A., Harris B., McLellan, J., Skotko, B., & Newton, R.A. (2001). Storybook based communication intervention for girls with Rett syndrome and their mothers. *Disability and Rehabilitation, 23,* 149–159.

Kovach, T., & Kenyon, P.B. (2003). Visual issues and access to AAC. In D.R. Beukelman & J. Reichle (Series Eds.) & J. Light, D. Beukelman, & J.

Reichle (Vol. Eds.), *Augmentative and alternative communication series: Communicative competence for individuals who use AAC* (pp. 277–319). Baltimore: Paul H. Brookes Publishing Co.

Liboiron, N., & Soto G. (2006). Shared storybook reading with a student who uses alternative and augmentative communication: An intervention session. *Child Language Teaching and Therapy, 22,* 69–95.

Light, J., Drager, K., McCarthy, J., Mellott, S., Millar, D., Parrish, C., et al. (2004). Performance of typically developing four- and five-year-old children with AAC systems using different language organization techniques. *Augmentative and Alternative Communication, 20,* 63–88.

Lund, S.K., & Light, J. (2003). The effectiveness of grammar instruction for individuals who use AAC systems: A preliminary study. *Journal of Speech, Language, and Hearing Research, 46,* 1110–1123.

Martinsen, H., & von Tetzchner, S. (1996). Situating augmentative and alternative language intervention. In S. von Tetzchner & M. Jensen (Eds.), *Augmentative and alternative communication: European perspectives.* New York: Whurr.

Marvin, C., Beukelman, D., & Bilyeu, D. (1994). Vocabulary-use patterns in preschool children: Effects of context and time sampling. *Augmentative and Alternative Communication, 10*(4), 224–236.

McCabe, A., & Bliss, L.S. (2003). *Patterns of narrative discourse: A multicultural life span approach.* Boston: Pearson Education.

McCabe, A., Bliss, L., Barra, G., & Bennett, M. (2008). Comparison of personal versus fictional narratives of children with language impairment. *American Journal of Speech-Language Pathology, 17,* 194–206.

McCabe, A., & Rollins, P.R. (1994). Assessment of preschool narrative skills. *American Journal of Speech-Language Pathology: A Journal of Clinical Practice, 3,* 45–56.

Nagy, W.E. (1988). *Teaching vocabulary to improve reading comprehension.* Urbana, IL: National Council of Teachers of English.

Nelson, N.W. (1992). Performance is the prize: Language competence and performance among AAC users. *Augmentative and Alternative Communication, 8*(1), 3–18.

Nelson, N.W., & Van Meter, A.M. (2005). Finding the words: Vocabulary development for young authors. In T.A. Ukrainetz (Ed.), *Contextualized language intervention: Scaffolding preK–12 literacy achievement* (pp. 95–143). Greenville, SC: Thinking Publications.

Olswang, L., & Bain, B. (1991). Intervention issues for toddlers with specific language impairments. *Topics in Language Disorders, 11,* 69–86.

Paul, R. (1997). Facilitating transitions in language development for children using AAC. *Augmentative and Alternative Communication, 13*(3), 141–148.

Paul, R. (2007). *Language disorders from infancy through adolescence: Assessment and intervention* (2nd ed.). Philadelphia: Mosby.

Peterson, C., & McCabe, A. (1983). *Developmental psycholinguistics: Three ways of looking at a child's narrative.* New York: Plenum.

Porter, G. (2000). *Low-tech dynamic displays: User friendly multi-level communication books.* Paper presented at the ISAAC conference, Washington, DC.

Porter, G., Kirkland, J., & Dunne, L. (1998). *Multilevel communication books.* Poster presented at the ISAAC conference, Dublin, Ireland.

Preece, A. (1987). The range of narrative forms conversationally produced by young children. *Journal of Child Language, 14,* 353–373.

Redmond, S.M., & Johnston, S.S. (2001). Evaluating the morphological competence of children with severe speech and physical impairments. *Journal of Speech, Language, and Hearing Research, 44,* 1362–1375.

Rider, J.D., Wright, H.H., Marshall, R.C., & Page, J.L. (2008). Using semantic feature analysis to improve contextual discourse in adults with aphasia. *American Journal of Speech Language Pathology, 17,* 161–172.

Romski, M.A., & Sevcik, R.A. (2003). Augmented input: Enhancing communication development. In D.R. Beukelman & J. Reichle (Series Eds.) & J. Light, D. Beukelman, & J. Reichle (Vol. Eds.), *Augmentative and alternative communication series: Communicative competence for individuals who use AAC* (pp. 147–162). Baltimore: Paul H. Brookes Publishing Co.

Rosenshine, B., & Stevens, R. (1986). Teaching functions. In M.C. Wittrock (Ed.), *Handbook of research on teaching* (3rd ed.). New York, Macmillan.

Silliman, E.R., & Wilkinson, L.C. (1991). *Communication for learning: Classroom observation and collaboration.* Gaithersburg, MD: Aspen Publications.

Smith, M. (2006). Literacy instruction and AAC: A mysterious mosaic. *Perspectives on Augmentative and Alternative Communication, 15*(2), 2–7.

Soto, G., & Dukhovny, E. (2008). The effect of shared book reading on the acquisition of expressive vocabulary of a 7 year old who uses AAC. *Seminars in Speech and Language, 29,* 133–145.

Soto, G., & Hartmann, E. (2006). Analysis of narratives produced by four children who use augmentative and alternative communication. *Journal of Communication Disorders, 39,* 456–480.

Soto, G., Yu, B., & Henneberry, S. (2007). Supporting the development of narrative skills of an eight-year old child who uses an augmentative and alternative communication device. *Child Language Teaching and Therapy, 23*(1), 27–45.

Soto, G., Yu, B., & Kelso, J. (2008). Effectiveness of multifaceted narrative intervention on the stories told by a 12-year-old girl who uses AAC. *Augmentative and Alternative Communication, 24*(1), 76–87.

Stahl, S.A. (1991). Beyond the instrumentalist hypothesis: Some relationships between word meanings and comprehension. In P. Schwanenflugel (Ed.), *The psychology of word meanings* (pp. 157–178). Hillsdale, NJ: Lawrence Erlbaum Associates.

Stahl, S.A. (1999). *Vocabulary development.* Cambridge, MA: Brookline Books.

Stahl, S.A. (2004). Vocabulary and the child with learning disabilities. *Perspectives of the International Dyslexia Association, 30*(1), 1–4.

Stuart, S., Beukelman, D., & King, J. (1997). Vocabulary use during extended conversations by two cohorts of older adults. *Augmentative and Alternative Communication, 13,* 40–47.

Sutton, A., & Gallagher, T. (1993). Verb class distinctions and AAC language-encoding limitations. *Journal of Speech and Hearing Research, 36,* 1216–1226.

Sutton, A., Gallagher, T., Morford, J., & Shahnaz, N. (2000). Relative clause sentence production using augmentative and alternative communication systems. *Applied Psycholinguistics, 21,* 1216–1226.

Sutton, A., Soto, G., & Blockberger, S. (2002). Grammatical issues in graphic symbol communication. *Augmentative and Alternative Communication, 18*(3), 192–204.

Swanson, L.A., Fey, M.E., Mills, C.E., & Hood, L.S. (2005). Use of narrative-based language intervention by children who have specific language impairment. *American Journal of Speech Language Pathology, 14,* 131–145.

Tarver, S.G. (1996). Direct instruction. In W. Stainback & S. Stainback (Eds.), *Controversial issues confronting special education: Divergent perspectives* (2nd ed., pp. 143–165). Boston: Allyn & Bacon.

Udwin, O., & Yule, W. (1987). Augmentative communication modes taught to cerebral palsied children: Findings from a longitudinal study. *International Journal of Rehabilitation Research, 10*(2), 202–206.

Udwin, O., & Yule, W. (1990). Augmentative communication systems taught to cerebral palsied children-A longitudinal study: 1. The acquisition of signs and symbols, and syntactic aspects of their use over time. *British Journal of Disorders of Communication, 25,* 295–309.

Vanderheiden, D.H., & Grilley, K. (1976). (Eds.). *Non-vocal communication techniques and aids for the severely physically handicapped.* Baltimore: University Park Press.

Vicker, B. (1974). Advances in nonoral communication system programming: Project summary 2. In B. Vicker (Ed.), *Nonoral Communication System Project 1964–1973.* Iowa City, Iowa: Campus Stores.

Waller, A., O'Mara, D.A., Tait, L., Booth, L., Brophy-Arnott, B., & Hood, H.E. (2001). Using written stories to support the use of narrative in conversational interactions: A case study. *Augmentative and Alternative Communication, 17,* 221–232.

Westby, C.E. (1985). Learning to talk—talking to learn: Oral-literate language differences. In C.S. Simon (Ed.), *Communication skills and classroom success: Therapy methodologies for language-learning disabled students* (pp. 181–218). San Diego: College-Hill Press.

Wilkinson, K.M., & Albert, A. (2001). Adaptations of fast mapping for vocabulary intervention with augmented language users. *Augmentative and Alternative Communication, 17,* 120–132.

Williams, M. (2005, Nov. 18). *How far we've come, how far we have to go: Tales from the trenches.* Edwin and Esther Prentke Distinguished Lecture, Philadelphia.

Wood, L., & Hood, E. (2004). Shared storybook readings with children who have little or no functional speech: A language intervention tool for students who use augmentative and alternative communication. *Perspectives in Education, 22,* 101–111.

9

Addressing the Literacy Demands of the Curriculum for Beginning Readers and Writers

Karen A. Erickson and Sally A. Clendon

Literacy is an integral part of the general education curriculum. The literacy demands of the general education curriculum in the areas of English and language arts are obvious, but there are literacy demands inherent in other core curriculum areas such as science, social studies, and math. Without literacy, students can learn isolated skills and information across the curriculum, but they will not learn important lifelong skills that allow them to revisit and build on that information without direct attention to literacy.

The Individuals with Disabilities Education Act Amendments of 1997 (IDEA 1997; PL 105-17) required that students with disabilities have access to the general education curriculum, as it is defined at the state or local level. These amendments also required that all students with disabilities be included in general and district-level assessment programs with appropriate alternate assessments for students who could not participate in the general assessments. These requirements were further refined with the passage of the No Child Left Behind Act (NCLB) of 2001 (PL 107-110), a reauthorization of the Elementary and Secondary Education Act of 1965 (PL 89-10). NCLB required states to establish challenging standards aligned with the general education curriculum, develop an assessment program that measures student progress against those standards in the areas of reading/language arts and math, and hold schools accountable for ensuring that students achieve the standards. An important part of NCLB is the regulation that all children, including those with the most significant cognitive impairments, make adequate yearly progress (AYP) toward achieving grade-level standards (Title 1, 2003). For many students who use augmentative and alternative communication (AAC), achieving grade-level standards is not the same as meeting grade-level expectations because their instructional program addresses extensions or access points related to the grade-level standards. Furthermore, they often fall within the very small portion of the general student population whose progress is monitored using alternate assessments reflecting alternate achievement standards or modified achievement standards (see Chapter 1).

Whether students are gaining access to the general curriculum and demonstrating progress through standard, modified, or alternate achievement standards, literacy, in particular reading, has a central role. For students with AAC needs, the role of literacy extends beyond traditional access to content and demonstrating understanding to communication in general. Although symbols can meet a wide range of communication needs, the alphabet is the only symbol set that allows an individual to communicate precisely across environments and partners.

This chapter describes individuals with AAC needs who are beginning readers and writers and offers specific approaches and strategies that can be employed to help them meet the demands of the curriculum *while* building reading and writing skills that will develop over time. In contrast to the approaches and strategies to support participation in literacy activities that are described in a number of other resources (e.g., Browder & Spooner, 2006; Downing, 2005), the approaches and strategies described in this chapter are intended to build core skills and understandings across reading, writing, and communication so that students can move toward conventional uses of literacy to convey meaning to others.

KEY ISSUES

There are a number of issues to consider when trying to address the literacy demands of the curriculum for beginning readers and writers. In the following section, the population of learners with AAC needs who are beginning readers and writers is described, and emergent literacy is defined.

Who Are Beginning Readers and Writers?

The beginning readers and writers described in this chapter are a heterogeneous group of learners, including children who are just beginning school and are beginning readers and writers as a result of age and experience. With appropriate early literacy learning experiences during kindergarten and the primary grades, many of these young children make the transition from emergent literacy through early literacy and on to conventional literacy. Most of these children come to kindergarten with AAC systems that are language rich and flexible and have been taught well during the preschool years. Children with AAC needs who arrive at school without a comprehensive AAC system often find it difficult to engage in literacy learning in a way that allows them to successfully achieve more sophisticated levels of reading and writing abilities.

Some beginning readers and writers have language, cognitive, sensory, and other impairments that make it difficult for them to develop as readers and writers. As a result, they continue to be beginning readers and writers well into adolescence and beyond. It is possible for these students to eventually develop conventional literacy skills (see, e.g., Erickson, Koppenhaver, Yoder, & Nance, 1997), but progress is markedly slower. Another subgroup of beginning readers and writers described in this chapter includes adolescents who have not had adequate access to appropriate instruction to develop literacy skills. For many of these older beginning readers and writers, their underdeveloped literacy skills are the direct results of educational programs that have focused on the acquisition of basic skills or functional life skills without an opportunity to develop reading and writing skills and gain a greater understanding of the world around them (Downing, 2006).

Finally, there are students who have been fully included in general education settings, who have had full access to the content of the general education curriculum, and who remain beginning readers and writers because the emphasis of their education has been on keeping up with the curriculum. Their books are typically read to them. They often respond only to multiple-choice, yes-no, and fill-in-the-blank tasks, and adequate time has not been devoted to building reading and writing skills. Melinda provides an excellent example.

_____   When Melinda was 12 years old, she used a dynamic display communication device with dozens of well-organized pages along with dysarthric speech and gestures to communicate. She drove a power wheelchair with a joystick and used her right pointer finger to directly select items on her communication device and on a computer keyboard. No one doubted that Melinda was a very capable student. She was academically competitive all the way through school as a full member of a general education setting. Melinda was also a beginning reader and writer. Throughout her school career, Melinda had been able to keep up with her classmates by listening to a teaching assistant or her parents read texts aloud to her. These individuals enhanced the rate of her writing by providing her with slot-filler writing activities and word banks. They supported her participation in classroom interactions by programming her AAC device with activity and unit-specific vocabulary that they pretaught her so that she would be prepared.

On the surface, Melinda was a success, but Melinda longed to learn to read and write. Until a clear plan was developed to provide Melinda with intensive, high-quality reading and writing instruction, she remained a beginning reader and writer.   _____

What Is Emergent Literacy?

In this chapter, *literacy* is defined quite simply as reading and writing to convey meaning. Examples of reading and writing in this definition would include reading the newspaper, writing a letter to a friend, or using initial letter cueing to support dysarthric speech in face-to-face communication. Literacy is often defined much more broadly to include such things as listening or viewing, but in the context of this chapter, listening and viewing are presented as separate competencies that may affect one's ability to acquire literacy skills, but are not sufficient to ensure the development of literacy skills.

The focus of this chapter is on beginning readers and writers who are emerging in their understandings of literacy. This emergent literacy comprises nonconventional, and often idiosyncratic, behaviors and understandings that beginning readers and writers exhibit prior to achieving conventional literacy (see, e.g., Teale & Sulzby, 1986). As a function of experience rather than development, emergent literacy is not linked to a particular age level or level of cognitive or linguistic skill. Young children are necessarily beginning readers and writers engaging in emergent rather than conventional literacy because they have not had the experience required to be conventional in their demonstrations of reading and writing. At the same time, older children, adolescents, and adults can be beginning readers and writers demonstrating emergent literacy understandings because they have not had adequate literacy learning experience for a variety of reasons.

Emergent and conventional literacy as described in this chapter are not unitary constructs that are achieved at particular points in time. Instead, they exist along a continuum. This continuum has been described by many as a three-stage model that includes prereading, learning to read, and reading to learn (see, e.g., Chall, 1983; Ehri, 1998). There is significant overlap between emergent literacy as it is described in this chapter and prereading as it is described in the stage model, but the continuum better describes the recursive and interrelated development of reading and writing that is characteristic of emergent literacy than does a stage model (Teale & Sulzby, 1986).

Beginning readers and writers who are emerging in their understandings of literacy can be taught conventional literacy skills in isolation. In fact, the literature is replete with studies demonstrating that individuals with significant cognitive impairments who are beginning readers and writers can learn to identify sight words in isolation (see Browder & Xin, 1998) long before they have developed basic concepts about print, alphabet knowledge, oral language understandings, or phonological awareness. The problem with this approach is that development of these other basic concepts, skills, and understandings are required for word-identification skills to be used meaningfully in reading with comprehension (Dickinson, McCabe, Anastasopoulos, Peisner-Feinberg, & Poe, 2003; Nation & Snowling, 2004; Storch & Whitehurst, 2002). When sight words are taught in isolation without careful attention to the development of these other concepts, skills, and understandings, beginning readers and writers struggle to use their word-reading skills to support their attempts to read for meaning or use writing to communicate with others.

Through the Individuals with Disabilities Education Improvement Act of 2004 (IDEA 2004; PL 108-446) and the subsequent emphasis on access to the general curriculum for all students, there has been a call to define literacy more broadly so that idiosyncratic, nonconventional, and often symbol-based behaviors of students with the most significant disabilities can be described as literate behaviors (Downing, 2005). There is no doubt that these behaviors have value as students develop their abilities to communicate meaningfully with others and participate in print-based activities, but these are emergent literacy behaviors, and there is a danger in describing them as literate behaviors. The danger is that these learners would be denied meaningful, intensive, ongoing opportunities to further develop emergent and then conventional literacy skills and understandings because the skills and behaviors they are already demonstrating are viewed as sufficient. As Koppenhaver stated,

> Unfortunately, our field has often treated emergent literacy as an end goal rather than a starting place. That is, practitioners have been quicker to accept emergent literacy and nonconventional performance than to consider how to move the children on to conventional reading and writing. (2000, p. 273)

More About Emergent Literacy   Emergent literacy is defined here with reference to a model of emergent literacy proposed by Sénéchal, LeFevre, Smith-Chant, and Colton (2001). The model encompasses existing holistic understandings of emergent and early literacy that incorporate all aspects of written and oral language (Clay, 1966, 1979; Teale & Sulzby, 1986). In addition, it provides a description of the constructs underlying emergent and early literacy rather than a description of the behavioral indicators or components of emergent literacy that are described in other models (as per Mason & Stewart, 1990, or Whitehurst & Lonigan, 1998). This distinction is important given that individuals with AAC needs, particularly those with physical impairments, will have behavioral differences in demonstrating increasing literacy knowledge.

Sénéchal et al.'s (2001) model (see Figure 9.1) proposes three separate constructs: emergent literacy, oral language, and metalinguistic skills. We call the first construct *print/literacy knowledge* rather than emergent literacy to minimize confusion when we use Sénéchal et al.'s model to describe all of the constructs involved in emergent reading and writing. The print/literacy knowledge construct includes conceptual (knowledge about the functions of print, self-perception of learning to read, emergent reading in context) and procedural knowledge about literacy (phonetic spelling, alphabet knowledge, letter–sound knowledge). The oral language construct comprises knowledge of the world, vocabulary, and narrative language. Finally, the metalinguistic skills construct includes both phonological and syntactic awareness.

The interrelationships among the constructs comprising early and emergent literacy are well documented (Dickinson et al., 2003; Dickinson & Snow, 1987; Scarborough, 2001; Tabors, Roach, & Snow, 2001), but the three constructs can also be observed, measured, developed, and described separately. Oral language is a separate construct in the model because it is "biologically primary" and develops for most children in the absence of any formal instruction or particular opportunities. In contrast, print/literacy skills are "biologically secondary" and require specific exposure to experiences or instruction in order to develop (Geary, 1995; Jordan, Snow, & Porche, 2000; Sénéchal et al., 2001; Snow, 1983). Statistical models demonstrate that the three constructs (in contrast to one or two) best explain children's developing literacy skills (Lonigan, Burgess, & Anthony, 2000; Sénéchal et al., 2001; Whitehurst et al., 1994). Furthermore, early childhood oral language abilities explain variance

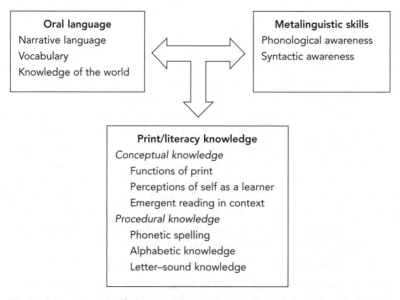

Figure 9.1.   A model of the constructs comprising emergent and early literacy. (*Source:* Sénéchal, LeFevre, Smith-Chant, & Colton, 2001.)

in later reading achievement that is unique from metalinguistic skills or literacy knowledge as separate constructs (Biemiller, 1999; Cunningham & Stanovich, 1997; Dickinson & Tabors, 2001; Sénéchal & LeFevre, 2002). Likewise, metalinguistic abilities are individually strong predictors of later reading achievement (Scarborough, 1998; Sénéchal & LeFevre, 2002).

The relationship among the three components is less clear when considering individuals with AAC needs as a result of a limited research base. Research does confirm that the three constructs are operating on some level to influence the emergent literacy development of these individuals. The oral language abilities of individuals with AAC needs vary across individuals (Berninger & Gans, 1986). Many individuals with AAC needs have significantly impaired vocabulary skills (Udwin & Yule, 1990). This impaired vocabulary knowledge is influenced by restricted experiences and background knowledge (Carlson, 1981; Light, 1997) and may be the result of difficulties fast mapping (Romski, Sevcik, & Robinson, 1996), which is the process of linking a word to a novel object in the absence of overt definitions (Carey, 1978). The oral language abilities of individuals with AAC needs are also characterized by delays in phonology (Berninger & Gans, 1986; Vandervelden & Siegel, 1999); difficulty producing morphemes (Binger & Light, 2002; Kelford Smith, Thurston, Light, Parnes, & O'Keefe, 1989); and a prevalence of simple clause structures, atypical word order, omitted syntactic structures (Soto, 1997, 1999; van Bolkom & Welle Donker-Gimbrere, 1996), and impaired pragmatic skills (Light, Collier, & Parnes, 1985; O'Keefe & Dattilo, 1992; von Tetzchner & Martinsen, 1996).

Efforts to understand the metalinguistic skills of individuals with AAC needs have produced conflicting results (Clendon, Gillon, & Yoder, 2005). Dahlgren Sandberg and Hjelmquist (1996, 1997) found no significant differences between children who used AAC and matched controls. In contrast, Vandervelden and Siegel (1999) found significant deficits in the metalinguistic skills of children with AAC needs in comparison with reading age-matched control groups of children without disabilities. It is apparent, however, that students with AAC needs can improve their metalinguistic skills when provided with systematic instruction targeting these skills (Clendon et al., 2005).

The construct of *literacy knowledge* is used in this chapter to reflect all of the processes, skills, and understandings in emergent and early literacy that relate directly to print or its equivalent (e.g., braille). For many individuals with AAC needs, limited access to print may result in underdeveloped literacy knowledge (Koppenhaver & Yoder, 1993). When children with AAC needs are provided with regular opportunities to engage in print-based interactions, there is evidence that they make progress toward the development of these important skills. For example, a group of young children identified as having autism spectrum disorders (ASDs) demonstrated increasingly sophisticated understandings of print when provided with twice weekly opportunities to engage in child-directed, adult-supported, print-based interactions (Koppenhaver & Erickson, 2003). A group of young girls with Rett syndrome demonstrated improved literacy knowledge when their mothers engaged in repeated book sharing with them using simple communication technologies (Skotko, Koppenhaver, & Erickson, 2004). Also, adolescents with multiple disabilities, including deafblindness and AAC needs, demonstrated more sophisticated literacy knowledge when provided with alternative writing tools and regular opportunities to write about self-selected topics (Hanser, 2006). James provides an excellent example of this interrelationship between emergent literacy and communication development for children who use AAC.

James has significant intellectual, physical, visual, hearing, and communication impairments. At the age of 15, he smiled broadly when people interacted with him and vocalized to protest and otherwise gain the attention of others, but he was unable to use symbols to communicate in any way. During the school year, his team started implementing many of the emergent literacy and communication strategies described in this chapter. Over the course of the next several years, James developed emergent literacy and communication skills in an interrelated and integrated manner. As he began using symbols to communicate, he engaged more effectively in book-sharing interactions and developed more sophisticated concepts about print.

As his concepts about print developed, he began applying his understandings of written language in his own efforts to communicate. As he began using the alphabet to engage in writing, his increased knowledge of letters and sounds improved his word reading. And, as his word reading improved, his communication improved. It was clear throughout that what James was learning about symbols for communication was supporting his literacy development, and what he was learning about print use in literacy was supporting his communication. After 4 years of hard work, James now has a high-end communication device that he uses to communicate, and he is reading and spelling words to convey meaning. ─────────

Why Should Literacy Be an Integral Component of an Academic Program for Beginning Readers and Writers Who Use AAC?

In the late 1970s, education for students with significant disabilities underwent what has been called a transformation from a developmental to a functional approach (Spooner & Browder, 2006). This transformation dramatically changed the way individuals with significant disabilities were taught. Instead of focusing on mental age and using preexisting instructional approaches that matched that age (regardless of the chronological age of the individual), instruction started to focus on the skills individuals required to function effectively across current and future environments (Brown, Nietupski, & Hamre-Nietupski, 1976). Because of IDEA 2004 and NCLB, there are increased demands and expectations that all students will have access to the general curriculum and instruction that emphasizes academic growth.

Some argue that sight word instruction is a functional skill that separates it from other forms of reading and writing instruction. For example, in describing options for addressing both functional sight word instruction and broader literacy instruction, Browder, Courtade-Little, Wakeman, and Rickelman wrote,

> The first [option] is to provide two concurrent forms of reading instruction—one that focuses on promoting literacy and the other on the systematic instruction of sight words in the context of daily living as a "safe-guard" for having some functional reading if the student doesn't learn to read. A second option is to provide extensive literacy instruction in the elementary grades and transition to a functional reading approach if progress is not made by late middle school or high school. A third option is to make sight-word instruction part of the literacy program. (2006, p. 66)

In practice, we would advocate to make sight word instruction an integral part of any comprehensive literacy program. In fact, the ability to recognize words with automaticity is a critical component of fluent reading (Meyer & Felton, 1999) and cannot be ignored if we are to help students learn to read conventionally. We disagree, however, with the characterization of sight word reading as functional and all other forms of literacy as something else.

For individuals with AAC needs, particularly those who also experience significant physical impairments, literacy is the most important functional skill we can address. Literacy will provide these individuals with the voice they require to direct their own lives. It will provide these individuals with a means of establishing and maintaining relationships. Literacy is an essential life skill that is far more important than rehearsing partial participation in the activities of daily living.

───────   Jordan was 11 years old when he began his journey toward literacy in earnest. Prior to that, he had participated eagerly in the numerous literacy activities that occurred daily in his inclusive classroom setting. He often used laminated picture symbols to make choices between two items, used photographs to interact with peers during lessons, and used picture banks to write in errorless activities created by his team. The alphabet and systematic word study instruction took on great importance in developing Jordan's literacy skills rather than supporting his participation in activities with modifications that eliminated reading and writing demands. Through years of focused instruction, Jordan learned to spell and use word prediction well enough to communicate all of his thoughts and feelings with people across environments and events. By the time Jordan was a young adult, his family faced difficult choices about managing his health, and he could write well enough to play a central role in the decision making about his own health care. ———————

How Is Emergent Literacy Related to the General Education Curriculum?

As noted in the beginning of this chapter, the emphasis that is being placed on literacy for individuals with significant disabilities, including those with AAC needs, is in large part due to IDEA 1997 and NCLB. First, IDEA 1997 mandated that all students have access to the general curriculum. Then, NCLB required that states have challenging standards with assessments that measure student performance against them while holding schools accountable for student achievement in reading, math, and science. The assessments for accountability that fall under NCLB begin in the third grade and continue through high school.

Most beginning readers and writers participating in assessments for accountability are, by definition, older students. They may be third-grade students who are just beginning to read and write or they might be high school seniors who demonstrate very emergent understandings of oral language, metalinguistic skills, and literacy knowledge. Whatever the case, they are individuals with emergent literacy understandings gaining access to a curriculum filled with skills that are at least three grade levels higher than those they currently possess. Often, the result is that instruction emphasizes isolated skills that are deemed most appropriate given the ability gap.

Individual states are working to guide educational teams in meeting the demands of IDEA 2004 and NCLB by identifying alternative access or entry points that are aligned with the general curriculum (e.g., North Carolina, Florida, California). These access or entry points provide specific examples of the ways in which students with varying degrees of severe disabilities might gain access to the general curriculum and demonstrate achievement or progress over time. Educational teams should take great care to create instructional programs based on either the general curriculum or these alternate access or entry points to ensure that students are developing new skills from year to year.

During 2008, we saw two extreme examples of providing older beginning readers and writers who use AAC with access to the general curriculum. In one case, the state alternative assessment process provided an educational team with specific tasks or skills that a student was expected to demonstrate through the alternative assessment process. This team created an intervention program through which they taught the skills directly using a system of most-to-least prompts. The student spent a significant portion of his school day engaged in massed trials of the skills to ensure his successful performance of the skills on the assessment.

In contrast, another team received a similar set of tasks and skills. Instead of teaching them in isolation, the team taught them across environments and with a variety of materials and activities. Instead of devoting hours of instructional time to a narrow set of skills, the team taught the skills as part of instruction that also targeted communication and interaction skills, fostered initiation and problem solving, and eventually led to generalized understanding and application of the skills.

The first team went into the alternate assessment with a great deal of confidence that the student would perform quite well. They had weeks of data to support their belief that the student could consistently complete the tasks and demonstrate the skills on demand. The second team had a different type of confidence going into the alternate assessment. They, too, had data, but their data supported their confidence that the student could make decisions about when the skill would serve him well. In the end, both students did very well on the alternate assessment, but the second young man achieved far more than proficiency on the end-of-grade test. His team was committed to providing him with access to the general curriculum and to demonstrating achievement without sacrificing his development as a reader and writer, and it served him well. In contrast, the first team was so focused on ensuring high performance on the assessment that they missed opportunities that would have helped him develop as a reader and writer beyond the skills identified for the assessment.

Current Efforts To Make Text
Accessible to Beginning Readers and Writers

Developing accessible materials is part of providing access to the general curriculum. In reading, materials have to be physically, linguistically, and cognitively accessible. Physical access can be achieved through increasing the size of the font, adding tabs to pages to make them easier to turn, or acquiring an electronic version of the text. Linguistic access can be achieved by simplifying the language to a level that the student can understand when it is read to him or her. This might involve revising the vocabulary, simplifying the sentence structure, or decreasing the overall length. Cognitive access might be provided by offering additional graphic elements, addressing vocabulary and other issues related to background knowledge at the beginning of the text, and linking the text directly to the student's life experiences. Although there are many issues to consider when making text accessible, these represent a few strategies that can increase a student's opportunities to learn and develop literacy skills while gaining access to the general curriculum.

There are several efforts underway to provide students with disabilities with more comprehensive access to materials for learning. One primary example is the National Instructional Materials Accessibility Standards (NIMAS), which seeks to drive textbook publishers to make available a digitized version of all materials they produce to be used by individuals with print-related disabilities. The materials that will be produced as a result of NIMAS will not, in themselves, be accessible. Instead, the materials will be provided in a file format that is compatible with numerous accessibility software programs (e.g., screen readers) that can be used to present the content in an accessible format. Although the prospect of having all general education materials available in a format that can be presented in a number of accessible ways to students is appealing, there are important issues to consider, particularly with beginning readers and writers.

For example, there are many beginning readers and writers who will not be able to understand grade-level content just because it is read to them by a screen reader, presented in large font with extra spacing, or otherwise made physically accessible. These students require that the text be simplified or enhanced to address their linguistic and cognitive needs. One method that is being used extensively to address this need is the creation of picture-supported text that pairs picture symbols with every, or almost every, word in a text. To ensure that this method supports access to and comprehension of the text, AAC teams should first determine that the language level of the text is such that the student could understand the text if it was read to him or her. If this is not checked, then the risk is that the student will successfully call each word with the support of the picture but will not understand the text as a whole.

APPLICATION

Educational teams can address the literacy learning needs of beginning readers and writers through multiple means. In the following section, several specific approaches and issues to consider regarding communication and literacy instruction for beginnings readers and writers are described.

Identifying the Literacy Demands of the Curriculum

A lack of knowledge regarding the literacy demands of the curriculum is a primary barrier to achieving positive literacy learning outcomes for individuals who use AAC. The general education system has been recommended as a useful reference point when AAC teams are endeavoring to create educational environments that truly foster literacy learning for children who use AAC (Sturm et al., 2006). Research documenting literacy demands across grade levels has generated a wealth of useful information for AAC teams.

Obviously, the studies that are most relevant to improving the emergent and early literacy abilities of individuals who use AAC are those that have focused on the literacy demands inherent in preschools and the early primary grades (e.g., Morrow, Tracey, Woo, & Pressley, 1999; Sturm et al., 2006; Wharton-McDonald, Pressley, & Mistretta Hampston, 1998). In a study, Sturm et al. (2006) surveyed 141 first- and third-grade teachers and identified the literacy learning activities that were emphasized at each grade level. Examples of learning activities that occurred frequently during first grade included reading out loud to children, providing independent reading opportunities, building background knowledge, and teaching children to manipulate sounds. Figure 9.2 illustrates where these activities would fall within Sénéchal et al.'s (2001) model, provides examples of the literacy goals that are addressed in each, and gives possible solutions to support children who use AAC as they engage and learn in these instructional activities. Using the information from studies such as these in conjunction with classroom-based observations of children who use AAC can assist AAC teams to determine the teaching strategies and technology tools that are required in order for children to participate in learning opportunities that are as commensurate as possible to those experienced by their speaking peers (Sturm et al., 2006).

Addressing the Communication and Vocabulary Requirements Related to the Literacy Demands

A key outcome from the research that has examined the literacy demands of the curriculum has been an increased awareness of the range, depth, and quantity of communication that is needed for individuals to fully participate in and learn from literacy-related events (Sturm et al., 2006). Children who use AAC need access to tools and strategies that allow them to communicate about literacy. Just like their speaking peers, they must be able to express their ideas, thoughts, and opinions about books; make predictions about how stories will end; and tell their friends what they are writing about during emergent writing activities. "They need access to novel techniques and tools that support them in sharing what they know and connecting this knowledge to new information" (Sturm et al., 2006, p. 33). Some of the key issues surrounding communication in literacy for children who use AAC are discussed in the section that follows.

Core versus Fringe Vocabulary
Technological advances have lead to increases in memory capacity, and now most high-tech AAC systems are able to store a large number of symbols (Sutton, Morford, & Gallagher, 2004). This is obviously a positive development as it means that limited space can no longer be regarded as a barrier to providing children with AAC needs with access to comprehensive vocabularies; however, it also means that issues relating to vocabulary organization have moved to the forefront and are of considerable concern.

One major objective of the AAC team is to organize vocabulary in such a way that children with AAC needs have efficient access to core and fringe vocabulary. *Core vocabulary* refers to words and messages that are used with high frequency, by a variety of individuals (Beukelman & Mirenda, 2005), and across a number of different language contexts. An investigation suggests that there is a great deal of overlap between the core vocabulary children use in oral and written communication (Clendon, 2006). *Fringe vocabulary* refers to words and messages that are content rich, topic related (McGinnis & Beukelman, 1989), and specific to the individual (Beukelman & Mirenda, 2005). In the context of reading and writing, fringe vocabulary words are typically the focus of meaning vocabulary instruction and are divided into two tiers of words: *Tier 2* words are those that are found across demands of knowledge and are used with relatively high frequency by mature language users; *Tier 3* words are low-frequency words that are limited in use to specific knowledge domains (Beck, McKeown, & Kucan, 2002). It is important to consider frequency of use when determining which core and fringe vocabulary to store on a device to support both oral and written language development.

Activity	Target LK	Target OL	Target ML	Possible learning goals	Possible solutions
Shared reading and guided reading		✓		To discuss new vocabulary	Method for student to quickly indicate that he or she has something to say
		✓		To make predictions	AAC system with easy access to core vocabulary
		✓		To identify the main idea	Access to new vocabulary that has been integrated meaningfully into the student's AAC system
		✓		To relate the book to personal experiences	Remnant book or photo album for relating book to personal experiences
	✓			To recognize high-frequency words	Plausible multiple choice responses that limit expressive communication demands while maximizing opportunities for interaction after a choice is made
	✓			To recognize book characteristics (e.g., authors/illustrators, titles, front/back page)	
	✓			To understand print concepts (e.g., directionality, the difference between letters and words)	
		✓		To describe the main character, setting, or other story features	
Independent reading	✓			To select a book from a range of narrative and informational genres	Accessible books PowerPoint books (Microsoft) My Own Bookshelf (SoftTouch) Start-to-Finish Literacy Starters (Don Johnston) BookWorm (Ablenet)
	✓			To engage in sustained study of book pages, pictures, and words	Books without speech feedback—just pictures and words
	✓			To read books independently	Choice from a large selection of books

Figure 9.2. High-frequency literacy learning activities in first-grade classrooms: Examples of literacy activities, literacy learning goals, and potential adaptive technologies. (Key: LK, literacy or print knowledge; OL, oral language; ML, metalinguistics.)

	LK	OL	ML	Learning goals	Examples of literacy activities and potential adaptive technologies
Story retelling		✓		To list story events in chronological order	AAC device with easy access to core vocabulary (e.g., first, then, after) and common narrative structures (e.g., once upon a time, the end)
		✓		To tell a story with a clear beginning and end	Models of adults and other students using the AAC system to retell the story
		✓		To remember the most important information across the text	Sentence strips with one story event written on each for the student to place in order
Reading/reciting nursery rhymes			✓	To recognize words that rhyme	AAC device with easy access to core vocabulary and preprogrammed messages: "THOSE WORDS RHYME." "THAT RHYMES WITH _____."
	✓			To develop one-to-one correspondence between spoken and written words	Use talking word processors that highlight word-by-word in addition to charts
Counting and manipulating word sounds			✓	To identify the first sound in words	AAC device with easy access to alphabet, core vocabulary, and preprogrammed messages: "THAT WORD STARTS WITH _____;" "I HEAR _____ SOUNDS IN THAT WORD."
			✓	To blend sounds together to make words	Add letters to phonological awareness instruction from the beginning

205

Some AAC professionals feel that in order for children to be successful at school, they must have access to all of the vocabulary that they will encounter across the school day. This includes access to curriculum-related vocabulary, such as words from storybooks or science textbooks. Some words occur so infrequently in the English language that they are only used during the week of school when they are the focus of reading materials, discussion, or assessment (Erickson & Clendon, 2005). Other words occur more frequently, however, and the sheer volume often means they are buried so deep in children's AAC systems that when they are needed at a later date, children are unable to retrieve them (Erickson, 2003). Children need access to AAC systems that facilitate fast access to core vocabulary and logical access to fringe vocabulary when using AAC across reading, writing, and the curriculum.

For children who have low-tech devices or devices that have limited storage capacity, it is also important to consider both core and fringe vocabulary when making decisions regarding vocabulary selection for particular literacy activities. It is fairly common practice in the AAC field, for instance, for children to be provided with story-specific vocabulary for shared reading activities. The teacher or speech-language pathologist (SLP) will examine the vocabulary that is in the selected story and provide the same vocabulary to the child who uses AAC. Every time the teacher selects a new story, the process is repeated so that the child is constantly presented with new sets of words. The lack of a consistent core vocabulary that can be used across multiple storybooks may lead to decreased vocabulary learning and limited generalization across contexts. Furthermore, providing these children with access to only text-specific vocabulary may prevent them from being able to relate the book to extra-textual experiences such as a field trip they participated in or another book they have read.

The book *Brown Bear, Brown Bear* (Martin, 1983) provides an excellent example of the two approaches. Teams who follow a book-specific approach to selecting vocabulary would create a communication board that includes each of the animals in the book including the blue horse and purple cat. The children would use the board during book reading and perhaps some other activities that were a part of a unit of study related to the book. Unfortunately, the children would have very little long-term use for the communication board when the class was done with the book and unit of study. In contrast, a team selecting vocabulary from the perspective of core and fringe vocabulary would be more likely to add new vocabulary to an existing AAC system (or use them to start a system). The vocabulary would include the names of the individual animals clustered in an animal category plus the primary colors the child needs to describe or talk about the animals in the book. Then, the child can participate in early book-sharing activities by labeling the individual animals or labeling the colors while the teacher models the expanded form of color plus animal. This process supports children in learning more about language, provides them with practice using vocabulary they can use across environments, and teaches them to begin linking symbols long before they may be successful doing so on their own.

Efficient versus Precise Communication

Individuals who use AAC need to develop the ability to communicate both efficiently and precisely within the context of oral and written communication. Efficient communication strategies are important because they speed up the rate of message transmission and allow individuals who use AAC to participate in language and literacy activities in a timely manner (Harris, Doyle, & Haaf, 1996). Precise communication is also critical for individuals who use AAC. Being able to construct messages that are grammatically correct and complete is necessary for the prevention of communication breakdowns and misunderstandings, for the communication of complex ideas, and for literacy development (Lund & Light, 2003; Sutton, Soto, & Blockberger, 2002).

Efficient communication and precise communication are not necessarily mutually exclusive. They have, however, frequently been treated as such by researchers, clinicians, and manufacturers in the AAC field. For instance, most of the AAC devices that have been available to date have been either word based or utterance based. The word-based devices have enabled individuals with complex communication needs to construct novel messages and, therefore, communicate precisely what they wish to say (Bedrosian, Hoag, & McCoy, 2003). In contrast, the utterance-based devices have focused on increasing communication efficiency by including a range of prestored utterances. None of the devices, however, have been flexible and dynamic enough to allow individuals who use AAC to be both efficient and precise.

Devices are increasingly being designed to address the need for precise and efficient AAC communication through the inclusion of phrases or grammatically complete utterances into their language systems. The AAC field is making a transition into a new and exciting phase of research and development as we face the challenge of providing access to language systems that support a dynamic balance between both efficient and precise AAC communication.

There has been some hesitancy in the AAC field about providing individuals who use AAC, particularly children, with access to prestored utterances. Many professionals have expressed concern that providing children with such messages may be detrimental to children's language development. Specifically, these professionals have questioned the effect of providing children with access to utterances that are syntactically and morphologically more advanced than those that they are able to produce independently (Gerber & Kraat, 1992). They have also expressed concern that acquiring language in the context of prestored messages may prevent these children from learning to construct their own novel messages (Bedrosian, 1997; Nelson, 1992).

These are valid concerns that warrant further investigation; however, studies conducted outside the field of AAC suggest that the use of prestored messages is not a characteristic that is unique to individuals with complex communication needs. Adults and children who use spoken language as their primary mode of communication also rely heavily on prefabricated language forms (Erman & Warren, 2000; Wray, 2002). A study of the vocabulary used by typically developing beginning writers revealed that many children in the earliest stages of written language development used particular phrases (e.g., I see, I like) with sufficiently high frequency that AAC teams might consider storing them as whole units within children's AAC systems (Clendon, 2006, Clendon & Erickson, 2007).

First Letter Cueing and Word Prediction   First letter cueing and word prediction are both strategies that can be used to facilitate the communication abilities of individuals who use AAC. Until these individuals learn to spell conventionally, they are limited by the vocabulary stored in their AAC systems. Unfortunately, often the vocabulary that is stored in their AAC systems is inadequate to meet their communication needs (Light, 1997). Even if an individual has access to a very large vocabulary, there are still likely to be words that they encounter on a regular basis that they do not have access to in their AAC system. As mentioned previously, it is simply impossible to provide individuals who use AAC with access to all of the words that they could possibly need without seriously compromising the usability of their AAC systems (Erickson & King DeBaun, 2006).

First letter cueing is a strategy that individuals who use AAC can utilize when they want to assist communication partners to guess words that they are trying to communicate. The strategy involves individuals using an alphabet display to point to the first letters of words. The strategy builds on their emerging alphabet knowledge. Teachers can model first letter cueing throughout the school day. Natural opportunities to use this strategy occur when the teacher is prompting children to recall a specific word (e.g., "I am thinking of a new word we learned yesterday. It's an action word. It starts with *J.*") or concept (e.g., "Who remembers the name of the shape that has eight sides? It begins with the letter *O.*") (Erickson & King DeBaun, 2006). Individuals can learn to use first letter cueing long before they are able to read and spell conventionally.

Successful use of first letter cueing requires that children know letter names and letter sounds and apply that knowledge to initial consonant recognition. We begin to teach children letter names by reading alphabet books with them and by intentionally pointing out the letters in their names whenever we encounter them. At the same time, we pair letter names with actions (*K* is for kick) or foods (*M* is for mustard) that will help the children remember the letter names. To increase the likelihood that children will remember the associations, we work with the children and get them to make choices in determining the final pairing for each letter. Those associations are written on charts, and we regularly review and use the letters children are having the most difficulty learning. We can also work on the phonological awareness skill of identifying the initial consonant informally through management routines ("Line up if your name starts with /s/.") and formally through rhyming and other activities that strip or otherwise isolate the initial consonant from a word.

Word prediction is another strategy that can be used with beginning writers. Word prediction software was initially developed to increase typing speed for individuals with physical disabilities. It is now used with a wide variety of individuals, however, and has been found to be particularly beneficial for individuals who experience spelling and handwriting difficulties (Macarthur, 1999).

Word prediction software is used in conjunction with an individual's word processing program. It works as follows: the writer types the first letter of the word that he or she would like to spell, and the software predicts the word that the writer is intending to type and presents a list of alternatives that the writer can choose from (Erickson & Koppenhaver, 2007). The software can vary in its degree of complexity with the more sophisticated programs presenting choices based on complicated algorithms that take into consideration word frequency (Erickson & Koppenhaver, 2007), spelling, syntax, and the patterns of use exhibited by the individual writer (Macarthur, 1999).

If the writer is unable to read the choices that the software presents, then the writer can have the computer read the choices out loud. If the word that the writer wants is on the list, then he or she can select it. If the desired word is not on the list, then he or she can type the second letter of the word and read the new choices. If the word is still not on the list, then the writer should be encouraged to spell the word based on how he or she thinks the word sounds (Erickson & Koppenhaver, 2007).

Sometimes AAC team members express concern about using this software to support beginning writers. They are worried that it will have a negative effect on spelling development because there will not be as many opportunities for individuals to engage in invented spelling. There are a number of advantages to using the software, however. It is particularly beneficial for individuals who are unable to read their own spelling attempts. The software helps them to produce enough correctly spelled words to support them in reading and remembering the other words (Erickson & Koppenhaver, 2007). Secondly, it exposes individuals to new words and can provide a rich learning context for discussions regarding how choices are similar or different in terms of their phonology, orthography, and word meanings.

Although spelling itself is one approach to building phonics skills, specific spelling-based approaches to phonics instruction can support both reading and spelling development. Although we encourage teams to begin using word prediction as early as possible to maximize successful participation in the general education curriculum, we also recognize that explicit instruction is required. We use a combination of phonics instructional approaches that include the important, spelling-based strategy called Making Words (Cunningham & Cunningham, 1992). The research supports the use of this approach with children with and without disabilities (Stahl, Duffy-Hester, & Stahl, 1998) as well as children who use AAC (Hanser & Erickson, 2007). Because the strategy works with a limited letter set, it decreases access demands and leads to more efficient intervention. It is particularly useful with AAC users because the original strategy requires no speaking, but provides continuous evidence of student understanding. In this approach, children are given a handful of letters including only a single vowel in the beginning. The teacher then guides the child through making 1-, 2-, 3-, and 4-letter words, making minimal changes from one word to the next. This increases student success and also enables students to recognize and understand within-word spelling patterns more efficiently. At each point in the lesson, the student first attempts to use the letters to make a word as directed. After the attempt has been made, a visual model of the correct spelling is provided. The attempt is then compared with the correct version, and the student makes corrections as needed. In order to best support careful student examination of within-word spelling patterns, it is important that students be guided in comparing their words letter by letter with the target word rather than merely copying the model from scratch. After all of the words are made, the student is then directed to sort the words based on common letters, length, and spelling patterns, Finally, the child is directed to use words that were made during the lesson to spell a word or words that were not yet taught.

Determining Literacy Learning Goals

In addition to the guidance provided by the general curriculum, it is important that individualized education programs (IEPs) include carefully constructed goals that will support beginning readers and writers in improving their literacy skills and understandings. As described previously, this requires teams to go beyond mere rehearsal of the isolated skills to be assessed at the end of the year. It requires that beginning readers and writers have direct instruction designed to build their oral language, metalinguistic knowledge, and literacy knowledge while also having regular opportunities to apply those emerging understandings in self-directed reading and writing activities.

Providing direct instruction aimed at developing skills and understandings in these three areas can take a variety of forms. A specific goal that might be addressed in small-group book-sharing activities may read, "During shared reading activities, the student will use a 'I have a question' display with partner-assisted scanning to generate one or more questions on 4 out of 5 days." The communication display (high tech or low tech) might include question forms (what, who, when, where, why, how), common story grammar vocabulary (e.g., character, setting), and core vocabulary that could be used across shared reading materials. In this way, the student can be working on increasing communication, interaction, engagement, oral language, and literacy knowledge while learning the specific story-grammar vocabulary that is part of most general curricula.

At the same time, the student could be applying his or her developing knowledge about letters and letter sounds by writing with an alternative to a standard pencil or keyboard. For example, the partner could scan through the letters of the alphabet verbally while pointing to each letter. The student could use a single switch to indicate WRITE THAT LETTER DOWN FOR ME or two switches to direct the adult to GO TO THE NEXT ONE or WRITE THAT LETTER DOWN FOR ME. The goal addressed during this activity might read, "Given daily opportunities to write about self-selected, personally meaningful topics, the student will demonstrate increased sophistication in writing as indicated by changes in letter combinations and sequences as well as spaces and use of punctuation."

In addition to the individualized instruction provided as part of a student's IEP, many students will have regular access to the general curriculum in general education or other settings where groups of students are being taught at the same time. The pace of these group lessons often presents challenges to beginning readers and writers who use AAC because they cannot possibly compose responses or initiate interactions at a rate that allows them to be active participants. Two specific strategies to use in these settings are described next.

Use "Every Pupil Response" Whenever Possible   When working with a group of students, it is important to maximize engagement and participation for all of the students. Every pupil response supports this goal. The first step in employing every pupil response is to find some nonverbal gesture or movement that *all* of the students in the group can do, including using a thumbs up, looking in a designated direction (up, at the window, toward the door), closing eyes, nodding/shaking head, or raising an arm. Once the gesture or movement has been identified, it is up to the educator to pose questions or seek input in a way that allows the students to respond. For example, an educator might say, "Thumbs up if you think he is going to win."

Every pupil response decreases the demands on some students to generate a response independently and gives those who impulsively provide responses an alternative means of responding. It also provides the educator with ongoing information regarding the engagement and comprehension of the group.

Use Partner-Assisted Scanning Across the Day   Making a choice from the items on a list or on a communication board can be difficult for some students because they lack the ability to point, cannot see or read the choices, are positioned too far away (as in group activities), or have not developed sufficient switch access skills. Partner-assisted scanning addresses these issues by asking the communication partner (a teacher, paraprofessional, or child) to point to each of the options pausing long enough at each for the child with physical and communication impairments to respond "yes" if the item is their desired choice. Depending on the needs of the individual child, the partner can name each option when pointing or simply point. Partner-assisted scanning can be used with communication or alphabet boards designed for individual children, and it can also be used with large- or small-group instruction with the items printed on a chart or board. The teacher can couple every pupil response with partner-assisted scanning, and all children can use some agreed-on gesture (e.g., thumbs up) to indicate when the teacher points to and names the desired selection.

Speech-Language Pathologist's Role in Literacy

Since 2001, preschool- and school-based SLPs have been challenged to take on an increasingly active role in literacy assessment and intervention. Unfortunately, this has not been an easy transition for many SLPs who have struggled to apply the extensive knowledge base they have in spoken language to reading and writing development (Ehren & Ehren, 2001).

To date, most SLP literacy efforts have been reasonably narrow in their focus. Researchers and clinicians have embraced phonological awareness assessment and intervention with much fervor but have typically placed significantly less emphasis on other areas such as reading comprehension (Catts, Fey, Zhang, & Tomblin, 1999). The emphasis on phonological awareness is commendable given that it has been shown to be a strong predictor of literacy learning success (see Gillon, 2004, for a review of this research). Widespread, indiscriminate implementation of phonological awareness intervention, however, may be problematic.

Research has clearly demonstrated that children who go on to experience difficulty acquiring conventional literacy skills do not necessarily have a history of isolated phonological awareness problems. One study found that out of a group of 183 second graders who were classified as poor readers, 37% exhibited both language and phonological awareness difficulties in kindergarten, 22% exhibited language difficulties, and only 14% exhibited isolated deficits in phonological awareness (Catts et al., 1999). In current practice, some children may be exposed to phonological awareness intervention that they do not need, instead of being exposed to other types of interventions that they desperately do need. Children who use AAC are also likely to have diverse literacy learning profiles, and they, too, may be receiving interventions that are not multifaceted enough to address all of their learning needs. In addition, the SLP's knowledge base in comprehension and vocabulary is not being used.

Research suggests that the best defense for all children is the provision of excellent classroom instruction (Snow, Burns, & Griffin, 1998). Therefore, to have a significant effect on children's emergent literacy outcomes, SLPs need to deliver most of their services within the classroom environment, regardless of the age of the student. SLPs need to collaborate with teachers in planning interventions that support children's development of critical language targets within the context of classroom literacy lessons (Allington & Cunningham, 2002).

Ehren (2000) described how SLPs can maintain their therapeutic focus while at the same time sharing responsibility with teachers for student success. The SLP's role differs from the teacher's role in that the SLP's primary focus must be on the provision of services to children on their caseload. This means that particular activities within the classroom setting are more appropriate for an SLP to be involved in than others. For instance, it would be appropriate for the SLP working with a child who uses AAC to host an invitational group that focuses on a particular strategy or skill (e.g., building background knowledge for a story that the teacher is going to read tomorrow) (Keene & Zimmermann, 1997). The SLP would design the lesson to meet the IEP goals of the child who uses AAC but would open up spaces to other children who would also benefit from participating in the lesson. In contrast, an example of an inappropriate activity would be for an SLP to engage in coteaching a literacy lesson to an entire classroom of children when the lesson does not specifically address the IEP goals of the child who uses AAC (Ehren, 2000).

SLPs have an important role to play in developing a range of important emergent oral and written language skills. Building children's oral language abilities in the context of written language offers many advantages. For instance, it helps SLPs to prioritize therapy goals. Instead of feeling the weight of having to teach a child who uses AAC all of the vocabulary that he or she might need across every day and every environment, the SLP can focus on making sure that vocabulary is selected that will support the child's success in specific literacy lessons, with specific books, on specific days that has application across other environments, activities, and interactions.

The context of written language may also provide children who use AAC with increased cognitive clarity about why different language targets are important. SLPs often work on skills such as vocabulary, sequencing, and questioning; all of which are relevant to literacy learning success. If SLPs can show children who use AAC why these skills are important for literacy and how the skills will help them to read and write, then the children's increased metacognitive awareness may lead to greater therapy gains.

CONCLUSION

Addressing the demands of the general curriculum for beginning readers and writers presents numerous challenges for educational teams. There are challenges presented by the beliefs of practitioners who have historically taken a functional approach to intervention for students with severe disabilities without recognizing literacy as a valuable functional life skill. There are challenges presented by IDEA 2004, which requires access to the general curriculum, and NCLB, which requires access to the grade-level standards, even when older students are still beginning readers and writers. There are challenges presented by the need to address literacy learning relative to the end-of-grade assessments while also providing comprehensive opportunities to develop oral language, metalinguistic knowledge, and literacy knowledge through IEPs. This list goes on, but the challenges are not insurmountable. Efforts are being made across the country and throughout the assistive technology and augmentative communication industry to develop instructional programs that align with the general curriculum but address the unique learning needs of beginning readers and writers who use AAC. Research is being conducted that is demonstrating that beginning readers and writers who use AAC can emerge into conventional readers and writers all the way through their teenage years. But there is a great deal more work to do.

As states and schools work to develop systems that allow them to account for the progress that beginning readers and writers make, we must carefully monitor the contents of those systems. The AAC community has a responsibility to ensure that individuals who use AAC are provided with literacy programs that are as rich and comprehensive as those provided to their speaking peers. The challenge is for AAC teams to move beyond a focus on literacy participation to a true focus on literacy learning so that AAC users can maximize their potential along the continuum of literacy development and acquire the literacy skills that are needed for achieving independent self-expression and for gaining access to critical educational and vocational opportunities.

REFERENCES

Allington, R.L., & Cunningham, P.M. (2002). *Schools that work: Where all children read and write.* Boston: Allyn & Bacon.

Bedrosian, J.L. (1997). Language acquisition in young AAC system users: Issues and directions for future research. *Augmentative and Alternative Communication, 13,* 179–185.

Bedrosian, J.L., Hoag, L.A., & McCoy, K.F. (2003). Relevance and speed of message delivery trade-offs in augmentative and alternative communication. *Journal of Speech, Language, and Hearing Research, 46,* 800–817.

Beck, I.L., McKeown, M.G., & Kucan, L. (2002). *Bringing words to life: Robust vocabulary instruction.* New York: Guilford Press.

Berninger, V.W., & Gans, B.M. (1986). Language profiles in nonspeaking individuals of normal intelligence with severe cerebral palsy. *Augmentative and Alternative Communication, 2,* 45–50.

Beukelman, D.R., & Mirenda, P. (2005). *Augmentative and alternative communication: Supporting children and adults with complex communication needs* (3rd ed.). Baltimore: Paul H. Brookes Publishing Co.

Biemiller, A. (1999). *Language and reading success.* Brookline, MA: Brookline Books.

Binger, K., & Light, J. (2002). *Morphology and syntax in individuals who use AAC.* Seminar presented at the American Speech-Language-Hearing Association Convention, Atlanta, GA.

Browder, D.M., Courtade-Little, G., Wakeman, S., & Rickelman, R.J. (2006). From sight words to emerging literacy. In D.M. Browder & F. Spooner (Eds.), *Teaching language arts, math, and science to students with significant cognitive disabilities* (pp. 63–91). Baltimore: Paul H. Brookes Publishing Co.

Browder, D.M., & Spooner, F.H. (2006) *Teaching language arts, math, and science to students with significant cognitive disabilities.* Baltimore: Paul H. Brookes Publishing Co.

Browder, D.M., & Xin, P.Y. (1998). A meta-analysis and review of sight word research and its implications for teaching functional reading to individuals with moderate and severe disabilities. *Journal of Special Education, 32,* 130–153.

Brown, L., Nietupski, J., & Hamre-Nietupski, S. (1976). Criterion of ultimate functioning. In M.A. Thomas (Ed.), *Hey, don't forget about me! Education's investment in the severely, profoundly, and multiply handicapped* (pp. 2–15). Reston, VA: Council for Exceptional Children.

Carey, S. (1978). The child as word learner. In M. Halle, J. Bresnan, & G. Miller (Eds.), *Linguistic theory and psycholinguistic reality* (pp. 264–293). Cambridge, MA: MIT.

Carlson, F. (1981). A format for selecting vocabulary for the nonspeaking child. *Language, Speech, and Hearing Services in Schools, 12,* 240–245.

Catts, H.W., Fey, M.E., Zhang, X., & Tomblin, J.B. (1999). Language basis of reading and reading disabilities: Evidence from a longitudinal investigation. *Scientific Studies of Reading, 3*(4), 331–361.

Chall, J.S. (1983). *Stages of reading development.* New York: McGraw-Hill.

Clay, M.M. (1966). *Emergent reading behavior.* Unpublished doctoral dissertation, University of Auckland, New Zealand.

Clay, M.M. (1979). *The early detection of reading difficulties.* Auckland, New Zealand: Heinemann.

Clendon, S.A. (2006). *The language of beginning writers: Implications for children with AAC needs.* Unpublished doctoral dissertation, University of North Carolina at Chapel Hill.

Clendon, S.A., & Erickson, K.A. (2007). *The vocabulary of beginning writers: Implications for children with AAC needs.* Manuscript submitted for publication.

Clendon, S., Gillon, G., & Yoder, D. (2005). Initial insights into phoneme awareness intervention for children with AAC needs. *International Journal of Disability, Development, and Education, 52,* 7–31.

Cunningham, A.E., & Stanovich, K.E. (1997). Early reading acquisition and its relation to reading experience 10 years later. *Developmental Psychology, 33,* 934–945.

Cunningham, P., & Cunningham, J. (1992). Making words: Enhancing the invented spelling–decoding connection. *The Reading Teacher, 46,* 106–115.

Dahlgren Sandberg, A., & Hjelmquist, E. (1996). A comparative, descriptive study of reading and writing skills among non-speaking children: A preliminary study. *European Journal of Disorders of Communication, 31,* 289–308.

Dahlgren Sandberg, A., & Hjelmquist, E. (1997). Language and literacy in nonvocal children with cerebral palsy. *Reading and Writing: An Interdisciplinary Journal, 9,* 107–133.

Dickinson, D.K., McCabe, A., Anastasopoulos, L., Peisner-Feinberg, E.S., & Poe, M.D. (2003). The comprehensive language approach to early literacy: The interrelationships among vocabulary, phonological sensitivity, and print knowledge among preschool-aged children. *Journal of Educational Psychology, 95*(3), 465–481.

Dickinson, D.K., & Snow, C.E. (1987). Interrelationships among prereading and oral language skills in kindergarteners from two social classes. *Early Childhood Research Quarterly, 2,* 1–25.

Dickinson, D.K., & Tabors, P.O. (Eds.). (2001). *Beginning literacy with language: Young children learning at home and school.* Baltimore: Paul H. Brookes Publishing Co.

Downing, J. (2005). *Teaching literacy to students with significant disabilities.* Thousand Oaks, CA: Corwin Press.

Downing, J.E. (2006). Building literacy for students at the presymbolic and early symbolic levels. In D. Browder & F. Spooner (Eds.), *Teaching language arts, math, and science to students with significant cognitive disabilities* (pp. 39–61). Baltimore: Paul H. Brookes Publishing Co.

Ehren, B.J. (2000). Maintaining a therapeutic focus and sharing responsibility for student success: Keys to in-classroom speech-language services. *Language, Speech, and Hearing Services in Schools, 31,* 219–229.

Ehren, B.J., & Ehren, T.C. (2001). New or expanded roles for speech-language therapists: Making it happen in the schools. *Seminars in Speech and Language, 22*(3), 233–243.

Ehri, L.C. (1998). Grapheme-phoneme knowledge is essential for learning to read words in English. In J. Metsala & L. Ehri (Eds.), *Word recognition in beginning reading* (pp. 3–40). Mahwah, NJ: Lawrence Erlbaum Associates.

Elementary and Secondary Education Act of 1965, PL 89-10, 20 U.S.C. §§ 241 *et seq.*

Erickson, K. (2003). Reading comprehension in AAC. *The ASHA Leader, 8*(12), 6–9.

Erickson, K., & Clendon, S.A. (2005). Responding to individual needs: Promoting the literacy development of students who use AAC. *Perspectives on Augmentative and Alternative Communication, 14*(2), 11–16.

Erickson, K., & King DeBaun, P. (2006). *Adaptations to support inclusive instruction in the second grade reading workshop developed by The Reading and Writing Project, Teachers College, Columbia University.* Unpublished manuscript.

Erickson, K., & Koppenhaver, D. (2007). *Children with disabilities reading and writing the four blocks way.* Winston-Salem, NC: Carson Dellosa.

Erickson, K.A., Koppenhaver, D.A., Yoder, D.E., & Nance, J. (1997). Integrated communication and literacy instruction for a child with multiple disabilities. *Focus on Autism and Other Developmental Disabilities, 12*(3), 142–150.

Erman, B., & Warren, B. (2000). The idiom principle and the open-choice principle. *Text, 20,* 29–62.

Geary, D.C. (1995). Reflections of evolution and culture in children's cognition. *American Psychologist, 50,* 24–37.

Gerber, S., & Kraat, A. (1992). Use of a developmental model of language acquisition: Applications to children using AAC systems. *Augmentative and Alternative Communication, 8,* 19–32.

Gillon, G.T. (2004). *Phonological awareness: From research to practice.* New York: Guilford Press.

Hanser, G. (2006). Fostering emergent writing for children with significant disabilities: Writing with alternative pencils. *Technology Special Interest Section Quarterly, American Occupational Therapy Association, 16,* 1–4.

Hanser, G., & Erickson, K.A. (2007). Integrated word identification and communication instruction for students with complex communication needs: Preliminary results. *Focus on Autism and Developmental Disabilities, 22*(4), 268–278.

Harris, L., Doyle, E.S., & Haaf, R. (1996). Language treatment approach for users of AAC: Experimental single-subject investigation. *Augmentative and Alternative Communication, 12,* 230–243.

Individuals with Disabilities Education Act Amendments (IDEA) of 1997, PL 105-17, 20 U.S.C. §§ 1400 *et seq.*

Individuals with Disabilities Education Improvement Act (IDEA) of 2004, PL 108-446, 20 U.S.C. §§ 1400 *et seq.*

Jordan, G.E., Snow, C.E., & Porche, M. (2000). Project EASE: The effect of a family literacy project on kindergarten students' early literacy skills. *Reading Research Quarterly, 35,* 524–546.

Keene, E.O., & Zimmermann, S. (1997). *Mosaic of thought: Teaching comprehension in a reader's workshop.* Portsmouth, NH: Heinemann.

Kelford Smith, A., Thurston, S., Light, J., Parnes, P., & O'Keefe, B. (1989). The form and use of written communication produced by physically disabled individuals using microcomputers. *Augmentative and Alternative Communication, 5,* 115–124.

Koppenhaver, D.A. (2000). Literacy in AAC: What should be written on the envelope we push? *Augmentative and Alternative Communication, 16,* 267–277.

Koppenhaver, D.A., & Erickson, K.A. (2003). Natural emergent literacy supports for preschoolers with autism and severe communication impairments. *Topics in Language Disorders, 23*(4), 283–293.

Koppenhaver, D.A., & Yoder, D.E. (1993). Classroom literacy instruction for children with severe speech and physical impairments (SSPI): What is and what might be? *Topics in Language Disorders, 13*(2), 1–15.

Light, J. (1997). "Let's go star fishing": Reflections on the contexts of language learning for children who use aided AAC. *Augmentative and Alternative Communication, 13,* 158–171.

Light, J., Collier, B., & Parnes, P. (1985). Communicative interaction between young nonspeaking physically disabled children and their primary caregivers: Part III: Modes of communication. *Augmentative and Alternative Communication, 1,* 125–133.

Lonigan, C.J., Burgess, S.R., & Anthony, J.L. (2000). Development of emergent literacy and early reading skills in preschool children: Evidence from a latent-variable longitudinal study. *Developmental Psychology, 36,* 596–613.

Lund, S.K., & Light, J. (2003). The effectiveness of grammar instruction for individuals who use augmentative and alternative communication systems: A preliminary study. *Augmentative and Alternative Communication, 46,* 1110–1123.

Macarthur, C.A. (1999). Word prediction for students with severe spelling problems. *Learning Disabilities Quarterly, 22,* 158–172.

Martin, B. (1983). *Brown bear, brown bear, what do you see?* New York: Henry Holt.

Mason, J.M., & Stewart, J.P. (1990). Emergent literacy assessment for instructional use in kindergarten. In L.M. Morrow & J.K. Smith (Eds.), *Assessment for instruction in early literacy* (pp. 155–175). Upper Saddle River, NJ: Prentice Hall.

McGinnis, J.S., & Beukelman, D.R. (1989). Vocabulary requirements for writing activities for the academically mainstreamed student with disabilities. *Augmentative and Alternative Communication, 5,* 183–191.

Meyer, M.S., & Felton, R.H. (1999). Repeated reading to enhance fluency: Old approaches and new directions. *Annals of Dyslexia, 49,* 283–306.

Morrow, L.M., Tracey, D.H., Woo, D.G., & Pressley, M. (1999). Characteristics of exemplary first-grade literacy instruction. *Reading Teacher, 52,* 462–477.

Nation, K., & Snowling, M.J. (2004). Beyond phonological skills: Broader language skills contribute to the development of reading. *Journal of Research in Reading, 27*(4), 342–356.

Nelson, N.W. (1992). Performance is the prize: Language competence and performance among

AAC users. *Augmentative and Alternative Communication, 8,* 3–18.

No Child Left Behind Act of 2001, PL 107-110, 115 Stat. 1425, 20 U.S.C. §§ 6301 *et seq.*

O'Keefe, B.M., & Dattilo, J. (1992). Teaching the response recode form to adults with mental retardation using AAC systems. *Augmentative and Alternative Communication, 8,* 224–233.

Romski, M., Sevcik, R.A., & Robinson, B.F. (1996). Mapping the meaning of novel visual symbols by youth with moderate or severe mental retardation. *American Journal on Mental Retardation, 100,* 391–402.

Scarborough, H. (1998). Early identification of children at risk for reading disabilities: Phonological awareness and some other promising predictors. In B.K. Shapiro, P.J. Accardo, & A.J. Capute (Eds.), *Specific reading disability: A view of the spectrum* (pp. 75–119). Timonium, MD: York Press.

Scarborough, H. (2001). Connecting early language and literacy to later reading (dis)abilities: Evidence, theory, and practice. In S.B. Neuman & D.K. Dickinson (Eds.), *Handbook of early literacy research* (pp. 97–110). New York: Guilford Press.

Sénéchal, M., & LeFevre, J. (2002). Parental involvement in the development of children's reading skill: A five-year longitudinal study. *Child Development, 73*(2), 445–460.

Sénéchal, M., LeFevre, J., Smith-Chant, B.L., & Colton, K.V. (2001). On refining theoretical models of emergent literacy: The role of empirical evidence. *Journal of School Psychology, 39*(5), 439–460.

Skotko, B., Koppenhaver, D., & Erickson, K. (2004). Parent reading behaviors and communication outcomes in girls with Rett syndrome. *Exceptional Children, 70*(2), 145–166.

Snow, C.E. (1983). Literacy and language: Relationships during the preschool years. *Harvard Educational Review, 53,* 165–189.

Snow, C.E., Burns, M.S., & Griffin, P. (1998). *Preventing reading difficulties in young children.* Washington, DC: National Academies Press.

Soto, G. (1997). Multi-unit utterances and syntax in graphic symbol communication. In E. Björk-Åkesson & P. Lindsay (Eds.), *Communication... naturally: Theoretical and methodological issues in augmentative and alternative communication: Proceedings of the Fourth International Society for Augmentative and Alternative Communication Research Symposium* (pp. 26–32). Västerås, Sweden: Mälardalen University.

Soto, G. (1999). Understanding the impact of graphic sign use on the message structure. In F.T. Loncke, J. Clibbens, H.H. Arvidson, & L.L. Lloyd (Eds.), *Augmentative and alternative communication: New directions in research and practice* (pp. 40–48). London: Whurr.

Spooner, D.M., & Browder, F. (2006). Why teach the general curriculum? In D.M. Browder & F.

Spooner (Eds.), *Teaching language arts, math, and science to students with significant cognitive disabilities* (pp. 1–13). Baltimore: Paul H. Brookes Publishing Co.

Stahl, S.A., Duffy-Hester, A.M., & Stahl, K.A.L. (1998). Everything you wanted to know about phonics (but were afraid to ask). *Reading Research Quarterly, 33,* 338–355.

Storch, S.A., & Whitehurst, G.J. (2002). Oral language and code-related precursors to reading: Evidence from a longitudinal structural model. *Developmental Psychology, 38*(6), 934–947.

Sturm, J., Spadorcia, S.A., Cunningham, J.W., Cali, K.S., Staples, A., Erickson, K., et al. (2006). What happens to reading between first and third grade?: Implications for students who use AAC. *Augmentative and Alternative Communication, 22*(1), 21–36.

Sutton, A., Morford, J., & Gallagher, T. (2004). Production and comprehension of graphic symbol utterances expressing complex propositions by adults who use augmentative and alternative communication systems. *Applied Psycholinguistics, 25,* 349–371.

Sutton, A., Soto, G., & Blockberger, S. (2002). Grammatical issues in graphic symbol communication. *Augmentative and Alternative Communication, 18,* 192–204.

Tabors, P.O., Roach, K.A., & Snow, C.E. (2001). Home language and literacy environment: Final results. In D.K. Dickinson & P.O. Tabors (Eds.), *Beginning literacy with language: Young children learning at home and school* (pp. 111–138). Baltimore: Paul H. Brookes Publishing Co.

Teale, W.H., & Sulzby, E. (1986). Emergent literacy as a perspective for examining how young children become writers and readers. In W.H. Teale & E. Sulzby (Eds.), *Emergent literacy: Writing and reading* (pp. vii–xxv). Norwood, NJ: Ablex.

Title 1—Improving academic achievement of the disadvantaged: Final rule, 68 Fed. Reg. 236 (Dec. 2003).

Udwin, O., & Yule, W. (1990). Augmentative communication systems taught to cerebral palsied children: A longitudinal study. I. The acquisition of signs and symbols, and syntactic aspects of their use over time. *British Journal of Disorders of Communication, 25,* 295–309.

van Bolkom, H., & Welle Donker-Gimbrere, M. (1996). A psycholinguistic approach to graphic language use. In S. von Tetzchner (Ed.), *Augmentative and alternative communication: European perspectives* (pp. 153–170). London: Whurr.

Vandervelden, M., & Siegel, L. (1999). Phonological processing and literacy in AAC users and children with motor speech impairments. *Augmentative and Alternative Communication, 15,* 191–211.

von Tetzchner, S., & Martinsen, H. (1996). Words and strategies: Conversations with young children who use aided language. In S. von Tetzchner (Ed.), *Augmentative and alternative communication: European perspectives* (pp. 65–88). London: Whurr.

Wharton-McDonald, R., Pressley, M., & Mistretta Hampston, J.M. (1998). Literacy instruction in nine first-grade classrooms: Teacher characteristics and student achievement. *Elementary School Journal, 99*(2), 101–128.

Whitehurst, G.J., Epstein, J.N., Angell, A.L., Payne, A.C., Crone, D.A., & Fischel, J.E. (1994). Outcomes of an emergent literacy intervention in Head Start. *Journal of Educational Psychology, 86,* 542–555.

Whitehurst, G.J., & Lonigan, C. (1998). Child development and emergent literacy. *Child Development, 69*(3), 848–872.

Wray, A. (2002). *Formulaic language and the lexicon.* New York: Cambridge University Press.

10

Addressing the Literacy Demands of the Curriculum for Conventional and More Advanced Readers and Writers Who Require AAC

Janice C. Light and David McNaughton

The development of literacy skills has a profound positive effect on all aspects of life—educational, vocational, social, and personal. Given the fundamental importance of literacy skills, it is not surprising that reading and writing occupy pivotal roles in the school curriculum, from the early elementary grades, where the focus is on learning to read and write, to the later school years, where the focus is on developing more advanced reading and writing skills to support learning in other areas of the curriculum (National Reading Panel [NRP], 2000). Unfortunately, historically, many individuals with augmentative and alternative communication (AAC) needs have not had the opportunity to participate in effective and appropriate literacy instruction within the schools (Koppenhaver, 1991; McNaughton, Light, & Arnold, 2002; Mirenda, 2003). Although there are adults who use AAC who have developed high-level literacy skills (Koppenhaver, Evans, & Yoder, 1991), most individuals who require AAC perform well below their typically developing peers in reading and writing (e.g., Berninger & Gans, 1986; Kelford Smith, Thurston, Light, Parnes, & O'Keefe, 1989; Koppenhaver, Steelman, Pierce, Yoder, & Staples, 1993; Lund & Light, 2006). Many have not acquired even basic literacy skills (Koppenhaver & Yoder, 1992).

In order to reap the full educational, vocational, social, economic, and personal benefits of literacy, individuals who require AAC must move well beyond the stage of emergent literacy and must acquire conventional and more advanced literacy skills. In light of this requirement, the goal of this chapter is to delineate procedures and tools for effective evidence-based instruction to teach conventional literacy skills (i.e., learning to read and write) and more advanced literacy skills (i.e., reading and writing to learn) to individuals who require AAC. In delineating appropriate procedures and tools, we have drawn on the best evidence available as suggested by Schlosser and Rhagavendra (2004). There is a small but growing body of experimental research studies that provide important evidence of effective interventions to teach the initial acquisition of conventional literacy skills to individuals with AAC needs. We have used these studies to define appropriate tools and procedures for this early stage of literacy acquisition. To date, there is a paucity of experimental research focused on interventions to teach more advanced literacy skills to individuals who require AAC.

The authors are grateful to the many individuals who use AAC and their families who have helped us to learn about effective literacy instruction. The research by Light and McNaughton described in this chapter was funded in part by the Communication Enhancement Rehabilitation Engineering Research Center (AAC-RERC). The AAC-RERC is a virtual research center that is funded by the National Institute on Disability and Rehabilitation Research (NIDRR) of the U.S. Department of Education under grant number H133E030018. The opinions contained in this publication are those of the grantees and do not necessarily reflect those of the U.S. Department of Education. For additional information on the AAC-RERC, see http://www.aac-rerc.com.

Therefore, the procedures and tools proposed for this later stage of literacy development rest on the evidence provided by a number of anecdotal and case study reports in the AAC field, as well as the research on effective interventions to teach more advanced literacy skills to students who speak but are at risk for the development of reading and writing skills (e.g., Adams, 1990; Graham & Perin, 2007; NRP, 2000), with adaptations proposed to accommodate students with AAC needs. There remain many unanswered questions. It is our hope that this chapter will serve as an impetus for researchers to systematically investigate techniques to improve literacy outcomes for individuals who require AAC.

KEY ISSUES AND CHALLENGES

The development of conventional literacy skills is a complex process that is affected by a wide range of intrinsic factors (i.e., characteristics of the learner who requires AAC) and extrinsic factors (i.e., environmental variables). Some of these factors are under the direct control of interventionists (e.g., instructional content and techniques); others may be outside the direct control of interventionists and not easily amenable to change (e.g., the learner's oculomotor function, head and hand control). Adaptations, strategies, and instructional supports may be required to compensate for limitations.

Intrinsic Factors that May Affect Literacy Development

There are a wide range of intrinsic factors that may put individuals who require AAC at risk for problems in the development of conventional reading and writing skills, including: 1) visual impairments that may affect perception and processing of written text; 2) motor deficits that may limit access to reading and writing materials; 3) difficulties with phonological awareness skills that may limit their ability to blend phonemes into words and to segment words into phonemes; 4) pragmatic, semantic, syntactic, and morphological limitations that may affect understanding and production of written texts; 5) working memory limitations that may negatively affect their ability to hold information in their mind and work with it; and 6) deficits in executive functions such as planning and monitoring performance that may affect reading comprehension and writing. One or more of these intrinsic factors may negatively affect the development of the orthographic, phonological, contextual, and meaning processing skills required by students to read and write (Adams, 1990).

Children with AAC needs who come from diverse cultural and linguistic backgrounds face additional challenges in developing conventional literacy skills. In addition to the linguistic code of their AAC systems, they must learn at least two languages or dialects—the language/dialect of their family and that of the broader social community. These languages may differ significantly with respect to their pragmatics, phonology, semantics, syntax, and morphology as well as with respect to the culture of language and literacy and the relationship between the characteristics of the oral language and the written orthography (Geva & Wang, 2001; Harrison-Harris, 2002). To date, we have only a limited understanding of how to support the development of communication, language, and literacy skills for children with AAC needs who come from diverse cultural and linguistic backgrounds (Harrison-Harris, 2002). There is a critical need for additional research in this area.

Extrinsic Factors that May Affect Literacy Learning

In addition to these types of intrinsic factors, there are also a wide range of environmental factors that may put individuals who require AAC at risk for developing conventional reading and writing skills. For example, individuals who require AAC, especially those with significant motor impairments, may have limited access to printed materials and writing activities. Their partners may dominate interactions so that they may have limited opportunities to participate in communicative interactions and reading activities, and they may not have access to their AAC systems during literacy activities, severely limiting their participation (Light, Binger, & Kelford Smith, 1994; Light & Kelford Smith, 1993). Furthermore, parents and teachers may have low expectations for the development of literacy skills (Light & McNaughton, 1993; McNaughton et al., 2002; Mirenda, 2003). Parents may be overwhelmed by care routines and may consider literacy learning a lower priority compared with other more immediate needs (Light & Kelford Smith, 1993). Furthermore, parents and teachers may have little reason to think that the development of literacy skills is an attainable goal if they do not have access to effective evidence-based curricula adapted to meet the needs of students who require AAC. When expectations are inappropriately low, they may negatively affect the quantity and quality of time spent in literacy-related activities. Furthermore, they may indirectly affect the student's own expectations for success, reducing motivation for learning (Light & McNaughton, 1993).

The literacy environments of students with AAC needs may vary significantly depending on a variety of factors such as socioeconomic status and cultural background. In some cases, environmental factors may provide important supports for students who are acquiring literacy skills; in other cases, environmental factors may be such that they negatively affect literacy learning opportunities.

Intervention is critical to address the wide range of intrinsic and extrinsic variables and to support students with AAC needs in developing conventional and more advanced literacy skills. The development of literacy skills is not an innate process; most students require organized and consistent instruction to learn to read and write (NRP, 2000). Literacy instruction for individuals with AAC needs should be embedded within a comprehensive plan for intervention that provides adaptations, strategies, and instruction to maximize motor, sensory perceptual, language, and cognitive skills. Effective literacy intervention requires the commitment and involvement of a skilled and knowledgeable multidisciplinary team (e.g., special education teacher, reading specialist, speech-language pathologist [SLP], occupational therapist, vision specialist, paraprofessional), as well as the student with AAC needs and the family.

It is especially important to ensure that appropriate seating and positioning is in place (as required) to maximize motor function and that appropriate access techniques have been determined for the student to maximize participation in instructional tasks. Furthermore, because reading and writing depend on visual and auditory skills, it is essential to ensure that appropriate vision and hearing assessments are completed and the required supports and adaptations are in place to maximize auditory and visual perceptual function (e.g., assistive listening devices, appropriate location of instructional materials, size of print, color contrast).

INSTRUCTIONAL VARIABLES THAT AFFECT LITERACY OUTCOMES

Historically, the lack of effective evidence-based instruction adapted to meet the needs of students who require AAC has been one of the major contributing factors to poor literacy outcomes (Browder, Wakeman, Spooner, Ahlgrim-Delzell, & Algozzine, 2006; Mirenda, 2003; Sturm et al., 2006). Literacy instruction must be well designed to positively affect the reading and writing skills of individuals who require AAC. There are a number of variables related to instruction that may affect literacy outcomes, including 1) the time devoted to instruction, 2) the appropriateness of the content/instructional goals that are targeted, 3) the effectiveness of the instructional techniques employed to teach this content, 4) the adaptations provided to meet the needs of individuals with significant speech (and motor) impairments who require AAC, and 5) the evaluation procedures employed to monitor progress (Light & McNaughton, 2007; Pressley et al., 2001).

Time Devoted to Literacy Instruction

To date, there has been limited research to investigate the amount of literacy instruction typically provided to students with AAC needs. Many individuals with AAC needs report that they had limited, if any, opportunity to participate in literacy instruction (McNaughton et al., 2002). In a study of the classroom experiences of three students with AAC needs, Koppenhaver (1991) reported that only 17–29 minutes per day were allocated for reading instruction and only 7–15 minutes were allocated to writing instruction; furthermore, less than half of the allocated time was actually spent in instruction. This amount of instruction is woefully inadequate given the complexity of learning conventional reading and writing skills.

Recommended practice is that all students in Grades 1–3 receive a minimum of at least 90 minutes of literacy instruction per day and that students who are at risk should receive an additional 40–60 minutes, for a total of 130–150 minutes of literacy instruction per day (IRIS Center, 2007; Vaughn, Wanzek, Woodruff, & Thompson, 2007). Students with AAC needs may require additional instructional time because they often have very slow rates of communication and may, therefore, require more time to participate than their peers. In order to ensure that students with AAC needs receive the appropriate quantity (and quality) of reading instruction, a collaborative approach may be required involving the general education teacher, the special education teacher, the SLP, the paraprofessional or classroom volunteer, and the family (Ehren, 2006; Mather, Bos, & Babur, 2001). Additional research is needed to identify effective models of instructional delivery to ensure successful literacy outcomes for students with AAC needs.

Instructional Content

Consistent with recommendations of the NRP and others for literacy instruction with students without disabilities (e.g., Adams, 1990; NRP, 2000; Pressley et al., 2001), students with AAC needs require instruction in the following skills: language skills, phonological awareness skills, letter–sound correspondences, single-word decoding skills, application of decoding skills in book reading, recognition of sight words, reading and understanding connected text, and building writing skills (e.g., Coleman-Martin, Heller, Cihak, & Irvine, 2005; Erickson, 2003; Light & McNaughton, in press; Sturm & Clendon, 2004; Truxler & O'Keefe, 2007).

Once students have acquired conventional literacy skills, instruction should continue to build more advanced literacy skills by fostering more complex language skills; developing world knowledge and domain-specific knowledge; building fluency and automaticity in sight word recognition, decoding, and encoding skills; learning the conventions of written language (e.g., spelling, punctuation, capitalization); developing executive functions to facilitate reflection, planning, and monitoring of performance; and developing more specific cognitive strategies (i.e., planning, revising, editing) to support reading comprehension and writing (e.g., Copeland, 2007; Graham & Perin, 2007; NRP, 2000; Peterson, Caverly, Nicholson, O'Neal, & Cusenbary, 2000; Sturm & Clendon, 2004). At this advanced stage, the focus is not simply on the acquisition of simple skills, but rather on building fluency in these basic skills and learning cognitive strategies or multistep procedures to accomplish more complex tasks such as comprehension of more complex reading materials or writing essays and other genres.

Specific goals, materials, and procedures to teach basic and advanced literacy skills and strategies are discussed in further detail later in this chapter along with evidence of the effectiveness of the techniques described. Instruction in these skills and strategies should be complemented by regularly reading interesting texts from a range of genres to students and by talking about these texts. By reading and talking about more complex, interesting texts, instructors and/or parents achieve the following goals: They 1) establish the meaningfulness of reading and writing; 2) provide access to a range of models of effective writing and models of the reading process; 3) increase student motivation for learning literacy skills; 4) provide important opportunities for students to build comprehension and learn to understand, interpret, and talk about texts, and 5) offer a means for students to develop more advanced language skills, extend their world knowledge, and build domain-specific knowledge (Ivey & Broaddus, 2001; Kucan & Beck, 1997).

Instructional Techniques

The NRP (2000) recommended that students at risk for literacy learning difficulties be taught following the principles of effective instruction, with numerous opportunities to apply new skills in the context of meaningful and motivating reading and writing activities. Specifically, instruction should address both direct teaching of basic skills (e.g., letter–sound correspondences, phonological awareness, decoding skills) as well as opportunities to develop vocabulary knowledge and acquire text comprehension skills (NRP, 2000). Light, McNaughton, Fallon, Millar, and colleagues applied this recommendation to literacy instruction in the AAC field, proposing direct instruction in basic skills that adheres to the following steps: 1) model the skill, 2) use guided practice, and 3) provide opportunities for independent practice (Fallon, Light, McNaughton, Drager, & Hammer, 2004; Light & McNaughton, 2007, in press; Millar, Light, & McNaughton, 2004). See Table 10.1 for explanations of the instructional steps. The "model, guided practice, independent practice" instructional procedures have been used effectively to teach a wide range of skills to learners with and without disabilities (e.g., Kame'enui & Simmons, 1990; Rosenshine & Stevens, 1986). They have been applied successfully to teach conventional reading and writing skills to students with AAC needs (e.g., Fallon et al., 2004; Light & McNaughton, 2007, in press; Millar et al., 2004). Once students acquire conventional literacy skills, similar instructional procedures can be adapted and applied to teach more advanced reading comprehension and writing strategies as well. (See the section on advanced literacy skills for more detailed discussion of strategy instruction.)

As learners acquire skills, they should be provided with numerous opportunities to apply these skills in meaningful and motivating literacy activities (NRP, 2000). For example, as soon as students begin to acquire basic decoding skills, they should be provided with opportunities to apply these skills in the context of motivating and functional shared reading activities (Light & McNaughton, in press).

Adaptations for Individuals with AAC Needs

Most of the available literacy curricula for students with reading disabilities require students to produce oral responses in order to fully participate. Adaptations are required to allow students with AAC needs to participate fully in instructional activities. Specifically, adaptations are required to address three issues: 1) eliminate the need for oral or handwritten responses and facilitate more efficient and less fatiguing participation in instruction, 2) provide insight into areas of difficulty for the student that may require additional instruction, and 3) compensate for the student's lack of access to oral rehearsal/production.

Table 10.1. Instructional procedures to teach basic literacy skills to students with augmentative and alternative communication needs

Step	Instructional procedures
Model	The instructor demonstrates the skill for the student.
Guided practice	The instructor provides scaffolding support/prompting to help the student perform the skill successfully.
	The instructor gradually fades the support as the student develops competence.
Independent practice	The student completes the skill independently.
	The instructor monitors performance and provides feedback.
Feedback	If the student performs the skill accurately, then the instructor provides appropriate positive feedback.
	If the student is incorrect, then the instructor directs the student's attention to the error, models the correct response, provides guided practice for the student, and then provides additional opportunities for independent practice.

Source: Light & McNaughton (in press).

A number of researchers have described techniques to adapt literacy instruction so that students who require AAC do not need to respond orally in reading activities or use handwriting for writing activities (e.g., Bedrosian, Lasker, Speidel, & Politsch, 2003; Blischak, 1995; Coleman-Martin et al., 2005; Fallon et al., 2004; Heller, Fredrick, Tumlin, & Brineman, 2002; Light & McNaughton, in press; Millar et al., 2004). Typically, instructional tasks are modified so that students with AAC needs can respond using alternative modes (e.g., pointing or eye pointing to AAC symbols, words, or letters provided specifically for instructional tasks; using listener-assisted scanning of response options; selecting AAC symbols on a speech-generating device [SGD] or communication board; selecting letters from a standard or adapted keyboard). Examples of specific task adaptations to bypass the need for oral responses in literacy instruction are provided in subsequent sections. It is critical to evaluate these curricular adaptations to ensure their effectiveness.

In typical literacy instruction, the instructor uses the students' oral responses to gauge their understanding and competence, utilizing errors to determine areas that require further instruction. When students are not able to produce oral responses, the instructor may have more difficulty pin-pointing areas of difficulty (Heller et al., 2002). Fallon et al. (2004) and Light and McNaughton (in press) described procedures for carefully controlling response options and providing systematic error analysis to allow the instructor to pinpoint areas of difficulty. For example, if students are learning to decode consonant-vowel-consonant (CVC) words, they may be presented with the written target word (e.g., *map*) and then provided with four AAC symbols or pictures as possible responses with one of the four options representing the correct response (e.g., symbol for MAP), one representing an initial letter–sound substitution (e.g., NAP), one a final letter–sound substitution (e.g., MAT), and one a substitution of the medial vowel (e.g., MOP; see Figure 10.1). By analyzing response patterns over multiple trials, the instructor can identify areas of strength (e.g., initial letter sounds) as well as areas where the student may demonstrate repeated errors and require focused instruction (e.g., confusion with medial vowels).

Finally, students with AAC needs may require adaptations to compensate for their lack of access to oral production during literacy activities. When typically developing children are learning to decode novel words, they often say the sound for each letter in the word orally or subvocally and then blend the sounds to decode the word (Adams, 1990). Conversely, when they are learning to write, they may say a word slowly (either orally or subvocally) to segment out the sounds that form the word and then select the letters for each sound that they hear. Students who have AAC needs may be unable to orally produce some or all of the sounds in the target word, and they may have difficulty with sub-vocal rehearsal. As a result, they face increased demands on their working memory and increased chal-lenges in learning to decode and encode words (Dahlgren Sandberg, 2006; Millar et al., 2004).

Students with AAC needs may benefit from external scaffolding support in the initial stages of instruction to compensate for their lack of access to oral rehearsal and to help them build subvocal

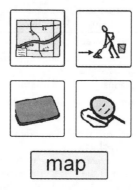

Figure 10.1.   Response plate for decoding the word *map* with augmentative and alternative communication symbols for the target word and foils representing initial, final, and medial substitutions. The Picture Communication Symbols © 1981–2008 by Mayer-Johnson LLC. All Rights Reserved Worldwide. Used with permission.

rehearsal. The instructor may model saying the sounds aloud for the student while encouraging the student to say the sounds in his or her head subvocally. As the student develops competence, the instructor gradually fades the oral scaffolding support until the student is able to perform independently. Research by Fallon et al. (2004) and Light and McNaughton (2007, in press) demonstrated the effectiveness of the application of this type of scaffolding support in reading instruction; research by Millar et al. (2004) demonstrated application in writing instruction.

Progress Monitoring and Evaluation of Student Skills

Regular monitoring and evaluation of student skills is required in order to ensure that instruction is as effective and efficient as possible. Witt, Elliot, Daly, Gresham, and Kramer (1998) argued for the direct observation and measurement of student performance within the curriculum to assess learning and gather information to make valid decisions about instruction. Essentially, assessment probes are developed using the books and materials that comprise the student's literacy curriculum; related curricular materials can be used to assess generalization of skills as well. Data are collected on student performance within these probes to evaluate the student's progress and to determine the effectiveness of instruction (Fuchs, Deno, & Mirkin, 1984). This teach–test process ensures 1) that instructors know when students have successfully acquired skills so that new skills can be introduced and 2) that instructors identify difficulties with specific skills that may require additional instruction or adjustments in the instructional program.

INSTRUCTION IN CONVENTIONAL READING AND WRITING SKILLS

Instruction in conventional literacy skills is a primary focus of the curriculum during the early elementary years (Sturm et al., 2006). Ideally, students with AAC needs will have the opportunity to participate in conventional literacy instruction with their typically developing peers during these years. Given the importance of literacy skills for students with AAC, there is significant justification for getting students who require AAC started on instruction in conventional literacy skills as early as possible, even before they start elementary school. Research by Light and McNaughton (in press) found that, with appropriate instruction, four preschool students with AAC needs (ages 3–5) demonstrated significant gains learning conventional literacy skills. All entered kindergarten able to read and compose simple texts. This had a significant effect on their communication skills, as well as a powerful positive influence on the expectations of their educational team.

Of course, some individuals with AAC needs may be older when they first have the opportunity to participate in conventional literacy instruction, either because they missed out on these instructional opportunities at a younger age or because they required additional time to develop basic communication skills. There is evidence that individuals with AAC needs can benefit from literacy instruction at any age (Light & McNaughton, 2006, in press). For individuals who start instruction at older ages, it is important to ensure that materials are age appropriate and interesting to ensure motivation.

The following section discusses 1) the importance of each of the skills required for the development of basic conventional literacy skills, 2) materials and procedures for effective instruction in these skills, and 3) evidence of the effectiveness of the instruction described. The subsequent section discusses instruction in more advanced literacy skills.

In general, the instruction described is based on research by Light and McNaughton (in press) as well as earlier research on single-word decoding completed with Fallon (Fallon et al., 2004) and earlier research on early writing skills completed with Millar (Millar et al., 2004). Many of the instructional materials and procedures discussed are illustrated in a web cast (Light & McNaughton, 2006) that can be accessed at http://www.aac-rerc.com.

To date, most of the research on literacy instruction with students who require AAC has investigated the effectiveness of one-to-one instruction in school and home settings (e.g., Fallon et al.,

2004; Light & McNaughton, in press; Millar et al., 2004). Future research is required to investigate the effectiveness of instructional strategies to support the participation of students with AAC needs in small-group reading instruction with their speaking peers in general education classrooms (Koppenhaver, Spadorcia, & Erickson, 1998).

Although this chapter, out of necessity, presents skill instruction in a linear sequence starting with the basic underlying skills and building to more complex skills, it should be noted that, in most cases, students will be involved in instruction to address multiple skills concurrently. For example, in the very early stages of instruction, students may be involved in instruction in sound blending, phoneme segmentation, and letter–sound correspondences. Later in the instructional process, as students develop their skills, they may be involved in instruction in single-word decoding, sight word recognition, shared reading, reading comprehension, and early writing, as well as continued practice in phonological awareness skills and letter–sound correspondences to build automaticity.

Language Intervention

According to Sturm and Clendon (2004), language is the cornerstone of literacy learning. Unfortunately, many individuals with AAC needs lag behind their peers in the development of pragmatic, semantic, syntactic, and morphological skills (see Blockberger & Sutton, 2003; Light, 1997; and Smith & Grove, 2003 for further discussion). Individuals with AAC needs may also struggle with developing the narrative skills that are used to structure early writing (Soto & Hartmann, 2006; Soto, Hartmann, & Wilkins, 2006). AAC interventions often focus solely on the development of functional communication and may neglect the pragmatic, semantic, syntactic, and morphological skills required to support reading comprehension and functional writing. It is beyond the scope of this chapter to discuss in detail interventions to support language development; readers are referred to Chapters 7 and 8 for further discussion.

Instruction in Phonological Awareness Skills

In addition to pragmatic, semantic, syntactic, and morphological skills, students also require phonological awareness skills to support the acquisition of conventional literacy skills (Adams, 1990; Stanovich, 1986). *Phonological awareness* is defined as an individual's understanding or awareness of the sound structure of language; it involves the ability to notice, think about, and manipulate the phonemes of words (Torgesen, Wagner, & Rashotte, 1994). Phonological awareness tasks include rhyming, segmenting words into component sounds, blending individual sounds to produce words, identifying beginning or final sounds in words, and so forth. There is a growing body of research that supports the following conclusions: Individuals with AAC needs can develop phonological awareness skills despite severe speech impairments; however, many demonstrate deficits in phonological awareness compared with their typically developing peers (e.g., Bishop, 1985; Bishop & Robson, 1989; Card & Dodd, 2006; Dahlgren Sandberg, 2006; Foley, 1993; Foley & Pollatsek, 1999; Vandervelden & Siegel, 1999).

Given the positive correlation between phonological awareness skills and literacy learning (NRP, 2000) and the evidence that individuals with AAC needs are at risk in the development of phonological awareness skills, it is important to provide focused instruction in these skills as part of any literacy intervention. As discussed by Erickson and Clendon (see Chapter 9), intervention to promote the development of phonological awareness skills should be initiated during the emergent literacy stage before the introduction of conventional literacy skills. Many students with AAC needs, however, may not have had effective instruction in phonological awareness skills during the emergent literacy stage and may require this instruction as they are introduced to instruction in conventional literacy skills. Even if students with AAC needs have had some prior instruction in phonological awareness skills, it is important that instruction continues past the point of simple acquisition of these skills to the point at which skills are automatic, requiring minimal (if any) conscious processing. Without automaticity, students will need to devote considerable cognitive resources to these component skills, thus increasing working memory demands and leaving limited cognitive resources available for actual reading and writing processes.

Sound blending and phoneme segmentation skills are two phonological awareness skills that are strongly associated with positive literacy outcomes (Hatcher, Hulme, & Ellis, 1994; Lovett & Steinbach, 1997).

Instruction in Sound Blending   Sound blending involves the ability to build words from individual phonemes and is essential to the process of decoding novel words. Fallon et al. (2004) and Light and McNaughton (in press) evaluated instruction in sound blending designed to teach students who use AAC to 1) listen to target phonemes in a word presented orally by the instructor with each phoneme extended 1–2 seconds, 2) blend these sounds in sequence, 3) determine the target word, and 4) indicate the word by pointing to the appropriate AAC symbol out of a field of four or more options provided specifically for the task or by indicating the correct response using their AAC systems (e.g., sign, communication board, SGD). Participants in both studies acquired sound blending skills successfully.

Instruction in Phoneme Segmentation   Whereas sound blending is essential to the reading process, phoneme segmentation is essential to the writing process. Phoneme segmentation involves the ability to break words down into individual sounds. Several studies have targeted intervention in phoneme segmentation skills designed to teach students who use AAC to match a target phoneme, presented orally by the instructor, to the picture/AAC symbol of a word that begins with the target phoneme from an array of symbols selected specifically for instruction or from their AAC systems (e.g., Fallon et al., 2004; Light & McNaughton, 2007, in press). Typically, instruction focuses first on segmentation of initial sounds or onset of one-syllable words because these tend to be stressed and are easier to learn to segment (Millar et al., 2004; Vandervelden & Siegel, 1995). Later, once the student attains competence with initial phoneme segmentation, instruction may target segmentation of final and/or medial sounds as required (Millar et al., 2004; Vandervelden & Siegel, 1995).

The single-subject multiple baseline research studies by Fallon et al. (2004) and Light and McNaughton (2007, in press) demonstrated the effectiveness of this type of intervention in teaching phonological awareness skills (specifically sound blending and initial phoneme segmentation) to a wide range of individuals with AAC needs including those with cerebral palsy, Down syndrome, autism, developmental apraxia, and multiple disabilities. Results of the studies were consistent: All of the participants demonstrated significant gains in their phonological awareness skills as the result of direct instruction. Blischak, Shah, Lombardino, and Chiarella (2004) also targeted phonological awareness training in a study with two children with severe speech impairments. They used a most-to-least prompting hierarchy to teach the students to segment and manipulate phonemes in CVC pseudowords. The children acquired the targeted skills, demonstrated improved skills in the encoding of pseudowords, and generalized to improved encoding of untrained words and pseudowords as well.

Instruction in Letter–Sound Correspondences

In addition to phonological awareness skills, learning conventional reading and writing skills requires knowledge of the code of written language—specifically the correspondence between the phonemes or sounds of speech and the graphemes or letters of the written language that encodes speech. Learning letter–sound correspondences requires both phonological processing and orthographic processing by the student. Phonological awareness and knowledge of letter–sound correspondences are the basic building blocks of conventional literacy skills; research suggests that these skills are strong predictors of how well children learn to read (Adams, 1990). Through instruction in letter–sound correspondences, students learn to match target phonemes presented orally by the instructor to the correct letter from an array of letters provided for the task or from a keyboard designed to meet the student's needs.

Several researchers have investigated instruction in letter–sound correspondences. For example, Fallon et al. (2004) and Millar et al. (2004) targeted a subgroup of letters and sounds in their intervention studies. Light and McNaughton (2007, in press) targeted a greater array of letter–sound correspondences (e.g., *a, m, t, s, i, f, d, r, o, g, l, h, u, c, b, n, k, v, e, w, j, p, y, x, q, z*) following guidelines proposed by Carnine, Silbert, Kame'enui, and Tarver (1997): 1) lower case letters were taught first because these occur more frequently in written text than upper case letters, 2) letters that occur more frequently were taught first so that the students were able to read more words earlier in the instructional process, 3) letters that were similar aurally and visually were separated in the instructional sequence to minimize confusions, and 4) short vowel sounds were taught before long vowels because words with short vowels (e.g., *bus*) are more likely to follow simple decoding procedures. Letter names were not taught because these are not required for successful decoding. Letter–sound correspondences were taught incrementally following a most-to-least prompting hierarchy (i.e., model, guided practice, independent practice). As the students mastered one letter–sound correspondence, a new one was introduced with regular review of previously learned letter–sound correspondences. All of the participants in the studies by Fallon et al. (2004), Light and McNaughton (2007, in press), and Millar et al. (2004) demonstrated gains in letter–sound correspondences as a result of these instructional procedures, although instruction with some students took longer than others depending on a variety of intrinsic and extrinsic factors.

Blischak et al. (2004) taught 10 letter–sound correspondences to children with severe speech impairments using different instructional procedures. Specifically, they provided a speech sound orally and asked the children to select the correct letter from an array of 10 letters, providing corrective feedback if student responses were incorrect using the following prompting hierarchy: repeat the sound, name the letter and the sound, and model the correct selection. Two of the three children acquired the targeted letter–sound correspondences during the instructional period. The third child (age 5) demonstrated consistent progress in learning the letter–sound correspondences; however, he did not reach criterion within the instructional period, and his participation in the research project was discontinued. His performance might have improved if the letter–sound correspondences had been introduced incrementally and/or he had received additional instruction.

Instruction in Single-Word Decoding

Learning to decode single words requires knowledge of at least some letter–sound correspondences and skills in blending sounds. Several researchers have targeted instruction in single-word decoding with individuals who require AAC. For example, Fallon et al. (2004) and Light and McNaughton (2007, in press) targeted instruction in decoding regular CVC, vowel-consonant (VC), and consonant-vowel (CV) words. Specifically, students were taught to decode/read a single written word and then select the AAC symbol representing the word by pointing to the appropriate AAC symbol out of a field of four or more options provided for the instructional task (see Figure 10.1). The study by Fallon et al. (2004) targeted single-word decoding of 50 regular CVC and VC words using 14 letter–sound correspondences with five students with AAC needs (ages 9–14). All participants learned to read the 50 target words, and three demonstrated generalization to decoding of untrained words. Research by Light and McNaughton (2007, in press) demonstrated the effectiveness of this approach to decoding instruction across a wider range of individuals with AAC needs, including those with cerebral palsy, autism, developmental apraxia, and Down syndrome, using a greater number of letter–sound correspondences and a much larger corpus of words. Heller et al. (2002) used a direct instruction approach to teach three individuals (ages 9–22) who knew all of the letter–sound correspondences to use sound blending to decode 10 words. Coleman-Martin et al. (2005) evaluated a modified replication of the intervention using computer-assisted instruction and demonstrated the effectiveness of the program in teaching 15 words to three students (ages 11–16).

Applying Decoding Skills in Book Reading

As soon as students demonstrate that they are acquiring the skills to decode a few single words reliably in isolation, they should be encouraged to apply these skills to book reading. This is an important step because it allows students to apply the basic skills that they have acquired in the context of meaningful and motivating reading activities (Browning, 2002). Furthermore, it enhances generalization of decoding skills across reading materials and activities. When students are just learning to decode words, the process is still effortful, requiring significant cognitive resources and conscious processing. Therefore, at this early stage, it may be most appropriate to encourage students to apply decoding skills to read targeted single words within shared reading activities mediated by literate partners (Light & McNaughton, 2007, in press). In this type of task, the instructor reads the text of the book out loud and tracks the words with a finger while reading; the instructor pauses within the sentence at the words targeted for the student to read. The goal is for the student to decode the word and select the AAC symbol representing the word from a communication board or SGD with appropriate vocabulary, from the pictures included in the book (e.g., the *I Spy* series by Marzollo & Wick, 1999), or with a sign or speech approximation if intelligible in context. Unlike storybook activities at the emergent stage of literacy instruction (see Chapter 9), at this stage, students are actually decoding words.

A variety of materials can be used for this shared reading activity to build generalization of reading skills (e.g., the *I Spy* series, storybooks for early readers, books related to curricular content, books customized for individual students or classes with photos of personal experiences; Fallon et al., 2004; Light & McNaughton, 2007, in press). Figure 10.2 provides an example of an adapted book. In developing materials for shared reading activities, it is important to choose books that are motivating and interesting and are at an appropriate language level for the student (Light, McNaughton, Weyer, & Karg, 2008).

The study by Fallon et al. (2004) investigated the generalization of single-word decoding skills taught in isolation to book reading with the *I Spy* series; four of five participants demonstrated gen-

Mom , dad , and I
went on a train

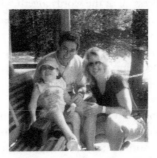

Figure 10.2.   An adapted book for shared reading with the target words highlighted for the student to decode.

eralization of decoding skills to these novel materials without instruction. Light and McNaughton (2007, in press) provided instruction in single-word decoding not only in isolation but also in a range of shared book-reading tasks using a variety of materials as described previously. All participants demonstrated competence decoding in these shared reading contexts. As the students in this study developed greater competence and fluency, the instructor targeted more words per page, gradually increasing the reading demands on the students.

Learning Irregular Words as Sight Words

In order to make the leap from single-word decoding to reading connected text, students will need to learn to read some frequently occurring irregular words as well as words governed by more complex rules that they have not yet learned to decode (e.g., *boy, the, eat, friend*). In addition, students may also be taught to recognize more complex, high-interest words to enhance their motivation for reading (e.g., *Spiderman, Darth Vader, dinosaur*). Teaching sight word recognition skills allows individuals with AAC needs to read irregular words that are too complex for them to decode. Browder, Wakeman, et al. (2006) cautioned, however, that literacy instruction should not be limited to teaching isolated sight word vocabulary or students with AAC needs will be severely restricted in their ability to read novel words and will be constrained in their ability to read a range of texts.

There are numerous studies that have demonstrated that students with moderate and severe cognitive impairments can learn to recognize sight words (e.g., Browder, Courtade-Little, Wakeman, & Rickelman, 2006; Browder & Xin, 1998; Collins & Griffen, 1996; Rehfeldt, Latimore, & Stromer, 2003; Sheehy, 2002). Furthermore, the strongest evidence supported instruction that utilized systematic prompting and fading, with repeated opportunities to practice skills (Browder, Wakeman, et al., 2006). Typically, interventions to teach sight words employ some type of paired associate learning: The target word is introduced to the student and is paired with the spoken word and/or AAC symbol representing the word (Coleman-Martin et al., 2005; Heller et al., 2002; Light & McNaughton, in press). Future research is required to evaluate the relative effectiveness of different instructional task adaptations and response procedures. As with decoding instruction, instruction in sight words should continue until students are fluent and responses are automatic.

Learning to Read and Understand Connected Text

Students are ready to read connected text once they are able to reliably and fluently decode a range of regular words (including novel ones) and recognize frequently used sight words. Learning to read connected text is much more complicated than simply decoding or recognizing single words in isolation (Erickson, Koppenhaver, Yoder, & Nance, 1997). In order to read connected text, students must 1) track through the entire sentence from left to right, in the correct sequence, and potentially across multiple lines; 2) decode or recognize each word in sequence in the sentence; 3) access the meaning of the words; and 4) process all of the words together in sequence to derive the full meaning of the sentence (or longer text). It is important that students are relatively automatic in their decoding of single words and their sight word skills before they are expected to read connected texts. If they are not relatively automatic with these component skills, then they will need to devote too many cognitive resources to the decoding process at the word level and will overtax working memory, leaving few, if any, resources to process and understand the meaning of the entire sentence or text (Jenkins, Fuchs, van den Broek, Espin, & Deno, 2003).

In order to make the transition from reading single words in isolation to reading full sentences, Light and McNaughton (in press) developed specific instructional procedures to ensure that students were reading and processing the entire sentence and not just focusing on decoding a key word or two in the sentence. Essentially, they developed sets of four or more written sentences that varied only slightly. Each set of sentences had a small communication board of response options, each representing slight variations so that the student had to attend to each word in the sentence to iden-tify the correct answer. For example, the target sentence might be, "The cat is in the bus," and the response options might include pictures of the following: a cat sleeping on top of a bus, a cat in a box, a cat in a bus, and a car parked beside a bus. Although this approach could be used with any type of pictorial materials, these researchers used sentences and funny pictures of animals for several reasons: 1) they allowed the presentation of unusual situations and thus minimized the students' ability to rely solely on world knowledge (rather than reading) to respond, 2) they were highly moti-vating and fun, and 3) they appealed to students across a wide range of ages. A wide range of sentences and materials were used to ensure that students were not simply memorizing responses. Case evidence (Light & McNaughton, in press) suggests that these procedures were effective; however, additional research is required in this area.

As soon as students demonstrate competence in reading sentences, they can begin to read books independently. The instructor should introduce the topic to the student prior to reading the book to activate the student's background knowledge and should teach any new vocabulary words (Musselwhite, 2005; Tierney & Cunningham, 1984). As students begin reading a range of books and stories, they face increased demands on reading comprehension. Strategies to improve reading comprehension are described in more detail in the subsequent section on more advanced literacy skills. These strategies should be introduced to students as soon as they start reading texts.

Teaching Basic Writing Skills

Writing skills are also critical in today's society to maximize participation in educational, vocational, and social environments. In fact, writing skills have assumed even greater importance in recent years with society's increased reliance on electronic and wireless communication (DeRuyter, McNaughton, Caves, Bryen, & Williams, 2007; Graham & Perin, 2007). Unfortunately, "writing remains the most neglected aspect of instruction, research, and experience in the lives of individuals who use AAC" (Millar et al., 2004, p. 165). Many students with AAC needs do not receive regular meaningful opportunities to write (Koppenhaver, 1991).

Learning to write is more difficult than learning to read. The writing process imposes addi-tional working memory demands because it requires students to dynamically encode the required sequences of letters and words while composing written text compared with decoding a static sequence as in reading (Ehri, 2000). The working memory demands are amplified even further for individuals who require AAC, especially those with motor impairments, because the process of selecting letters on a keyboard (or via other means) may be slow and effortful (Millar et al., 2004). The development of basic writing skills depends on the integration of knowledge and skills across a number of domains: 1) knowledge of basic narrative structure to organize stories; 2) language skills to structure sentences in the stories appropriately; 3) phoneme segmentation skills to break down the words in sentences into component sounds; 4) knowledge of letter–sound correspondences to code the sounds of language into written form; and 5) handwriting, keyboarding, or other access skills to produce or locate/select the required letters/words (Graham, Harris, & Larsen, 2001; Light & McNaughton, 2007).

In addition, students need access to the tools to write, including 1) a range of writing materials (with adaptations to assist with grip as required), 2) letters on their AAC systems with letter sounds as speech output to reinforce letter–sound correspondences, and 3) word banks of high-interest words (e.g., *Tyrannosaurus*, *Power Ranger*) that are challenging to write (Light & McNaughton, 2006).

Effective use of writing skills is predicated on the acquisition of letter–sound correspondences and phoneme segmentation skills. Once students know a number of letter–sound correspondences, demonstrate phoneme segmentation skills with at least 80% accuracy, and are able to decode a num-ber of words, they are ready to start more structured instruction in conventional writing skills. In order to avoid overwhelming students with too many new skill demands in the early stages of writing instruction, Light et al. (2005) proposed using familiar motivating storybooks to help struc-ture writing experiences. Initially, students may read simple storybooks with repeated lines (e.g., *Brown Bear, Brown Bear* [Martin, 1983]; *I Spy* series) and fill in selected slots in the story with their own text (e.g., *Red pig, red pig;* I spy a *bug*). Later, students may fill in short narrative sequences in longer storybooks with repeated plot lines (e.g., *PJ Funny Bunny* series). Finally, students may build simple narratives with a beginning, middle, and end based on their own experiences, familiar books, or picture prompts. In each of these writing activities, students first fill in the target slot/storyline or tell their story using their AAC systems (with vocabulary added as required). Then, the instructor helps the students encode the target words using the instructional procedures of modeling, provid-ing guided practice, and providing independent practice with corrective feedback as required. At the guided practice stage of instruction, the instructor provides oral scaffolding support that helps the student encode the text by saying each word slowly and segmenting the phonemes while the student listens and selects the appropriate letters from an accessible keyboard. Gradually, the instructor fades the oral scaffolding support until the student is encoding text independently.

The focus at this early stage of writing instruction is on sound spelling. The instructor recog-nizes the communicative intent of sound spelling attempts and provides models of conventional spellings as appropriate (Clarke, 1988). The conventional spellings of irregular words that are fre-quently occurring are taught later to students who use AAC, following the same sequence as the school curriculum. (See the section on advanced writing skills for further discussion of spelling skills.)

It is critically important that students have the opportunity to engage in frequent authentic writ-ing experiences to illustrate the meaningfulness of writing and build student motivation (Erickson & Koppenhaver, 1995; Erickson et al., 1997; Foley & Staples, 2003; Graves, 2003; Millar et al., 2004). The texts generated by students can be published as books and used for repeated readings with the students and their peers. These books can be scanned into the students' AAC systems if the systems are dynamic display systems that can support scanned images (Light & McNaughton, 2007). In this way, students have independent access to their stories and can share them with adults and peers.

Along with these authentic writing experiences, students may benefit from additional practice encoding words into written text. Millar and colleagues (Millar et al., 2004; Millar & Light, 2001) described a writing instruction program that provided direct instruction in encoding skills to com-plement writing workshop experiences. Specifically, the encoding instruction was designed to target: 1) first, the selection of the initial letters of words from an adapted keyboard; 2) then, the selection of initial and final letters; and 3) finally the full encoding of regular CVC words. The instruction uti-lized a most-to-least prompting hierarchy to facilitate errorless learning. Initially, the instructor pre-sented the target word orally, elongating and stressing the initial sound and segmenting it from the rest of the word using a pause. Once the student demonstrated competence at this level of prompt-ing, the instructor faded some of the scaffolding support, elongating and stressing the initial sound but not segmenting it from the rest of the word. Finally, the instructor eliminated the elongation and stress as well. Results of a study by Millar et al. (2004) demonstrated that these instructional proce-dures were effective teaching first-letter encoding to two of three students with AAC needs. The third student required additional instruction in letter–sound correspondences prior to instruction in encoding skills. Similar procedures were found to be effective teaching first- and final-letter encoding to two students who used AAC in a second study (Millar & Light, 2001). Blischak et al. (2004) also provided encoding instruction to three children with severe speech impairments, targeting letter–sound correspondences, phoneme segmentation and manipulation, and encoding of CVC pseudowords. Two of the three participants reached criterion in the encoding of trained pseudowords and demonstrated generalizaton of skills to untrained words and pseudowords. One participant did not reach criterion and discontinued participation, although some improvement in his skills was observed over time.

The use of evidence-based practices to teach conventional reading and writing skills to students with AAC needs can have a dramatic effect. Although these students have traditionally been excluded from literacy instruction and have experienced low expectations from others, research provides clear evidence that many students with AAC needs can "break the code" and acquire conventional literacy skills with systematic instruction adapted to meet their needs.

INSTRUCTION IN ADVANCED LITERACY SKILLS

Although tremendously significant, simply acquiring the skills to read and write is not sufficient if students with AAC needs are to derive the full benefits of literacy. Rather, they must develop more advanced literacy skills that extend beyond the basic skills targeted in the previous section. Once students acquire basic literacy skills in the early elementary years, then the curriculum in the later elementary years and secondary years focuses on building the reading and writing skills necessary to support learning in other domains (i.e., reading and writing to learn; Graham & Perin, 2007; NRP, 2000). This section describes procedures for building these more advanced literacy skills with individuals who require AAC, with a specific focus on reading comprehension and writing strategies. It should be noted that, as of 2008, there is little published research that has empirically evaluated interventions to teach advanced literacy skills to students who require AAC. Therefore, this section draws on research on teaching more advanced reading and writing skills to students who speak but are at risk for problems in the development of literacy skills (e.g., Graham & Perin, 2007; NRP, 2000). Adaptations are proposed to ensure that students who require AAC are able to participate actively in instruction based, at least in part, on anecdotal reports and case descriptions in the AAC literature (e.g., Bedrosian et al., 2003; Blischak, 1995). Future research is urgently required to investigate the effectiveness of the procedures proposed and to determine the effectiveness of other interventions.

Reading Comprehension

Comprehension is the ultimate goal of the reading process (Durkin, 1978–1979). Reading comprehension should be emphasized during emergent literacy instruction (see Chapter 9). As students begin to learn conventional literacy skills, instruction should focus not only on decoding but also on deriving meaning from the texts decoded. As students progress within school, there is an increasing emphasis on making use of what they read to extend their knowledge and experience across the curriculum (e.g., social studies, science). If students are going to be able to make use of what they read, then they must be able to not only decode texts but also construct meaningful representations of the texts as they read, relate these to their prior knowledge and experience, and use these representations to understand and make use of the information read for a variety of purposes across the educational curriculum (NRP, 2000).

Attaining successful comprehension of written texts is a highly complex process, dependent on the fluid integration of a wide range of skills. Copeland (2007) described four factors that are critical to any effort to assist students in successfully understanding written texts: 1) the ability to decode print and recognize sight words fluently; 2) the ability to comprehend the vocabulary and language structures of the text; 3) the ability to activate world knowledge and domain-specific knowledge; and 4) the metacognitive processes of monitoring comprehension and making adjustments as required to build understanding.

Building Fluency in Decoding and Sight Word Recognition Skills   It is essential that students with AAC needs develop fluency with their decoding and sight word recognition skills in order to maximize reading comprehension. Too often, AAC intervention extends only to the point where students acquire the targeted skills (Treviranus & Roberts, 2003). When skills are first acquired, they are still effortful and require conscious processing, leaving few cognitive resources to support reading comprehension. It is important that instruction continue until students develop fluency in their decoding/word recognition skills in order to free the necessary cognitive resources to allow students to process and understand the written text. Fluent readers recognize words automatically so they can focus their attention on making connections among the ideas and their background knowledge (Armbruster, Lehr, & Osborn, 2001). Traditionally, fluency is built through intervention that emphasizes oral reading rate (Fuchs, Fuchs, Hosp, & Jenkins, 2001). Clearly, this approach is inappropriate for students with AAC needs. Research suggests, however, that fluency or automaticity can also be built through continued skill instruction and multiple diverse experiences with reading and writing (Dowhower, 1987). In this approach, fluency is developed through repeated readings of familiar texts by the student both independently and in conjunction with a literate partner who reads aloud (NRP, 2000).

Building Language Comprehension Skills

Deficits in language skills can negatively affect reading comprehension, even if decoding skills are fluent. In this case, the student may be able to decode the word/sentence but has difficulty knowing what it means. Unfortunately, many individuals with AAC needs lag behind their peers in the development of pragmatic, semantic, syntactic, and morphological skills, especially the more advanced language skills needed in the later elementary and secondary school years (Smith, 2005). Ironically, the development of advanced language skills is facilitated by reading (Blachowicz & Fisher, 2000). The corollary is also true: The development of advanced language skills is impeded if the student does not read widely. Students who use AAC require more than haphazard, incidental opportunities for learning more advanced language skills. Rather, they may require concerted intervention that provides multiple and varied opportunities to learn specific vocabulary, language structures, and functions to support advanced literacy skills (e.g., intervention to teach the use of pronouns, text structures such as persuasive essays or narratives, cohesion and coherence of written texts; Sturm & Clendon, 2004).

Developing World Knowledge and Domain-Specific Knowledge

In addition to well-developed language skills, students must also have a base of world knowledge to help them understand the text. For example, if a student reads a sentence with a new word (e.g., He was going to the supermarket to purchase a pound of *sirloin*), then the student draws on knowledge of language to know that the boy or man is going to a food store and that he is intending to buy something. The student, however, requires some knowledge of how stores operate and about the types of items that are sold by weight in order to begin to construct hypotheses about the full meaning of this sentence. Prior to reading a text, it is important to set a clear purpose and to build or activate relevant background knowledge (Erickson, 2003). Prereading activities may include sharing relevant personal experiences, summarizing current knowledge or understanding, and brainstorming relevant vocabulary and concepts.

As students with AAC needs move further along in their education and progress deeper in the curriculum, they require not only general world knowledge but also domain-specific knowledge (e.g., world history, biology). As with language skills, ironically world knowledge and domain-specific knowledge are best built by reading widely (Peterson et al., 2000). Students who lag behind their peers in their reading skills face a conundrum: They have difficulty reading and understanding the curricular texts because they do not have a well-developed bank of world knowledge and domain-specific knowledge. They have difficulty building their world knowledge and domain-specific knowledge because they have difficulty reading widely to acquire this knowledge. Students with AAC needs may benefit from books/texts on tape, screen readers, or peer tutors to expose them to a wide range of sources/materials and to help them build world knowledge and domain-specific knowledge. Peterson et al. (2000) argued, however, that it is not enough to simply listen to texts or other sources to build knowledge, but rather it is essential that students also communicate what they have read to others and discuss the content to maximize the effects. In the case of students with AAC needs, it is important to ensure that they have access to the necessary tools (e.g., domain-specific vocabulary within their AAC systems) and the time and opportunities to engage in these types of discussions.

Regardless of efforts to build world knowledge and domain-specific knowledge, students with AAC needs will inevitably be in situations in which they are required to read and comprehend texts about unfamiliar topics. As the content becomes less familiar, readers need to rely more on inference to support their comprehension. Essentially, they must develop a mental model of the meaning (Graesser, Millis, & Zwaan, 1997) and then test out this hypothetical model. Inference may be required at a microlevel to derive, for example, word meaning, or at a macrolevel to infer the meaning of the entire paragraph or text. The student must apply metalinguistic/metacognitive skills and actively search for the most appropriate meaning given linguistic and contextual information (Smith, 2005). Students with AAC needs may be at risk in terms of developing the metacognitive functions required (Light & Lindsay, 1991), and they may have difficulty applying metacognitive strategies to enhance text comprehension without explicit instruction.

Instruction in Reading Comprehension Strategies

Students with AAC needs are at risk for difficulties with reading comprehension given potential deficits in decoding fluency, language skills, world knowledge, domain-specific knowledge, and metacognitive self-regulation. Reading comprehension may be further compromised because textbooks are often poorly organized, include distracting extraneous content, and make inappropriate assumptions about students' prior knowledge (Boone & Higgins, 2007). The NRP (2000) concluded that students who are at risk for deficits in reading comprehension benefit from explicit instruction in the conscious and controlled use of comprehension strategies. Comprehension strategies are "specific cognitive procedures that guide students to become aware of how well they are comprehending as they attempt to read and write" (NRP, 2000, p. 40). There is empirical evidence that students at all grade levels benefit from instruction in comprehension strategies, demonstrating significant gains in comprehension as a result (Gersten, Fuchs, Williams, & Baker, 2001; Rosenshine, Meister, & Chapman, 1996). The NRP (2000) identified seven specific strategies that have a firm scientific basis, including comprehension monitoring, summarization, graphic organizers, question answering, question generation, and cooperative learning. Each of these strategies is described in more detail in Table 10.2 along with potential adaptations for students with AAC needs.

Comprehension monitoring represents the critical first step for readers—determining whether readers understand each part of the text. This metacognitive process should become self-regulated so that students know to reprocess the text if problems are detected, utilize strategies to support comprehension, and revise their understanding as required (Pressley, 2002; Snow, Burns, & Griffin, 1998). If readers determine that they are having difficulty comprehending the text, then they should implement strategies to improve comprehension (see Table 10.2). Ideally, students learn to use more than one strategy to enhance their comprehension. There is considerable scientific support for the flexible use of multiple strategies (e.g., question generation, summarization) to enhance reading comprehension (NRP, 2000). Teaching reading comprehension strategies may have positive collateral effects on writing as well as reading. For example, graphic organizers provide a visual model of the structures of cohesive written texts. Students may learn to use graphic organizers to structure their own writings as they face more advanced writing demands.

It is possible to adapt most reading comprehension strategies for use by students with AAC needs (see Table 10.2). Whenever tasks are adapted, it is critical to assess the demands of the adapted task in relation to the original task. For example, some adapted tasks only require students to recognize the correct answer but not to recall and generate the correct answer based on memory of the text. Recognition does not require as much deep processing as recall does (Light & Lindsay, 1991). It is unknown if such differences in task requirements affect comprehension outcomes. Future research is required to determine the most appropriate adaptations to maximize the effects on comprehension for students who require AAC while minimizing task and time demands. Future research and development is also required to design new, more flexible AAC technologies that provide more efficient, seamless access to a wide range of curricular content as well as strategies to support reading comprehension and writing (e.g., graphic organizers, visual prompts for use of writing strategies; Sturm, Erickson, & Yoder, 2002).

Table 10.2.   Strategies to support reading comprehension and adaptations for students who require augmentative and alternative communication (AAC)

Strategy	Adaptation for students with AAC needs
Comprehension monitoring: Students stop periodically to check understanding of the text.	Use of written words or AAC symbols as visual prompts to stop reading and check understanding
Summarization: Students identify the main ideas of the text and eliminate details.	Use of written words or AAC symbols as visual prompts to summarize the main idea by answering "Who is it about?" or "What happened?" (Light et al., 2003)
	Selection of the best summary from three or more written summaries provided (Erickson, 2003)
	Selection of the sentence that best describes what happened from a list and selection of the sentence that best describes the cause from a list (Erickson, 2003)
	Selection of sentence strips in the correct sequence to summarize the story (Erickson, 2003)
Graphic organizers: Students map out the content of the text and illustrate visual construction of the text's meaning.	Use of hand-drawn graphic organizers with or without the collaboration of the peer recorder
	Use of computer-generated concept maps (operational and formatting requirements may present difficulties for some students)
Question answering: Students read the text, answer questions posed by the teacher, and receive feedback.	Use of AAC systems to generate responses to open-ended questions
	Use of multiple choice questions to increase efficiency and reduce fatigue
	Matching of questions presented on sentence strips (in left-hand column) with answers presented on sentence strips in random order (in right-hand column) (Erickson, 2003)
Question generation: Students generate questions (especially inferential ones) prior to reading and answer these questions as they read.	Use of AAC systems to generate questions
	Selection of appropriate questions of interest from a list of possible options
Cooperative learning: Students instruct and interact with peers about the meaning of the text; they often structure the interaction around one of the comprehension strategies.	Provide instruction or feedback for the peer in the use of appropriate interaction strategies to support effective communication
	Use of preprogrammed vocabulary in the AAC system to structure the interaction (Bedrosian et al., 2003)
	Use of written words or text as visual prompts to structure the interaction (e.g., story grammar map) (Bedrosian et al., 2003)

Instructional Procedures to Teach Reading Comprehension Strategies

The Kansas Institute for Research in Learning Disabilities developed a model to teach cognitive strategies and has applied this model effectively to teach a wide range of cognitive strategies (e.g., reading comprehension strategies) to individuals with and without disabilities (e.g., Deshler et al., 2001). Essentially, the instructional model includes the following components: 1) pretest and commitment to the instructional program, 2) description or definition of the strategy and discussion of its benefits, 3) modeling or demonstration strategy use by the instructor with think-aloud explanations of the steps performed, 4) practice naming the strategy steps, 5) guided practice implementing the strategy for the learner with support from the instructor as required, 6) fading of support as the student learns the strategy, 7) repeated opportunities for independent practice with corrective feedback as required, 8) ongoing opportunities to practice in increasingly more complex conditions, and 9) explicit planning to ensure generalization and maintenance (Deshler et al., 2001; Ellis, Deshler, Lenz, Schumaker, & Clark, 1991; Kent-Walsh & McNaughton, 2005). This model is built on the core instructional procedures (i.e., model, guided practice, independent practice) used to teach basic literacy skills. The strategy instruction model amplifies the core procedures by 1) providing greater discussion of goals, the rationale for these goals, and student commitment to these goals and 2) incorporating teacher think alouds in which teachers explain and demonstrate the cognitive processes they use to understand and construct meaning from the text. Essentially, these procedures are intended to make the processes underlying the cognitive strategies more explicit to students.

Cognitive strategy instruction has been adapted and applied successfully to teach individuals who require AAC and/or their partners a range of strategies, including communication skills (Light & Binger, 1998), sociorelational skills and collaborative problem-solving skills (Light et al., 2007), social problem solving (McCarthy, Light, & McNaughton, 2007), and partner interaction strategies (Kent-Walsh, Light, & McNaughton, 2008). Future research is required to evaluate its effectiveness in teaching strategies to promote more advanced literacy skills to students with AAC needs.

Instruction in More Advanced Writing Skills

Writing assumes greater importance as students with AAC needs progress within their education (Atanasoff, McNaughton, Wolfe, & Light, 1999). From third grade on, writing is the most common way of communicating information and conveying knowledge at school (Sturm et al., 2006). According to Graham and Perin, in the later grades, writing plays two distinct but complementary roles:

> First, it is a skill that draws on the use of strategies...to accomplish a variety of goals, such as writing a report or expressing an opinion with the support of evidence. Second, writing is a means of extending and deepening students' knowledge; it acts as a tool for learning subject matter. (2007, p. 17)

Although there are individuals who use AAC who demonstrate advanced writing skills (Koppenhaver et al., 1991), the majority seem to lag significantly behind their typically developing peers in developing advanced writing skills. Kelford Smith et al. (1989) investigated the written communication skills of six individuals (ages 13–22) who had cerebral palsy and used AAC. Results indicated that 1) the participants produced a limited amount of writing in a week (range of 0–6 samples); 2) they required significant amounts of time to plan, generate, and revise written texts (range of less than 1 word per minute [wpm] to approximately 3 wpm); 3) they demonstrated difficulties in using morphemes/functors; and 4) all but one participant experienced difficulties with sentence formulation. Clearly, intervention is warranted to improve writing outcomes for individuals who require AAC.

Skilled writing is not a simple linear process that results in the immediate production of a finished written product. Rather, it is an iterative process that requires 1) reflection (i.e., writers reflect on their ideas, experiences, and intent to plan the written text); 2) production (i.e., writers translate their ideas and produce the written text); and 3) interpretation (i.e., writers review what they have written, reflect on their goals, and make revisions; Hayes, 2000). As writing demands increase, students must integrate a complex array of knowledge and skills, including 1) discourse skills to structure written text appropriately (e.g., narrative, persuasive essay, expository writing); 2) pragmatic skills to determine the appropriate voice for the target audience; 3) semantic, syntactic, and morphological skills to generate the required language structures to convey meaning; 4) phoneme segmentation skills to break down the words in the sentences into components; 5) knowledge of letter–sound correspondences (and later of spelling conventions and exceptions) to code the language into written form; 6) knowledge of the conventions of writing (e.g., punctuation, capitalization, paragraphs); and 7) handwriting, keyboarding, or other access skills to produce or locate/select the required letters/words. Students require significant world knowledge, domain-specific knowledge, and/or meaningful personal experiences so that they have something to write about. Finally, students require frequent meaningful opportunities to write in order to develop their skills. Effective interventions are required with students who require AAC to address these issues.

To date, there have been no experimental studies that have investigated interventions to build advanced writing skills with students who require AAC. Graham and Perin (2007) completed a meta-analysis of the research on writing instruction for adolescents with and without disabilities in middle school and high school and identified several instructional approaches that reliably demonstrated significant positive effects on writing for these students. The two approaches that seem to offer the most promise for students with AAC needs are instruction in writing strategies and collaborative writing.

Writing Strategies   As with reading comprehension, students with AAC needs may benefit significantly from instruction to explicitly and systematically teach them writing strategies (i.e., the multistep procedures required for success at each stage of the writing process—planning, drafting, and revising; Graham, 2006; Graham & Perin, 2007). For example, Graham and colleagues described a strategy to teach the planning process that incorporates four steps, each represented by one of the letters in the acronym PLAN (i.e., Pay attention to the writing prompt, List the main idea, Add supporting ideas, Number your ideas; De La Paz & Graham, 2002; Graham & Perin, 2007; Harris & Graham, 1996). As with reading comprehension strategies, writing strategies can be effectively taught using the cognitive strategy instructional model (Graham & Perin, 2007). Students are also taught the self-regulation skills of goal setting, self-monitoring, self-instruction, and self-reinforcement to help them develop as independent, skilled writers. This is an area that requires future research given the empirical evidence of the benefits of strategy instruction with other groups of students with disabilities and the relative ease of adapting these strategies for use with students who require AAC.

Collaborative Writing   Collaborative writing is another intervention that offers promise to enhance the writing skills of students with AAC needs. According to Graham and Perin, collaborative writing "involves developing instructional arrangements whereby adolescents work together to plan, draft, revise, and edit their compositions" (2007, p. 42). Cooperative learning with peers encourages students to take greater responsibility for their learning. It results in increased learning of cognitive strategies, may increase motivation by building learning through social interaction, and may save time for teachers (NRP, 2000).

Bedrosian et al. (2003) described a writing intervention implemented with an adolescent with autism who used AAC and a speaking peer who had a mild cognitive impairment. The intervention combined elements of collaborative writing and instruction in writing strategies. Specifically, the intervention included 1) the provision of assistive technologies (i.e., an SGD with messages to facilitate interaction during joint story planning, writing, revising, and publishing; a story grammar map; storyboards listing story starters and vocabulary words; story-writing software); 2) explicit instruction; 3) modeling by the instructor and peer; 4) prompting; and 5) written support provided by peer scaffolding. The intervention had a positive effect on the quality of the students' writing. Moreover, the effects generalized to writing completed independently by the student with autism who used AAC. His postintervention story demonstrated marked improvement compared with his preintervention story in terms of length as well as the inclusion of the elements of story grammar. Unfortunately, it is not possible to tease out the relative contributions of collaborative writing and instruction in writing strategies in this study. Future research is required to investigate the effects of these two interventions separately with a wider range of students with different types of disabilities engaging in different genres of writing.

Instruction in Spelling and Writing Conventions   In addition to instruction to support the planning, drafting, and revising of texts, students with AAC needs also require instruction in spelling and the conventions of writing (e.g., punctuation, paragraphs). Spelling demands increase as students progress through school and seek employment. Despite the availability of spell check and linguistic prediction software, students with AAC needs still require some spelling skills to recognize correct orthographies and make full use of these assistive technologies. Hart, Scherz, Apel, and Hodson (2007) reported that some individuals with severe speech impairments experience difficulty applying their phonemic awareness knowledge to the spelling of words. If spelling approximations are not close matches for the target word, then technology supports such as spell checkers will not be effective. Other technological supports (e.g., speech output) may have a positive effect on spelling skills as well. Blischak and Schlosser (2003) reported that the use of speech feedback had positive effects on the spelling performance of some individuals with autism who had little or no functional speech. They concluded that speech output should be considered as a support for writing interventions.

To date, there has been only limited research on the effectiveness of instruction to teach spelling skills to individuals with AAC needs. McNaughton and Tawney (1993) described the benefits of a structured approach to spelling instruction for two adults who used AAC. Both participants demonstrated improved performance on high-interest vocabulary items, and continued improvement in spelling performance was observed after spelling instruction was completed. Future research is required to investigate the most effective interventions to teach conventional spelling skills and other writing conventions and to support students in making appropriate use of technological supports.

ASSISTIVE TECHNOLOGIES TO SUPPORT LITERACY

In addition to effective evidence-based instruction to teach conventional and more advanced literacy skills, it is also essential that students with AAC needs have the necessary tools available to allow them to become proficient readers and writers. Educational teams should consider assistive technologies that support three functions: AAC systems, assistive technologies for reading, and assistive technologies for writing. In some cases, students will require access to several different technologies to meet their needs. In other cases, it will be possible to integrate these supports in a single nondedicated system. It is beyond the scope of this chapter to provide a full review of available technologies, so readers are referred to Sturm, Beukelman, and Mirenda (2005) for further discussion.

AAC Systems

First and foremost, students with complex communication needs require appropriate AAC systems to allow them to communicate effectively with a wide range of partners to develop their language skills and learn a wide range of discourse functions (e.g., narratives, persuasive arguments). These systems serve as important communication tools in the social interactions that surround literacy activities. AAC systems not only serve as tools for expressive communication; they can also be used as cognitive prostheses that provide scaffolds or visual prompts to support reading and writing activities. For example, Light et al. (2003) described using AAC systems to prompt the use of a simple summarization strategy to promote reading comprehension. Bedrosian et al. (2003) described using AAC systems preprogrammed with appropriate questions (e.g., WHERE DOES THE STORY TAKE PLACE? WHAT HAPPENS FIRST?) to support the use of story grammar in written narratives. Finally, AAC systems provide a means to participate using alternative response modes during specific literacy instructional tasks (e.g., sound blending, single-word decoding, shared reading).

There are numerous AAC systems available, including unaided systems (e.g., signs, gestures) and aided ones (e.g., low-tech communication boards, SGDs). In brief, it is essential 1) that systems are selected on an individual basis to meet the needs of the student given his or her skills and capabilities; 2) that they provide access to appropriate vocabulary/language to meet the child's literacy needs; 3) that they are customized so that the representation, organization, display, selection, and output of language are appropriate to the individual's developmental needs; and 4) that they have the potential to grow seamlessly with the individual to address qualitative and quantitative developmental changes and to promote ongoing language and literacy learning (Light & Drager, 2007).

Assistive Technologies for Reading

In addition to appropriate AAC systems, some individuals with AAC needs may also benefit from assistive technologies to enhance reading. Technologies can serve two different functions: 1) provide computer-assisted instruction in reading and 2) provide a prosthesis to allow the student to bypass reading demands. Coleman-Martin et al. (2005) explored the use of computer-assisted instruction to build word-recognition skills and suggested that this approach may hold promise for individuals who require AAC. At present, however, we have only limited information on the use of drill and practice or learning game software on the reading performance of students with AAC needs (Sturm et al., 2005). In developing literacy instruction software, it is critical that the software addresses appropriate instructional goals and that it can be used effectively by students with motor impairments (Sturm et al., 2002).

Since the late 1990s, we have witnessed a significant increase in the availability of technologies that serve as reading prostheses, allowing the student to bypass reading demands. Texts in electronic format offer several potential advantages: 1) text can be presented in an appropriate format for the student (e.g., font size, color); 2) text can be read aloud; 3) oral presentation of texts can allow students to bypass the cognitive demands of decoding and free resources for higher-order processing of the text; 4) definitions and explanations can be provided for new concepts; 5) links can be provided to additional support materials; and 6) texts can be accessed via computers across locations (e.g., home, school; Anderson-Inman & Horney, 2007). Although digital texts may be easier for many students with disabilities, in fact, there are few examples of effective application of these texts in the classroom (Puckett & Brozo, 2004). Boone and Higgins (2007) cautioned that simply providing access to texts through electronic media and oral presentation does not necessarily translate into successful comprehension of these texts by students with disabilities. The shift in media from written to oral presentation does not necessarily reduce the comprehension demands. It simply shifts the focus of these demands, placing more emphasis on oral channels of input rather than visual orthographic ones. At present, we know very little about how to design and present texts in electronic format to minimize the processing demands and to maximize motivation and learning (Anderson-Inman & Horney, 2007). There remain many unanswered questions surrounding applications of digital texts with students with disabilities, including those who require AAC. For instance, researchers struggle with the appropriate balance between applications of assistive technologies to bypass decoding/reading requirements and implementation of evidence-based instruction to teach requisite literacy skills (Edyburn, 2007; McKenna & Walpole, 2007). As with other assistive technologies, applications of reading technologies will be most effective if they are mediated by effective instruction to support appropriate use by the student.

Assistive Technologies for Writing

Many students who use AAC require access to assistive technologies to participate in writing activities, including adapted writing materials (e.g., pencils with special grips) and communication boards or alphabet boards to dictate to transcribers, as well as high-tech systems that may offer more independent access to word processing, speech output, linguistic prediction, organizational tools (e.g., graphic organizers, concept maps), spell checking, dictionary/thesaurus, and so forth. As of 2007, there is only limited research that has investigated the effects of these types of technological supports on the writing of students with AAC needs. Although assistive technologies to support literacy are promising, future research is required to determine how best to support their effective use (Antonucci et al., 2006; Iacono, 2004).

Word of Caution

Although assistive technologies offer significant potential benefits for students with AAC needs, they are not a panacea. The implementation of assistive technologies may impose a significant cost of learning for students. Many assistive technologies are not designed appropriately to meet the needs of individuals who require AAC. As a result, they impose significant learning demands and may actually add to the metacognitive demands of instructional activities (Light & Drager, 2007; McKenna & Walpole, 2007). Time spent learning to operate assistive technologies may actually result in time taken away from literacy instruction. Future research and development is required to redesign assistive technologies to reduce the learning demands so that their operation is more transparent to students with AAC needs and their families and teachers (Light & Drager, 2007). Future research is also required to develop AAC systems that seamlessly integrate communication and curricular demands, allowing students to participate fully in instructional activities with easy and efficient curricular adaptations as required. In the meantime, it is incumbent on the educational team to ensure that the benefits of the assistive technologies prescribed outweigh the instructional costs (cf. Beukelman, 1991).

PRACTICAL CONSIDERATIONS

There is a growing body of AAC research that suggests effective practices to teach students conventional and more advanced literacy skills. Now we face the challenge of bridging the gap between research and practice to ensure that these evidence-based interventions are implemented consistently in schools with students with AAC needs. There are a number of challenges that teachers confront as they attempt to translate research to effective practice, including challenges related to 1) lack of training in AAC, 2) instructional adaptations required, and 3) delivery of instruction.

Training in AAC

General education teachers reported that training in AAC was one of the key factors in determining the success or failure of the inclusion of students with AAC needs in their classrooms (Kent-Walsh & Light, 2003; Soto, Müller, Hunt, & Goetz, 2001). Unfortunately, many educational personnel (e.g., general education teachers, special education teachers, SLPs, occupational therapists, paraprofessionals) lack training in AAC. Future research is required to investigate the most effective and efficient techniques to train educational personnel and parents in evidence-based literacy instruction. It is not sufficient to simply provide information to professionals and parents. Rather, training must result in professionals (and/or parents) actually changing their behaviors and adopting evidence-based practices in their classrooms (and/or homes).

Instructional Adaptations

The literacy curricula used in most schools require students to produce oral responses to participate. As discussed in this chapter, there are a number of ways to adapt these curricula to support alternative response modes and meet the needs of students who require AAC; however, these adaptations require preparation time. General education teachers who teach students with AAC needs reported that the time demands for classroom accommodations and curricular adaptations were a major barrier to the successful inclusion of students with AAC needs. These teachers recommended training for teachers in curriculum adaptation, ongoing classroom support and assistance with curriculum adaptations, and additional planning time (Kent-Walsh & Light, 2003). Clearly, there is an urgent need for a greater range of readily available curricular materials that meet the needs of students who require AAC. In the meantime, assistance with adapting curriculum materials may come from the student's educational team, family, school volunteers, older adults, peer buddies, and so forth. See Chapter 6 for further discussion of academic adaptations.

Delivery of Instruction

The third challenge is the scheduling and delivery of instruction. As much as possible, students with AAC needs should be included in general education classrooms and receive instruction with their typically developing peers (Beukelman & Mirenda, 2005). Many students with AAC needs may require additional instruction beyond what is typically provided in the classroom to ensure that they have sufficient time and opportunity to practice targeted skills. Future research is required to identify mechanisms for the delivery of this instruction (e.g., resource room instruction, additional skill practice at home, selective grade retention).

Although there are practical challenges in implementing evidence-based literacy instruction with students who require AAC, these challenges can typically be overcome if there is effective communication and collaborative problem solving by the student, the educational team, and family (Granlund, Steensson, Sundin, & Olsson, 1992; Soto et al., 2001). Clearly, the enormous benefits of literacy skills for students with AAC needs far outweigh the costs.

CONCLUSION

Significant progress has been made in understanding the development of literacy skills for students with AAC needs. We have investigated the effectiveness of interventions to teach conventional literacy skills to students with AAC needs and have begun to define appropriate content, instructional techniques, and adaptations. Future research is required to determine answers to the many questions that remain and to improve our understanding of literacy learning by students with AAC needs. Specifically, studies are required to 1) compare the relative effectiveness of different interventions to teach conventional literacy skills, 2) investigate the effect of strategy instruction on more advanced reading comprehension and writing skills, 3) explore the effects of different instructional approaches such as collaborative learning arrangements, 4) design new assistive technologies to better integrate communication and curricular content and provide instructional supports for literacy learning, and 5) evaluate the relative effectiveness of different approaches to training for parents and professionals to support the translation of research to effective evidence-based practice.

Realization of this research agenda will serve to improve literacy outcomes for individuals who require AAC. With the successful acquisition of literacy skills, individuals with AAC needs will reap many positive benefits—enhanced communication, improved education and employment opportunities, access to mainstream technologies, expanded social networks, enhanced personal expression, increased self-esteem, and positive societal attitudes and perceptions. Providing effective instruction in literacy skills is truly the single most important step in empowering individuals with AAC needs to meet their personal goals and attain their full potential (Lindsay, 1989).

REFERENCES

Adams, M.J. (1990). *Beginning to read.* Cambridge, MA: MIT Press.

Anderson-Inman, L., & Horney, M.A. (2007). Supported eText: Assistive technology through text transformations. *Reading Research Quarterly, 42,* 153–160.

Antonucci, M., Lancioni, G.E., Singh, N.N., O'Reilly, M.F., Sigafoos, J., Oliva, D., et al. (2006). Writing program with word prediction for a young man with multiple disabilities: A preliminary assessment. *Perceptual Motor Skills, 103,* 223–228.

Armbruster, B.B., Lehr, F., & Osborn, J. (2001). *Put reading first: The research building blocks for teaching children to read.* Jessup, MD: National Institute for Literacy.

Atanasoff, L., McNaughton, D., Wolfe, P., & Light, J. (1999). Communication demands of university settings for students using augmentative and alternative communication. *Journal of Postsecondary Education, 13,* 32–47.

Bedrosian, J., Lasker, J., Speidel, K., & Politsch, A. (2003). Enhancing the written narrative skills of an AAC student with autism: Evidence-based research issues. *Topics in Language Disorders, 23,* 305–324.

Berninger, V.W., & Gans, B.M. (1986). Language profiles in nonspeaking individuals of normal intelligence with severe cerebral palsy. *Augmentative and Alternative Communication, 2,* 45–50.

Beukelman, D. (1991). Magic and cost of communicative competence. *Augmentative and Alternative Communication, 7,* 2–10.

Beukelman, D., & Mirenda, P. (2005). *Augmentative and alternative communication: Supporting children and adults with complex communication needs* (3rd ed.). Baltimore: Paul H. Brookes Publishing Co.

Bishop, D.V. (1985). Spelling ability in congenital dysarthria: Evidence against articulatory coding in translating between phonemes and graphemes. *Cognitive Neuropsychology, 2,* 229–251.

Bishop, D.V., & Robson, J. (1989). Accurate nonword spelling despite congenital inability to speak: Phoneme-grapheme conversion does not require subvocal articulation. *British Journal of Psychology, 80,* 1–13.

Blachowicz, C.L.Z., & Fisher, P. (2000). Vocabulary instruction. In M.L. Kamil, P.B. Mosenthal, P.D. Pearson, & R. Barr (Eds.), *Handbook of reading research* (pp. 503–523). Mahwah, NJ: Lawrence Erlbaum Associates.

Blischak, D.M. (1995). Thomas the writer: Case study of a child with severe physical, speech and visual impairments. *Language, Speech, and Hearing Services in Schools, 26,* 11–20.

Blischak, D.M., & Schlosser, R.W. (2003). Use of technology to support independent spelling by students with autism. *Topics in Language Disorders, 23,* 293–304.

Blischak, D.M., Shah, S.D., Lombardino, L.J., & Chiarella, K. (2004). Effects of phonemic awareness instruction on the encoding skills of children with severe speech impairment. *Disability and Rehabilitation, 26,* 1295–1304.

Blockberger, S., & Sutton, A. (2003). Toward linguistic competence: Language experiences and knowledge of children with extremely limited speech. In D.R. Beukelman & J. Reichle (Vol. Eds.) & J.C. Light, D.R. Beukelman, & J. Reichle (Series Eds.), *Augmentative and alternative communication series: Communicative competence for individuals who use AAC: From research to effective practice* (pp. 63–106). Baltimore: Paul H. Brookes Publishing Co.

Boone, R., & Higgins, K. (2007). The role of instructional design in assistive technology research and development. *Reading Research Quarterly, 42,* 135–140.

Browder, D.M., Courtade-Little, G., Wakeman, S., & Rickelman, R.J. (2006). From sight words to emerging literacy. In D.M. Browder & F. Spooner (Eds.), *Teaching language arts, math, and science to students with significant cognitive disabilities* (pp. 63–91). Baltimore: Paul H. Brookes Publishing Co.

Browder, D.M., Wakeman, S., Spooner, F., Ahlgrim-Delzell, L., & Algozzine, B. (2006). Research on reading instruction for individuals with significant cognitive disabilities. *Exceptional Children, 72,* 392–408.

Browder, D.M., & Xin, P.Y. (1998). A meta-analysis and review of sight word research and its implications for teaching functional reading to individuals with moderate and severe disabilities. *Journal of Special Education, 32,* 130–153.

Browning, N. (2002). Literacy of children with physical disabilities: A literature review. *Canadian Journal of Occupational Therapy, 69,* 176–182.

Card, R., & Dodd, B. (2006). The phonological awareness abilities of children with cerebral palsy who do not speak. *Augmentative and Alternative Communication, 22,* 149–159.

Carnine, D.W., Silbert, J., Kame'enui, E., & Tarver, S.G. (1997). *Direct instruction reading.* Upper Saddle River, NJ: Prentice Hall.

Clarke, L. (1988). Invented versus traditional spelling in first graders' writings: Effects on learning to spell and read. *Research in the Teaching of English, 22,* 281–309.

Coleman-Martin, M.B., Heller, K.W., Cihak, D.F., & Irvine, K.L. (2005). Using computer-assisted instruction and the nonverbal reading approach to teach word identification. *Focus on Autism and Other Developmental Disabilities, 20,* 80–90.

Collins, B.C., & Griffen, A.K. (1996). Teaching students with moderate disabilities to make safe responses to product warning labels. *Education and Treatment of Children, 19,* 30–45.

Copeland, S.R. (2007). Reading comprehension. In S.R. Copeland & E.B. Keefe (Eds.), *Effective literacy instruction for students with moderate or severe disabilities* (pp. 79–94). Baltimore: Paul H. Brookes Publishing Co.

Dahlgren Sandberg, A.D. (2006). Reading and spelling abilities in children with severe speech impairments and cerebral palsy at 6, 9, and 12 years of age in relation to cognitive development: A longitudinal study. *Developmental Medicine and Child Neurology, 48,* 629–634.

De La Paz, S., & Graham, S. (2002). Explicitly teaching strategies, skills, and knowledge: Writing instruction in middle school classrooms. *Journal of Educational Psychology, 94,* 687–698.

DeRuyter, F., McNaughton, D., Caves, K., Bryen, D.N., & Williams, M. (2007). Enhancing AAC connections with the world. *Augmentative and Alternative Communication, 23,* 258–270.

Deshler, D.D., Schumaker, J.B., Lenz, B.K., Bulgren, J.A., Hock, M.F., Knight, J., & Ehren, B.J. (2001). Ensuring content-area learning by secondary students with learning disabilities. *Learning Disabilities Research and Practice, 16,* 96–108.

Dowhower, S.L. (1987). Effects of repeated reading on second-grade transitional readers' fluency and comprehension. *Reading Research Quarterly, 22,* 389–406.

Durkin, D. (1978–1979). What classroom observations reveal about reading comprehension instruction. *Reading Research Quarterly, 14,* 481–533.

Edyburn, D.L. (2007). Technology-enhanced reading performance: Defining a research agenda. *Reading Research Quarterly, 42,* 146–152.

Ehren, B.J. (2006). Partnerships to support reading comprehension for students with language impairment. *Topics in Language Disorders, 26,* 42–54.

Ehri, L.C. (2000). Learning to read and learning to spell: Two sides of a coin. *Topics in Language Disorders, 20,* 19–36.

Ellis, E.S., Deshler, D.D., Lenz, B.K., Schumaker, J.B., & Clark, F.L. (1991). An instructional model for teaching learning strategies. *Focus on Exceptional Children, 22*(9), 1–16.

Erickson, K. (2003). Reading comprehension in AAC. *The ASHA Leader, 8*(12), 6–9.

Erickson, K., & Koppenhaver, D. (1995). Developing a literacy program for children with severe disabilities. *The Reading Teacher, 48,* 676–684.

Erickson, K.A., Koppenhaver, D.A., Yoder, D.E., & Nance, J. (1997). Integrated communication and literacy instruction for a child with multiple disabilities. *Focus on Autism and Other Developmental Disabilities, 12,* 142–150.

Fallon, K.A., Light, J., McNaughton, D., Drager, K., & Hammer, C. (2004). The effects of direct instruction on the single-word reading skills of children who require augmentative and alternative communication. *Journal of Speech Language Hearing Research, 47,* 1424–1439.

Foley, B.E. (1993). The development of literacy in individuals with severe congenital speech and motor impairments. *Topics in Language Disorders, 13,* 16–32.

Foley, B.E., & Pollatsek, A. (1999). Phonological processing and reading abilities in adolescents and adults with severe congenital speech impairments. *Augmentative and Alternative Communication, 15,* 156–173.

Foley, B.E., & Staples, A.H. (2003). Developing augmentative and alternative communication (AAC) and literacy interventions in a supported employment setting. *Topics in Language Disorders, 23,* 325–343.

Fuchs, L.S., Deno, S.L., & Mirkin, P.K. (1984). The effects of frequent curriculum-based measurement and evaluation on pedagogy, student achievement, and student awareness of learning. *AmericanEducational Research Journal, 21,* 449–460.

Fuchs, L.S., Fuchs, D., Hosp, M.K., & Jenkins, J.R. (2001). Oral reading fluency as an indicator of reading competence: A theoretical, empirical, and historical analysis. *Scientific Studies of Reading, 5,* 239–256.

Gersten, R., Fuchs, L.S., Williams, J.P., & Baker, S. (2001). Teaching reading comprehension strategies to students with learning disabilities: A review of research. *Review of Educational Research, 71,* 279–320.

Geva, E., & Wang, M. (2001). The development of basic reading skills in children: A cross-language perspective. *Annual Review of Applied Linguistics, 21,* 182–204.

Graesser, A.C., Millis, K.K., & Zwaan, R.A. (1997). Discourse comprehension. *Annual Review of Psychology, 48,* 163–189.

Graham, S. (2006). Strategy instruction and the teaching of writing: A meta-analysis. In C. MacArthur, S. Graham, & J. Fitzgerald (Eds.), *Handbook of writing research* (pp. 187–207). New York: Guilford Press.

Graham, S., Harris, K.R., & Larsen, L. (2001). Prevention and intervention of writing difficulties for students with learning disabilities. *Learning Disabilities Research and Practice, 16,* 74–84.

Graham, S., & Perin, D. (2007). *Writing next: Effective strategies to improve writing of adolescents in middle and high schools. A report to Carnegie Corporation of New York.* Washington, DC: Alliance for Excellent Education.

Granlund, M., Steensson, A., Sundin, M., & Olsson, C. (1992). Inservice training in collaborative problem solving and goal setting for special education teacher consultants working with profoundly impaired persons. *The British Journal of Mental Subnormality, 38,* 94.

Graves, D.H. (2003). *Writing: Teachers and children at work.* Portsmouth, NH: Heinemann.

Harris, K.R., & Graham, S. (1996). *Making the writing process work: Strategies for composition and self-regulation.* Brookline, MA: Brookline Books.

Harrison-Harris, O. (2002). AAC, literacy, and bilingualism. *ASHA Leader, 7*(20), 4–5, 16–17.

Hart, P., Scherz, J., Apel, K., & Hodson, B. (2007). Analysis of spelling error patterns of individuals with complex communication needs and physical impairments. *Augmentative and Alternative Communication, 23,* 16–29.

Hatcher, P.J., Hulme, C., & Ellis, A.W. (1994). Ameliorating early reading failure by integrating the teaching of reading and phonological skills: The phonological linkage hypothesis. *Child Development, 65,* 41–57.

Hayes, J.R. (2000). A new framework for understanding cognition and affect in writing. In R. Indrisano & J.R. Squire (Eds.), *Perspectives on writing: Research, theory, and practice* (pp. 6–44). Newark, DE: International Reading Association.

Heller, K.W., Fredrick, L.D., Tumlin, J., & Brineman, D.G. (2002). Teaching decoding for generalization using the nonverbal reading approach. *Journal of Developmental and Physical Disabilities, 14,* 19–35.

Iacono, T.A. (2004). Accessible reading intervention: A work in progress. *Augmentative and Alternative Communication, 20,* 179–190.

IRIS Center. (2007). *Reading instruction: Response to intervention.* Retrieved July 12, 2007, from http://iris.peabody.vanderbilt.edu/rti03_reading/cwrap.htm

Ivey, G., & Broaddus, K. (2001). "Just plain reading": A survey of what makes students want to read in middle school classrooms. *Reading Research Quarterly, 36,* 350–377.

Jenkins, J.R., Fuchs, L.S., van den Broek, P., Espin, C., & Deno, S.L. (2003). Accuracy and fluency in list and context reading of skilled and RD groups: Absolute and relative performance levels. *Learning Disabilities Research and Practice, 18,* 237–245.

Kame'enui, E.J., & Simmons, D.C. (1990). *Designing instructional strategies: The prevention of academic learning problems.* Columbus, OH: Merrill.

Kelford Smith, A., Thurston, S., Light, J., Parnes, P., & O'Keefe, B. (1989). The form and use of written communication produced by physically disabled individuals using microcomputers. *Augmentative and Alternative Communication, 5,* 115–124.

Kent-Walsh, J., & Light, J. (2003). General education teachers' experiences with inclusion of students who use augmentative and alternative communication. *Augmentative and Alternative Communication, 19,* 104–124.

Kent-Walsh, J., Light, J., & McNaughton, D. (2008). *The effects of paraprofessional training on the communicative turns of students who use AAC during story reading interactions.* Manuscript submitted for publication.

Kent-Walsh, J., & McNaughton, D. (2005). Communication partner instruction in AAC: Present practices and future directions. *Augmentative and Alternative Communication, 21,* 195–204.

Koppenhaver, D.A. (1991). *A descriptive analysis of classroom literacy instruction provided to children with severe speech and physical impairments.* Unpublished doctoral dissertation, University of North Carolina at Chapel Hill.

Koppenhaver, D.A., Evans, D.A., & Yoder, D.E. (1991). Childhood reading and writing experiences of literate adults with severe speech and motor impairments. *Augmentative and Alternative Communication, 7,* 20–33.

Koppenhaver, D., Spadorcia, S., & Erickson, K. (1998). How do we provide inclusive early literacy instruction for children with disabilities? In S.B. Neuman & K.A. Roskos (Eds.), *Children achieving: Best practices in early literacy* (pp. 77–97). Newark, DE: International Reading Association.

Koppenhaver, D.A., Steelman, J.D., Pierce, P., Yoder, D.E., & Staples, A. (1993). Developing augmentative and alternative communication technology in order to develop literacy. *Technology and Disability, 2,* 32–41.

Koppenhaver, D.A., & Yoder, D.E. (1992). Literacy issues in persons with severe speech and physical impairments. *Issues and Research in Special Education, 2,* 156–201.

Kucan, L., & Beck, I.L. (1997). Thinking aloud and reading comprehension research: Inquiry, instruction, and social interaction. *Review of Educational Research, 67,* 271–299.

Light, J. (1997). "Let's go star fishing": Reflections on the contexts of language learning for children who use aided AAC. *Augmentative and Alternative Communication, 13,* 158–171.

Light, J.C., & Binger, C. (1998). *Building communicative competence with individuals who use augmentative and alternative communication.* Baltimore: Paul H. Brookes Publishing Co.

Light, J., Binger, C., & Kelford Smith, A. (1994). Story reading interactions between preschoolers who use AAC and their mothers. *Augmentative and Alternative Communication, 10,* 255–268.

Light, J., & Drager, K. (2007). AAC technologies for young children with complex communication needs: State of the science and future research directions. *Augmentative and Alternative Communication, 23,* 204–216.

Light, J., & Kelford Smith, A. (1993). Home literacy experiences of preschoolers who use AAC systems and of their nondisabled peers. *Augmentative and Alternative Communication, 9,* 10–25.

Light, J., & Lindsay, P. (1991). Cognitive science and augmentative and alternative communication. *Augmentative and Alternative Communication, 7,* 186–203.

Light, J., & McNaughton, D. (1993). Literacy and augmentative and alternative communication (AAC): The expectations and priorities of parents and teachers. *Topics in Language Disorders, 13*(2), 33–46.

Light, J., & McNaughton, D. (2006, November). *Maximizing the literacy skills of individuals who require AAC.* Retrieved July 5, 2007, from http://mcn.ed.psu.edu/dbm/Light_Reading/index.htm

Light, J., & McNaughton, D. (2007, November). *Evidence-based literacy intervention for individuals who require AAC.* Seminar presented at the annual convention of the American Speech-Language-Hearing Association, Boston.

Light, J., & McNaughton, D. (in press). *Accessible literacy learning: Evidence-based reading instruction for learners with autism, cerebral palsy, Down syndrome, and other disabilities.* Solana Beach, CA: Mayer-Johnson.

Light, J., McNaughton, D., Jansen, J., Kristiansen, L., May, J., Miller, L., et al. (2005, November). *Maximizing the literacy skills of individuals who require AAC.* Seminar presented at the annual convention of the American Speech-Language-Hearing Association, San Diego.

Light, J., McNaughton, D., Krezman, C., Williams, M., Gulens, M., Galskoy, A., et al. (2007). The AAC Mentor Project: Web-based instruction in sociorelational skills and collaborative problem solving for adults who use augmentative and alternative communication. *Augmentative and Alternative Communication, 23,* 56–75.

Light, J., McNaughton, D., Mohr, A., Bercaw, K., & Kristiansen, L. (2003, October). *Reading comprehension instruction for students using augmentative and alternative communication.* Presentation at the Pennsylvania Training and Technical Assistance Network, Pittsburgh.

Light, J., McNaughton, D., Weyer, M., & Karg, L. (2008). Evidence-based literacy instruction for individuals who require augmentative and alternative communication: A case study of a student with multiple disabilities. *Seminars in Speech and Language, 29,* 120–132.

Lindsay, P.H. (1989, April). *Literacy and the disabled: An unfulfilled promise or the impossible dream?* Presentation on at the Pacific Conference on Technology in Education and Rehabilitation, Vancouver, British Columbia.

Lovett, M.W., & Steinbach, K.A. (1997). The effectiveness of remedial programs for reading disabled children of different ages: Does the benefit decrease for older students? *Learning Disability Quarterly, 20,* 189–210.

Lund, S.K., & Light, J. (2006). Long-term outcomes for individuals who use augmentative and alternative communication: Part I: What is a "good" outcome? *Augmentative and Alternative Communication, 22,* 284–299.

Martin, B. (1983). *Brown bear, brown bear, what do you see?* New York: Henry Holt.

Marzollo, J., & Wick, W. (1999). *I spy treasure hunt.* Pueblo, CO: Cartwheel.

Mather, N., Bos, C., & Babur, N. (2001). Perceptions and knowledge of preservice and inservice teachers about early literacy instruction. *Journal of Learning Disabilities, 34,* 472–482.

McCarthy, J., Light, J., & McNaughton, D. (2007). The effects of internet-based instruction on the social problem solving of young adults who use augmentative and alternative communication. *Augmentative and Alternative Communication, 23,* 100–112.

McKenna, M.C., & Walpole, S. (2007). Assistive technology in the reading clinic: Its emerging potential. *Reading Research Quarterly, 42,* 140–145.

McNaughton, D., Light, J., & Arnold, K.B. (2002). "Getting your 'wheel' in the door": The successful full-time employment experiences of individuals with cerebral palsy who use augmentative and alternative communication. *Augmentative and Alternative Communication, 18,* 59–76.

McNaughton, D., & Tawney, J. (1993). Spelling instruction for adults who use augmentative and alternative communication. *Augmentative and Alternative Communication, 9,* 72–82.

Millar, D.C., & Light, J. (2001). *Exemplary practices in writing instruction for young children who use augmentative and alternative communication.* Grant report to the U.S. Department of Education. (ERIC Document Reproduction Service No. ED463614)

Millar, D.C., Light, J., & McNaughton, D. (2004). The effect of direct instruction and writer's workshop on the early writing skills of children who use augmentative and alternative communication. *Augmentative and Alternative Communication, 20,* 164–178.

Mirenda, P. (2003). "He's not really a reader…": Perspectives on supporting literacy development

in individuals with autism. *Topics in Language Disorders, 23*(4), 271–282.

Musselwhite, C. (2005). *Reading comprehension supports and AAC: Before, during, and after.* Retrieved July 12, 2007, from http://www.bridgeschool.org/aacbythebay/docs/cmusselwhilte_before-during-after.pdf

National Reading Panel (NRP). (2000). *Teaching children to read: An evidence-based assessment of the scientific research literature on reading and its implications for reading instruction: Reports of the subgroups* (NIH Publication No. 00-4754). Washington, DC: U.S. Government Printing Office, National Institute of Child Health and Human Development.

Peterson, C.L., Caverly, D.C., Nicholson, S.A., O'Neal, S., & Cusenbary, S. (2000). *Building reading proficiency at the secondary school level: A guide to resources.* Austin: Southwest Texas State University, Southwest Educational Development Laboratory.

Pressley, M. (2002). Comprehension strategies instruction: A turn-of-the-century status report. In M. Pressley & C.C. Block (Eds.), *Comprehension instruction* (pp. 11–27). New York: Guilford Press.

Pressley, M., Wharton-McDonald, R., Allington, R., Block, C.C., Morrow, L., Tracey, D., et al. (2001). A study of effective first-grade literacy instruction. *Scientific Studies of Reading, 5,* 35–58.

Puckett, K., & Brozo, W. (2004). Using assistive technology to teach content area literacy strategies to students with disabilities. In J.R. Dugan, P.E. Linder, M.B. Sampson, B.A. Brancato, & L. Elish-Piper (Eds.), *Celebrating the power of literacy* (pp. 462–479). Pittsburg, KS: College Reading Association.

Rehfeldt, R.A., Latimore, D., & Stromer, R. (2003). Observational learning and the formation of classes of reading skills by individuals with autism and other developmental disabilities. *Research in Developmental Disabilities, 24,* 333–358.

Rosenshine, B., Meister, C., & Chapman, S. (1996). Teaching students to generate questions: A review of the intervention studies. *Review of Educational Research, 66,* 181–221.

Rosenshine, B., & Stevens, R. (1986). Teaching functions. In M.C. Wittrock (Ed.), *Handbook of research on teaching* (3rd ed., pp. 376–391). New York: Macmillan.

Schlosser, R.W., & Rhagavendra, P. (2004). Evidence-based practice in augmentative and alternative communication. *Augmentative and Alternative Communication, 20,* 1–21.

Sheehy, K. (2002). The effective use of symbols in teaching word recognition to children with severe learning difficulties: A comparison of word alone, integrated picture cueing and the handle technique. *International Journal of Disability, Development and Education, 49,* 47–59.

Smith, M.M. (2005). The dual challenges of aided communication and adolescence. *Augmentative and Alternative Communication, 21,* 67–79.

Smith, M.M., & Grove, N.C. (2003). Asymmetry in input and output for individuals who use AAC. In D.R. Beukelman & J. Reichle (Vol. Eds.) & J.C. Light, D.R. Beukelman, & J. Reichle (Series Eds.), *Augmentative and alternative communication series: Communicative competence for individuals who use AAC: From research to effective practice* (pp. 163–195). Baltimore: Paul H. Brookes Publishing Co.

Snow, C.M., Burns S., & Griffin P. (1998). *Preventing reading difficulties in young children.* Washington; DC: National Academies Press.

Soto, G., & Hartmann, E. (2006). Analysis of narratives produced by four children who use augmentative and alternative communication. *Journal of Communication Disorders, 39,* 456–480.

Soto, G., Hartmann, E., & Wilkins, D.P. (2006). Exploring the elements of narrative that emerge in the interactions between an 8-year-old child who uses an AAC device and her teacher. *Augmentative and Alternative Communication, 22,* 231–241.

Soto, G., Müller, E., Hunt, P., & Goetz, L. (2001). Critical issues in the inclusion of students who use augmentative and alternative communication. *Augmentative and Alternative Communication, 17,* 62–72.

Stanovich, K.E. (1986). Matthew effects in reading: Some consequences of individual differences in the acquisition of literacy. *Reading Research Quarterly, 21,* 360–407.

Sturm, J., Beukelman, D.R., & Mirenda, P. (2005). Literacy development of children who use AAC. In D.R. Beukelman & P. Mirenda (Eds.), *Augmentative and alternative communication: Supporting children and adults with complex communication needs* (3rd ed., pp. 351–390). Baltimore: Paul H. Brookes Publishing Co.

Sturm, J.M., & Clendon, S.A. (2004). Augmentative and alternative communication, language, and literacy: Fostering the relationship. *Topics in Language Disorders, 24,* 76–91.

Sturm, J.M., Erickson, K., & Yoder, D.E. (2002). State of the science: Enhancing literacy development through AAC technologies. *Journal of Assistive Technology, 14,* 71–80.

Sturm, J.M., Spadorcia, S.A., Cunningham, J.W., Cali, K.S., Staples, A., Erickson, K., et al. (2006). What happens to reading between first and third grade? Implications for students who use AAC. *Augmentative and Alternative Communication, 22,* 21–36.

Tierney, R., & Cunningham, J. (1984). *Research on reading comprehension.* In P. Pearson (Ed.), *Handbook of reading research* (pp. 609–655). New York: Longman.

Torgesen, J.K., Wagner, R.K., & Rashotte, C.A. (1994). The development of reading-related phonological processing abilities: New evidence of bi-directional causality from a latent variable longitudinal study. *Developmental Psychology, 30,* 468–479.

Treviranus, J., & Roberts, V. (2003). Supporting competent motor control of AAC systems. In D.R. Beukelman & J. Reichle (Vol. Eds.) & J.C. Light, D.R. Beukelman, & J. Reichle (Series Eds.), *Augmentative and alternative communication series: Communicative competence for individuals who use AAC: From research to effective practice* (pp. 199–240). Baltimore: Paul H. Brookes Publishing Co.

Truxler, J., & O'Keefe, B.M. (2007). The effects of phonological awareness instruction on beginning word recognition and spelling. *Augmentative and Alternative Communication, 23,* 164–176.

Vandervelden, M., & Siegel, L. (1995). Phonological recoding and phoneme awareness in early literacy: A developmental approach. *Reading Research Quarterly, 30,* 854–875.

Vandervelden, M., & Siegel, L. (1999). Phonological processing and literacy in AAC users and students with motor speech impairments. *Augmentative and Alternative Communication, 15,* 191–211.

Vaughn, S., Wanzek, J., Woodruff, A.L., & Thompson, S. (2007). Prevention and early identification of students with reading disabilities. In D.H. Haager, J. Klingner, & S. Vaughn (Eds.), *Evidence-based reading practices for response to intervention* (pp. 11–27). Baltimore: Paul H. Brookes Publishing Co.

Witt, J.C., Elliot, S.N., Daly, E.J., III, Gresham, F.M., & Kramer, J.J. (1998). *Assessment of at-risk and special needs children* (2nd ed.). New York: McGraw-Hill.

11

Strategies to Support the Development of Positive Social Relationships and Friendships for Students Who Use AAC

Pam Hunt, Kathy Doering, Julie Maier, and Emily Mintz

"Every morning when the school children sleepily stepped off the bus and headed toward their classes, Nate was always waiting to greet Tim. Tim would often make a comment about the bus driving away or an airplane he heard above him, and his friend would wave to the bus or look up in the sky, too. He would take his hand, help him put his heavy backpack over his shoulders, and walk with him to class. Once inside their class, these two friends sought each other out during playtime or reading time to share their enjoyment of a favorite toy or to read a book together, finding familiar words on Tim's communication device as they were reading. It was clear that these two friends would enjoy each other's company for many years to come."

—*Julie Venuto, special education teacher*

We have several stories to share with you throughout this chapter that provide snapshots of friendships between students who use augmentative and alternative communication (AAC) and their schoolmates. These friendships developed because the students participated in educational settings that supported positive social relationships among children and adolescents with and without disabilities and because educational team members actively encouraged and systematically facilitated those relationships. These conditions serve as the premise for all that we have to offer in this chapter. The social support strategies that we describe were developed and validated in educational settings that provided membership and full social participation to students who used AAC. They were implemented by educational team members who considered the development of positive peer relationships to be a high-priority educational goal.

NATURE AND IMPORTANCE OF PEER RELATIONSHIPS

Positive peer relationships can vary along a continuum anchored by acquaintance relationships on one end to friendships on the other end (Janney & Snell, 2006). The continuum may be characterized by the degree of mutual "liking" (Bukowski, Newcomb, & Hartup, 1996) or the extent of closeness and intimacy (Bukowski et al., 1996; Falvey & Rosenberg, 1995; Janney & Snell, 2006). Acquaintances are peers whom a child may have known for some period of time and to whom they may have a social connection. Acquaintances may be members of the child's social network and provide a variety of social supports; however, the nature of acquaintance relationships is less investigated and defined than that of friendships.

Although the concept of friendship is familiar to all, definitions of friendship using natural language are typically ambiguous and "consist almost entirely of metaphors" (Bukowski et al., 1996,

p. 2). Researchers who have sought to define the friendship construct have relied on information from three sources: 1) what children and adolescents themselves tell them about these relationships (e.g., Berndt & Perry, 1986; Bukowski, Boivin, & Hoza, 1994; Parker & Asher, 1993; Staub, Schwartz, Gallucci, & Peck, 1994), 2) what parents and teachers report (e.g., Ladd, 1990; Parker & Asher, 1993), and 3) what trained observers identify in their observations of social behavior (e.g., Guralnick, 1980; Haring & Breen, 1992; Staub et al., 1994). Based on the results of their investigations, these researchers generally agree that the friendships of children and adolescents include the following characteristics: 1) *reciprocity*, that is, mutual regard, cooperation and conflict management, and equal sharing in the benefits that accrue from the social exchanges between the two friends; 2) *liking*, that is the desire to spend time with the friend; and 3) *affection and having fun* (Bukowski et al., 1996; Howes, 1996; Newcomb & Bagwell, 1996).

The nature of peer relationships change as children move from their preschool years to their elementary school years and finally to adolescence. Infants and toddlers' social interactions are primarily with caregivers. Developmental approaches stress the importance of parent–child bonding and attachment in infants, and a transactional model has been used to describe how the social-communicative development of infants and toddlers is facilitated through bidirectional, reciprocal interactions between the child and his or her social environment (McLean & Synder-McLean, 1978; Warren, Yoder, & Leew, 2002). During the preschool years, however, peer interactions become more dominant, particularly in the context of play. The social requirements of play can vary from the few demands associated with parallel play to the high, social-communicative demands of fantasy play including social coordination, role negotiation, and conflict resolution. In addition, fantasy play may provide a context for practicing roles and resolving fears (Goldstein & Morgan, 2002). Preschool relationships can change from day to day, but there is some evidence for the stability of friendship relationships (Gershman & Hayes, 1983).

Deeper friendships begin to emerge around the age of 8 or 9 as children become less egocentric and more conscious of and more affected by their peers (Goldstein & Morgan, 2002). Peer acceptance is of central concern to school-age children, and group membership is highly valued. When children become adolescents, they develop a need for interpersonal intimacy including self-disclosure, mutual trust and respect, commitment and loyalty, and the development of similar value systems to those of their peers. They explore their identities, feelings and beliefs, and frustrations and fears through discussions with their peers with these types of interactions serving as a "primary problem-solving strategy" for adolescents (Goldstein & Morgan, 2002, p. 8).

Although what children and youth seek in relationships with their peers may change as they move through these stages of their lives, their development and emotional well-being throughout their school years is significantly affected by the quality of their social relationships. Positive peer relationships and friendships provide them with nurturance, support, membership, and companionship and promote their self-confidence and self-esteem (Bukowski et al., 1996; Janney & Snell, 2006; Ladd, 1990; Light, Arnold, & Clark, 2003; Schwartz, Staub, Peck, & Gallucci, 2006; Staub et al., 1994). In addition, there is evidence that children who are accepted by their peers appear to develop more positive attitudes toward school and to integrate themselves into academic activities in ways that promote learning and achievement (Ladd, 1990; Ladd & Kochenderfer, 1996). Child development theorists with varying perspectives (e.g., Bruner, Flavel, Piaget, Vygotsky) suggest that successful child–child interactions provide both a context and a mechanism for developing interpersonal, communicative, and cognitive abilities. There is evidence that children who have positive relationships and friendships with peers are more socially competent and less troubled than children who do not (Hartup, 1996) and that friendship relationships promote social engagement, cooperation and conflict management, expression of personal thoughts and feelings, and task orientation in contexts that include a child's friends (Goldstein & Morgan, 2002; Newcomb & Bagwell, 1996).

BARRIERS TO DEVELOPING POSITIVE PEER RELATIONSHIPS AND FRIENDSHIPS

Several essential conditions have been identified for developing positive peer relationships for students with disabilities, including students who use AAC (Falvey & Rosenberg, 1995; Hunt, Farron-Davis, Wrenn, Hirose-Hatae, & Goetz, 1997; Janney & Snell, 2006; Kennedy, 2001; Schwartz et al., 2006).

- Opportunities to be with peers with diverse abilities, backgrounds, and interests
- Desire to interact with peers and the communicative means to do so
- Availability of informed and motivated peers who can serve as effective communication partners
- Organizational, emotional, and social supports to develop and maintain peer relationships

Opportunity

Students who use AAC may have limited opportunities to interact socially with a broad range of students. In the 1999–2000 school year, only 44% of the students with physical disabilities were placed in general education classes, 22% were served in separate educational settings for 21%–60% of the day, and 28% were placed in special classes. For students with cognitive disabilities, only 14% of the students were placed in general education classes, 29% were served in different educational settings for 21%–60% of the day, and 51% were placed in special classes (U.S. Department of Education, 2002).

In addition, students who receive educational services in separate classrooms may be further isolated from their peers by riding separate buses to school, having different recess schedules, and eating lunch only with their classmates from the separate classrooms. Obviously, students who use AAC cannot develop positive social relationships with peers with diverse abilities and interests if they are not participating in the same educational and social settings as those students (Fryxell & Kennedy, 1995).

Desire and Means

Students with AAC needs may not be motivated to interact socially with their peers because their earlier attempts to communicate with or be accepted by their peers were not successful (Lilienfeld & Alant, 2005). Other students who use AAC may have a desire to interact with their peers but do not have a communication system that supports social closeness and sustained reciprocal interactions (Light et al., 2003; Light, Parsons, & Drager, 2002). For example, a communication board may not include vocabulary relevant to social exchanges, or the student may not have been taught to use AAC to initiate or respond to greetings, make social comments, and engage in conversational exchanges (Light et al., 2002). Finally, students who use AAC may lack the social experiences needed to develop the sociorelational skills required for positive peer relationships because of their physical isolation from a variety of peers or because the settings and activities in which they participate are not structured to promote and support social interactions (Light et al., 2003).

Informed and Motivated Peers

The motivational level and attitude of peers can be an obstacle to establishing positive relationships for students who use AAC (Beck, Fritz, Keller, & Dennis, 2000; Goldstein & Morgan, 2002; Merges, Durand, & Youngblade, 2005). Positive peer relationships are based on a history of reinforcing interactions in which there are positive outcomes for both participants. Repeated experiences with dysfunctional, involuntary, or unsupported interactions with students with AAC needs produce negative peer attitudes and low motivation for future social interactions (Goldstein & Morgan, 2002; Merges et al., 2005). In addition, when peers lack the knowledge and skills to serve as effective communication partners with their schoolmates who use AAC, the students' attempts to interact socially are limited to brief exchanges (Kent-Walsh & McNaughton, 2005; Lilienfeld & Alant, 2005; Merges et al., 2005). Finally, mystification surrounding assistive technology (AT), AAC devices, specialized equipment, and curricular adaptations used by students with complex communication and educational needs can stigmatize or isolate the students unless their peers are given information specific to the need for and function of these supports as well as information related to ability and diversity awareness in general (Hunt, Alwell, Farron-Davis, & Goetz, 1996; Hunt et al., 1997; Janney & Snell, 2006).

Organizational, Emotional, and Social Supports

There is evidence that even if students who use AAC have access to integrated settings through general education placement; inclusion in general education classrooms; or integration opportunities during lunch, recess, and field trips, their physical presence alone is not sufficient. Planned and systematic support of positive student-to-student interactions through the collaborative efforts of creative and knowledgeable educational team members is needed for full social participation and the development of positive relationships and friendships (Beukelman & Mirenda, 2005; Hunt, Hirose-Hatae, Goetz, Doering, & Karasoff, 2000; Hunt, Soto, Maier, Müller, & Goetz, 2002; Kennedy, Cushing, & Itkonen, 1997; Soto, Müller, Hunt, & Goetz, 2001).

CHAPTER FOCUS

Discussion of strategies to address barriers related to educational placement and access to integrated settings for students with AAC needs is well beyond the scope of this chapter. Our chapter presents, however, a comprehensive social support model that is implemented collaboratively by educational team members to increase opportunities for students who use AAC to interact with their peers given their participation in integrated educational and social settings. In addition, it offers strategies to increase the motivation of students with and without disabilities to interact with each other and to provide them with the means to do so. Finally, it offers a set of organizational, emotional, and social supports designed to promote and sustain reciprocal relationships and friendships.

Our suggestions for social supports and contextual arrangements are based on our own research and our experience working with educational teams in inclusive settings over the years (Hunt et al., 1996; Hunt et al., 1997; Hunt, Soto, Maier, & Doering, 2003; Hunt et al., 2002) and on the input that we have received from team members on what is workable in school environments. We have also been guided by the criteria developed by Meyer, Park, Grenot-Scheyer, Schwartz, and Harry (1998) for developing usable interventions to promote positive peer relationships. These interventions are 1) practical and "doable" in average classroom contexts, 2) possible with available long-term resources, 3) sustainable over time, 4) created and implemented by school personnel and peers, and 5) culturally responsive and "intuitively appealing" to those implementing and those receiving support.

DESIGNING AND IMPLEMENTING SOCIAL SUPPORTS

The social support model that we describe includes three major building blocks (see Figure 11.1). The first building block is providing information to peers that will assist them in developing positive social relationships with their schoolmates who use AAC. The second building block is identifying and using a variety of interactive media (e.g., nonverbal communication; low-tech communication boards and books; high-tech AAC devices; interactive computer activities, toys, and

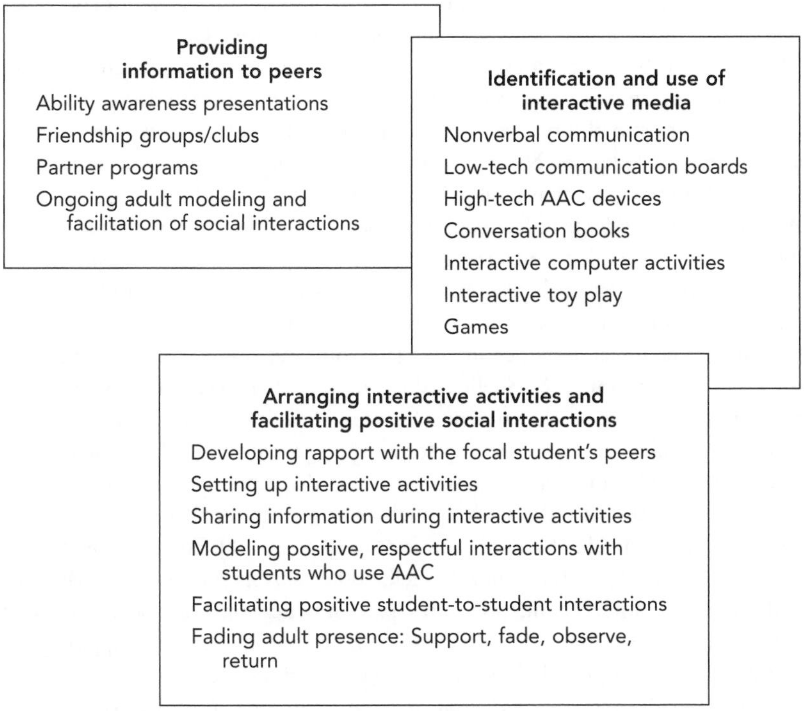

Providing information to peers	Identification and use of interactive media
Ability awareness presentations	Nonverbal communication
Friendship groups/clubs	Low-tech communication boards
Partner programs	High-tech AAC devices
Ongoing adult modeling and facilitation of social interactions	Conversation books
	Interactive computer activities
	Interactive toy play
	Games

Arranging interactive activities and facilitating positive social interactions

Developing rapport with the focal student's peers

Setting up interactive activities

Sharing information during interactive activities

Modeling positive, respectful interactions with students who use AAC

Facilitating positive student-to-student interactions

Fading adult presence: Support, fade, observe, return

Figure 11.1.   Three building blocks for designing and implementing social supports.

games) that serve as the basis for reciprocal, social interactions. The final building block is arranging interactive activities and implementing facilitation strategies to promote positive social interactions across activities and settings. All three components of the social support model are implemented through the collaborative efforts of core members of the educational team, and regularly scheduled team meetings serve as the vehicle for tailoring the intervention to meet the needs of individual students and for coordinating team member activities.

Providing Information to Peers

Information is provided to peers to assist them in developing positive social relationships with their schoolmates who use AAC (Beck & Fritz-Verticchio, 2003; Hunt et al., 1996; Janney & Snell, 2006; Kent-Walsh & McNaughton, 2005). The information and related activities are designed to help them understand and appreciate 1) cultural, language, and ability diversity (Derman-Sparks, 1989; Hunt et al., 1996; Hunt et al., 1997; Janney & Snell, 2006); 2) the qualities of friendship and ways to support others and ask others for support; 3) the means by which a student with AAC needs communicates, makes choices, initiates an interaction, and participates in a particular activity (Kent-Walsh & McNaughton, 2005; Lilienfeld & Alant, 2005); 4) the purpose and use of AAC devices and the means by which they can interact and socialize with schoolmates who use them (Beck & Fritz-Verticchio, 2003; Carter & Maxwell, 1998; Hunt et al., 1996; Lilienfeld & Alant, 2005); and 5) the ways in which AT and adapted curriculum and instruction assist students who use AAC to successfully participate in educational activities (Haring & Breen, 1992; Hunt et al., 1996).

Formats for Presenting Information   Multiple formats have been used to share information with peers. *Class lessons* that explore concepts related to cultural and ability diversity, equity and democracy, and cooperation and interdependence are incorporated into the classroom curriculum to increase students' sense of identity and self-worth and their capacity for cooperation; interdependence; and respect for cultural, language, and ability differences (Gibbs, 1994; Halvorsen & Neary, 2001; Hunt et al., 1996; Hunt et al., 1997; Janney & Snell, 2006). From this base, positive social relationships among students with varying backgrounds and characteristics can develop. Some schools provide diversity and ability awareness information through *schoolwide or grade-level events* (Halvorsen & Neary, 2001; Janney & Snell, 2006). During these events, information can be incorporated that increases peers' general awareness of types of disability and the accommodations, equipment, and AT used by the students to facilitate their social and educational participation in the school community. Regularly scheduled *class meetings* to discuss topics related to classroom rights, responsibilities and expectations, relationships among the students, and individual student concerns can serve as a context for brainstorming ways in which the student who uses AAC can more fully participate in educational and social activities in the classroom and other school settings (Hunt et al., 1996; Hunt et al., 1997; Janney & Snell, 2006; Salisbury, Gallucci, Palombaro, & Peck, 1995). *Friendship groups*—composed of the student who uses AAC, interested peers, and an adult facilitator—can provide a smaller, structured setting for all the participants to share their concerns or problems and receive feedback and support from their peers. Participants often brainstorm ways in which their peer who uses AAC can be more fully included in educational activities and participate in social events during and outside of school (Forest & Lusthaus, 1989; Frederickson & Turner, 2003; Hunt et al., 1996; Hunt et al., 1997; Janney & Snell, 2006). *Partner programs*—in which peers and the students who use AAC interdependently participate in educational and social activities—provide multiple, incidental opportunities for members of the educational team to support positive student-to-student interactions and provide information to peers (Hughes et al., 2002; Hunt et al., 1996; Hunt et al., 1997). Finally, ongoing *adult modeling and facilitation of social interactions*, especially when the student who uses AAC is initially building social relationships with peers, is an effective and important method for continually assessing the peers' need for information and providing that information in the context of naturally occurring interactions and social activities (Hunt et al., 1996; Hunt et al., 1997; Salisbury et al., 1995).

Ability Awareness Presentations Providing information that increases students' awareness of individuals with disabilities—their accomplishments, strengths, competencies, and educational supports—is known as *ability awareness*. For example, a third-grade class might receive information about a new student who uses AAC by learning about what his typical day looks like, how he uses AAC devices, what games he likes to play at recess, and how they can communicate and interact with him. Ability awareness presentations can be student specific, as in the previous example, or they can address general topics such as commonalities among students with and without disabilities, environmental adaptations, assistive devices, communicating with individuals who use AAC, and using people-first language and other respectful ways to refer to individuals or groups of people (Halvorsen & Neary, 2001; Janney & Snell, 2006).

Prior planning and preparation is essential. Initial plans are discussed with students and their families, other members of the educational team, and school administrators. Educational team members and students who will participate collaboratively develop the content of the presentation and the format and related activities. Questions are asked, such as the following:

- Is student-specific information needed?
- If so, what information is needed, and how will it be presented?
- Will an adult present the information, or will students participate?
- If the content is student specific, will the focal student participate in the presentation?

(*Note*: With older elementary and secondary students who use AAC devices, it is often very effective and powerful when the students are supported to present some of the information about themselves, including their interests, accomplishments, and the AAC aids that they use.)

When planning the activities, time is built in for group discussion after the presentation and activities are completed (Janney & Snell, 2006). In addition, follow-up activities in class or at home can also be included. For example, after a presentation focusing on communicating with school-mates who uses low-tech communication boards, students are assisted to construct their own communication boards by selecting symbols that support social exchanges with their peers. The students are then encouraged to try to use them to communicate with each other at lunch, at recess, and at home with their families.

Friendship Groups   Friendship groups, often referred to as *Circles of Friends* or *support circles*, are facilitated by a trained adult who uses a variety of formats to facilitate group discussion and problem solving (Forest & Lusthaus, 1989; Frederickson & Turner, 2003; Halvorsen & Neary, 2001; Haring & Breen, 1992; Hunt et al., 1996; Hunt et al., 1997; Janney & Snell, 2006). Some friendship groups meet once per week during lunch; other groups meet during a specified class period each week that does not interfere with academic instruction. Friendship groups may be formed around a common interest or characteristic, such as a girls-only group or a sign language club; however, the overriding purpose is to expand social connections and mutual support among the members of the group. The activities should be fun, socially interactive, and instructive for all participants. Although it is important for adults to develop and initially implement and facilitate the meetings, a primary goal is to establish student control of discussions and group activities with adults providing facilitation and support. For example, students may lead the weekly discussions of topics selected by group members, the brainstorming process to address issues of concern shared by group members, and the selection of discussion topics and activities for future meetings.

_____   Adam, a student who uses AAC, and some of his classmates were members of a Circles of Friends Club (Hunt et al., 1996). The group met once per week for approximately 40 minutes while the rest of the class had a study period. The inclusion support teacher facilitated the meeting. Approximately eight to nine classmates participated on a regular basis. The meeting routine included the following: 1) an opening activity such as a game or ice breaker; 2) a review of the agenda with a chance to add items; 3) individual student reports on incidences in which support was provided to Adam or another classmate during the week; 4) discussion of issues of concern in the students' lives, including issues related to Adam's opportunities to participate fully in classroom activities; 5) group problem solving in which suggestions were generated that addressed each concern discussed (e.g., "What could Maya do to get along better with her brother?" "How can Adam be more involved in social studies lessons?"); and 6) a final review of any commitments made by the students (e.g., offers to accompany Adam to recess). The students assumed the roles of facilitator, recorder, time keeper, and snack server. The reporter informed the general education teacher of topics discussed and actions taken. By the end of the school year, the students ran their own meetings with the inclusion teacher in attendance as a member. Adam participated in a variety of ways. For example, he took turns sharing with the other students using both partner-assisted scanning and his computer. In addition, a list of games the students liked for opening activities was stored on his computer, and the students reviewed the list with Adam to generate ideas for the meeting's opening activity. Finally, the students sometimes audio recorded meeting notes on Adam's computer so that he could take a turn being the reporter. _____

Partner Programs   When students who use AAC and their peers interdependently participate in educational and social activities through structured partner programs, there are multiple, incidental opportunities for members of the educational team to support positive student-to-student interactions; facilitate interdependent participation; and share information or answer questions about AT, specialized equipment, and adapted educational activities. In addition, partner programs provide the chance for the students to get to know each other better and develop deeper social relationships (Carter & Kennedy, 2006; Hughes et al., 2001; Hughes et al., 2002; Hughes et al., 1999; Hunt et al., 1996; Hunt et al., 1997; Janney & Snell, 2006).

Partner programs typically include four components: student recruitment and selection, peer training, peer-delivered support, and adult monitoring (Carter & Kennedy, 2006). At the elementary level, the student who uses AAC might have a "partner for the day" who sits by him or her in a general education class and assists with academic materials or activities. The peer is also a social partner during recess, lunch in the cafeteria, and other school activities (Hunt et al., 1996; Hunt et al., 1997). Students in the class are asked if they are interested in being a peer partner (it has been our experience that this is a very popular role). To help manage the partner schedule, a calendar is posted in the classroom that identifies the partner for the day. Class size dictates that if most students want to participate, each one is given a turn approximately once every 5 weeks. Educational staff 1) provide information to peers at naturally occurring opportunities on the communication system, adaptive equipment, and educational activities of the student who uses AAC; 2) facilitate peer support and interdependent participation and social interaction; and 3) ensure that partners also complete their work for the day and follow the same routine, for the most part, as their classmates.

At the secondary level, *peer buddies* might help their partners who use AAC to be included within general education classes and in the extracurricular activities that occur in a typical middle school or high school day. Hughes and her colleagues collaborated with educators and students in 11 local high schools to implement a peer buddy program that was centered around a credit course that provided information on various types of disabilities and learning problems, instructional techniques, and strategies to help peers with significant disabilities participate in school activities (Hughes et al., 2001; Hughes et al., 2002; Hughes et al., 1999). The elective course also allowed the peer buddies to spend one period each day with their partners to support them in and out of class. They helped their partners complete class projects and communicate with their instructors and classmates. They also introduced their partners to their own friends, and some peer buddies socialized with their partners outside school (e.g., going to the mall, attending community events, visiting each other's homes). During the 3 years in which the program was systematically evaluated, friendships developed, and the students with disabilities increased their participation in the mainstream of high school life including classes, recreational activities, after-school sports, student council, and school clubs.

Identification and Use of Interactive Media as the Basis for Reciprocal, Social Interactions

"Although Thomas only spoke one or two words, he was a great communicator. In seventh grade, he was just beginning to learn to use his new communication device, but he also had picture displays that he used. He loved his joke cards, a series of cards he handed to a friend to tell a joke. Soon his comedic talents expanded, especially in the area of physical comedy. One day he was telling an elaborate story to his friend Avery. Avery and Thomas viewed school through a similar lens—a great place to have fun and, once in a while, to study. I came upon the two of them during the break just before English class. Thomas was acting out the story and directing another boy in the staging of the tale. I was never completely clear on the details because they were all unable to stop laughing, but it did involve what appeared to be the portable telephone from Thomas's home, someone getting spooked by Thomas, and a great deal of flailing about. Once things had calmed down and Thomas's teacher came to take him and the portable telephone to the office for a call home in case it had been missed, Avery became very quiet. After a moment she said, 'Most of the time I forget that Thomas doesn't talk because he's always saying so much!'"

—*Mary Wrenn, speech-language pathologist (SLP)*

Students with AAC needs are often at risk for social exclusion because they and their peers lack the means and opportunity to develop a shared history of positive social interactions (Light et al., 2003; Merges et al., 2005). A variety of interactive media (e.g., nonverbal communication, low-tech communication boards, high-tech AAC devices, conversation books, interactive computer activities, interactive toy play, games) can be used across ages, cognitive differences, and communication ability to support sustained interactions between students who use AAC and their peers (Beukelman & Mirenda, 2005; Hunt et al., 1996; Hunt et al., 1997; Light et al., 2003; Light et al., 2002; Millar, 2001).

Nonverbal behaviors, including facial expressions (e.g., smiling, frowning), gestures (e.g., reaching, touching, pointing, waving, clapping, giving a high-five), body movements (e.g., nodding, orienting toward a communication partner), and vocalizations, account for more than 65% of any communicative exchange between verbal individuals (Downing, 2005b). Students who are skilled at using complex AAC devices and communicating abstract messages often prefer nonsymbolic communication to interact socially because the message can be communicated more quickly and is more likely to generate an immediate response from peers (Downing, 2005b; Murphy, Markovà, Moodie, Scott, & Boa, 1995). For example, a high school student who uses an electronic AAC device might respond to a funny comment made by a peer in the cafeteria with a smile and a high-five. Students, such as Thomas, who use low-tech communication books and boards to communicate, can greatly enrich, expand, and enliven their communicative interactions with peers by supplementing them with gestures, facial expressions, and body movements. For students who have not yet developed symbolic communication, these nonsymbolic, yet highly communicative, behaviors can serve as the primary means by which they engage their peers in a reciprocal social exchange (Downing, 2005b; Hunt et al., 1996). For students with significant disabilities, however, forms of nonsymbolic communication may be highly individualized, less universally understood, and more difficult to interpret. For example, some students may use gestures such as reaching or grabbing to gain a peer's attention. When educational team members help peers understand the intent of the message and respond accordingly, then the student's initiation is reinforced, and, therefore, more likely to occur again. In addition, peers begin to develop sensitivity to the nonverbal social initiations of their schoolmates and the ability to accurately interpret the messages that they express.

AAC aids, from low-tech communication boards to high-tech AAC devices, can serve as a medium through which students initiate and participate in social interactions and achieve social closeness with their peers (Beukelman & Mirenda, 2005; Hunt et al., 1996; Hunt et al., 2002; Light et al., 2003; Light et al., 2002; Merges et al., 2005; Mirenda, 2005). Vocabulary words can be incorporated that not only allow the students to participate in educational activities by making comments and asking and answering questions related to the lesson or activity but also to share information with another student, provide assistance to and ask for assistance from peers, and compliment peers on their work. Vocabulary can also be included that supports social interactions in unstructured, social contexts by enabling the students to greet peers, comment on topics of mutual interest (e.g., music, sports, movies, school events, friends), ask partner-focused questions (e.g., "What did you do this weekend?" "What did you think of the new *Harry Potter* movie?"), use social interjections in response to peers' comments or jokes (e.g., "right on," "sweet," "cool"), and make farewell statements (e.g., "See you later."). Finally, vocabulary can be included that enables students to follow the conventions of social etiquette as they interact with peers (e.g., communicating *please* and *thank you*).

Conversation books and a turn-taking structure were developed by Hunt and her colleagues to promote and support sustained and balanced conversational turn taking for students who use AAC and their peers (e.g., Hunt, Alwell, & Goetz, 1991). The intervention was designed for students who 1) used speech to communicate but did not articulate clearly so they were often misunderstood; 2) initiated verbal exchanges with greetings, comments, or questions but did not maintain the interactions beyond two to three conversational turns; and 3) communicated in simple sentences and may have used repetitive phrases in an attempt to extend the interaction. Poor articulation, limited vocabularies, and restricted ability to initiate topics for discussion are obstacles to conversation that are removed by the use of a conversation book. The books were small albums filled primarily with color photographs of people, activities, and places of high interest to the focal students and their peers (e.g., photos of schoolmates, teachers, school events, and field trips, as well as photos of the focal students' family, home events, and pets), a few pictures from magazines (e.g., pictures of athletes and movie stars), and remnants from trips or special events (e.g., tickets from a concert, postcards from a trip). The photos provided numerous cues for things to talk about and were readily accessed by the student with a point to a picture and a word or phrase. In addition, articulation difficulties were overcome because the photos provided a visual referent that helped to clarify the student's comment or question. Finally, the focal students and their classmates were taught to use a specific conversation structure that supported extended and balanced conversation turn taking.

Interactive toy play, games, and interactive computer activities that allow the participants to focus on each other and require turn taking and reciprocity can also serve as media for peer-to-peer social interactions (Hunt et al., 1996; Hunt et al., 1997; Light et al., 2002). These activities are designed to be age appropriate and occur in natural school environments; be pleasurable for both students; and have a clear, repetitive structure that is sustainable over time (Light et al., 2002). For beginning communicators who are presymbolic, interactive toy play (e.g., building a tower of blocks with a peer), simple games (rolling a ball back and forth), or cause-and-effect computer games played with a peer partner can serve as primary social connectors by supporting extended, reciprocal, and balanced social interactions with peers. For students who are symbolic communicators, interactive toy play, games, and interactive computer activities also serve as interactive media and allow for sustained, mutually enjoyable social interactions without the need for low-tech or high-tech AAC aids.

ARRANGING INTERACTIVE ACTIVITIES AND FACILITATING POSITIVE SOCIAL INTERACTIONS

"Tyrone was a friend of Adam's. He was an athletic kid who had a hard time with academics and sitting still. Socially, he was outspoken and 'poked his nose' into everyone else's business. He could be mean at times, but for some reason he looked out for Adam. He used to give me a hard time when I came in to check on things. He'd say to me, 'Ooooo—you left Adam all alone doin' nothin'!' grinning at me and accusing me at the same time. I'd say, 'What do you mean? You're here, aren't you? And what about all the other kids?' Then I'd help to set Adam up in some activity, help adapt some materials, or 'trouble shoot' any problems with the [computer]. Later in the year when I'd come in, Tyrone would either be near Adam or he'd come over when he saw me. He'd smile and say to me, 'We got Adam. He's fine. You can go now,' gesturing for me to leave. And he was right. They did have Adam—supported, involved, and fine."

—*Morgen Alwell, special education teacher*

Educational team members act as *social facilitators* who support the development of positive social interactions between students who use AAC (who will be referred to as *focal students*) and their peers. Six interventions will be described that are essential for effectively supporting positive peer-to-peer interactions and developing meaningful relationships. All members of the educational team must have access to information, training, and support to implement these strategies effectively.

Strategy 1: Developing Rapport with the Focal Student's Peers

It is important for educational team members to develop rapport with the focal student's peers by learning the names of as many of the students as possible and making meaningful connections with them. The first step is to get to know the peers by asking them questions about their hobbies and interests, pointing out their strengths, and complimenting their achievements (Causton-Theoharis & Malmgren, 2005; Turnbull, Pereira, & Blue-Banning, 2000). This personal knowledge enables team members to identify and highlight the experiences and interests that peers have in common with the focal student, which can create a bond between them and potentially lead to developing positive social relationships and friendships (Chadsey & Han, 2005; Merges et al., 2005; Stainback & Stainback, 1990). The initial personal connection with peers is strengthened when special education team members expand their specialist role to one that allows them to interact with and provide support to *all* students engaged in integrated educational activities (e.g., becoming part of the instructional team by leading small-group or whole-class lessons, providing individual support to any student in the class who could benefit from it, knowing and enforcing the classroom rules; Vandercook & York, 1990). When educational team members establish friendly and supportive relationships with peers, they can more effectively foster the development of positive social relationships between them and the focal student by pointing out common interests; facilitating social interactions; and structuring cooperative activities, partner programs, and friendship clubs.

Strategy 2: Setting Up Interactive Activities

Partner activities and interactive, small-group educational activities provide an important context for developing positive social relationships because they offer multiple opportunities for social exchanges, turn taking, interdependent participation to complete a task, and sharing of materials and information (Hunt et al., 1996; Hunt et al., 1997; Janney & Snell, 2006; Merges et al., 2005; Schwartz et al., 2006; Soto & von Tetzchner, 2003; Turnbull et al., 2000). Social facilitators structure the activities, prepare AAC aids, and provide the adaptations and peer supports necessary to ensure that the focal student is actively engaged and interacting with other students.

_____   When David went to his computer to work with his partner, an adult facilitator checked to see that all necessary materials were available, the computer was on, and appropriate software was open and operating. With brief reminders to the peer partner on the purpose of the activity (e.g., "David will use his communication board to tell you what he wants to write about, and then you can help him type a sentence. Then, it's your turn to write a sentence."), the facilitator left the students to work together, checking back occasionally to make sure that everything was working smoothly.

Aaron was given the stapler that was needed for his group's task of making lanterns during an art lesson. The students in the group shared materials and ideas for individualizing each lantern with creative designs and bright colors. Aaron offered his suggestions using vocabulary available on his AAC device and joined in as students complimented each other's creations with a smile and high-five to peers whose artwork he particularly admired. When it was time for the last steps of lantern making—that is, putting the pieces together—each member of the group sought out Aaron's assistance as "keeper of the stapler." _____

Structured recess games such as "Red Light, Green Light," "Red Rover," and "Mother May I?" are motivating, interactive social contexts that support sustained, positive social interactions among all of the participants (Hunt et al., 1996). It has been our experience that recess games organized and lead by an adult facilitator are very popular. Adult facilitators ask the peers to suggest ways in which the focal student can fully participate, including the type of direct support the peers might provide, and will sometimes structure the game to give the focal student a leadership role (e.g., recording "green light, red light" on the voice output communication aid so that the student can direct the activity).

Many middle school and high school academic courses may be lecture based with some to little opportunity for interactive, small-group activities. Yet, other courses such as physical education and many elective classes such as art, photography, and cooking still can provide rich contexts for social interactions, partner activities, and interdependent participation. In addition, extracurricular and recreational activities such clubs, pep rallies, sporting events, and recess games can serve as interactive social contexts if adult facilitators prepare AAC aids and put adaptations and peer supports in place to ensure that the focal student is actively engaged in the activity and interacting socially with other students (Haring & Breen, 1992; Hunt et al., 1996; Hunt et al., 1997; Janney & Snell, 2006).

Strategy 3: Sharing Information During Interactive Activities

Interactive activities provide multiple, naturally occurring opportunities for educational team members to provide information to peers about the focal student's communication system and the AT, equipment, and adaptations that the student may use (Causton-Theoharis & Malmgren, 2005; Hunt et al., 1996; Hunt et al., 1997; Lilienfeld & Alant, 2005; Merges et al., 2005). Peers' questions are answered in a straightforward but sensitive manner, and the information they are given is suited to their level of understanding (Janney & Snell, 2006). Information or modeling is provided that helps them interpret the nonsymbolic communicative behavior of the focal student (e.g., "Oh, I see that you are trying to get Jamal's attention. Use your device to tell him what you want.") or to be effective communication partners (e.g., "Wait, be sure to give Maria enough time to tell you. The Dynavox helps her to talk to you, but it takes a bit longer for her to communicate everything that she wants to say."). Adult facilitators also anticipate possible unspoken questions peers may have and provide information directly (e.g., "Could you understand what Antonio was saying? Antonio asked if someone could help him.") or indirectly ("Antonio, thank you for asking for help.").

Adult facilitators also give information to both the peer and the focal student on how to participate interdependently to accomplish a task such as playing a game, completing an educational activity, or taking turns to play a computer game. Without adequate knowledge, peers may not approach the student with AAC needs or they may take on a "helper" role rather than participating with the student through give-and-take interactions. Throughout the activity, adult facilitators highlight the competency of all the students by praising their progress and successes and encouraging them to acknowledge each other's accomplishments.

Strategy 4: Modeling Positive, Respectful Interactions with Students Who Use AAC

Peers will be watching educational team members as they interact with students who use AAC (Janney & Snell, 2006; Stainback & Stainback, 1990; Schwartz et al., 2006; Turnbull et al., 2000). The extent to which they see respect, warmth, and compassion modeled by team members will affect "their own interpretation of being 'different' in the classroom not only for their peer with disabilities but also for themselves" (Schwartz et al., 2006, p. 390). In addition, adult facilitators model strategies to communicate with and support students who use AAC (e.g., engaging in conversations with them, offering choices, respectfully providing physical support, adding needed symbols to a communication aid; Janney & Snell, 2006; Kent-Walsh & McNaughton, 2005; Merges et al., 2005; Schwartz et al., 2006). Finally, adult facilitators ensure that the focal student is the focus of any social interaction they have with peers and the primary receiver of information. When peers approach the adult and make a comment or ask a question, the adult takes this opportunity to redirect the conversation to the focal student by saying, for example, "Why don't you ask Caden?" or they involve the focal student in the conversation by saying, for example, "Caden, haven't you seen the *Spider Man* movie that Rachel is talking about? What did you think about it?"

Strategy 5: Facilitating Positive Student-to-Student Interactions

Arranging motivating, interactive activities and providing information to peers does not guarantee that meaningful social interactions will occur naturally. Facilitation is often required, at least initially.

An adult facilitator can act as a social bridge by teaching the focal student and peers how to interact with one another when necessary and by prompting interactions during naturally occurring opportunities (Hunt et al., 1996; Hunt et al., 1997; Merges et al., 2005; von Tetzchner, Brekke, Sjøthun, & Grindheim, 2005). Although they are well intentioned, adult facilitators who provide excessive prompting, constantly hover, help too much, and solve problems unilaterally interfere with student-to-student interactions (Causton-Theoharis & Malmgren, 2005; Giangreco, Edelman, Luiselli, & MacFarland, 1997). Effective social facilitators do the following:

- Support versus dominate student-to-student interactions
- Wait to see what happens versus interrupting peers' attempts to communicate with the focal student
- Step away to allow peers to step in with comments and feedback
- Ask the focal student's questions versus speaking for the student
- Allow the focal student to advocate for him- or herself by ensuring that the student has opportunities and the means to express preferences

Social facilitators determine the type and amount of support that is needed by first observing students to identify which peers the focal student gravitates toward, how peers interact with one another, the comfort level of all participants in the activity, and how peers naturally support the focal student. Indirect facilitation strategies can be used, such as modeling social interactions with the focal student or asking the peers to generate ideas for more fully including him or her (e.g., "It looks like Liam is having a hard time getting started. What could you do to help him?"). Asking students to share their ideas gives them a voice and promotes reflection and creative problem solving (Chadsey & Han, 2005; Jorgensen, 2006; Schwartz et al., 2006). Adult facilitators also praise students for their shared accomplishments and their efforts in supporting and encouraging one another.

When indirect facilitation does not give enough support, facilitators can provide more structure and direct instruction (Carter & Hughes, 2005; Chadsey & Han, 2005; Janney & Snell, 2006; Merges et al., 2005; Sapon-Shevin, 1990). Although this direct approach can increase the probability of a successful interaction, and the support may be necessary for a period of time, the ultimate goal is for students to initiate and maintain interactions without frequent adult intervention.

Strategy 6: Fading Adult Presence: Support, Fade, Observe, and Return

An effective social facilitator knows when to help and when to step back (Causton-Theoharis & Malmgren, 2005; Giangreco et al., 1997; Hunt et al., 1996; Hunt et al., 1997; Janney & Snell, 2006). Support staff must fade their physical presence in order to avoid helping too much, creating adult dependency, and interfering with student-to-student social interactions. This is an important goal, and yet care must be taken that the support is not withdrawn too quickly. We recommend an approach called support, fade, observe, and return (if necessary).

Support   Social facilitators ensure that AAC aids, adaptations, and AT are in place, and the students are given a clear set of directions for participating in the educational or social activity. They provide the information, prompting, instruction, encouragement, feedback, and praise needed to support the active engagement of the focal student and frequent positive student-to-student interactions.

Fade   Adults fade their support and their physical presence once it becomes apparent that social interactions between students are occurring spontaneously and that the focal student is participating independently or receiving adequate support from his or her peers. At first, the facilitator remains on the periphery of the work or social area, closely monitoring the students' activities and intervening when necessary. As relationships evolve and all students are successfully engaged in the activity, the social facilitator begins to support or supervise other students.

Observe and Return   As facilitators work with other students, they frequently observe the activity from a distance to monitor the need for more support. Periodically, or when they see that support is needed, they return to the activity to give the students additional information, instruction, or feedback and encouragement. When all the students are actively engaged and interacting positively with each other, the facilitator once again moves away to support others.

COLLABORATIVE TEAMING AS THE INTERVENTION VEHICLE

A collaborative effort of core members of the educational team is needed to develop and implement the three building blocks of social support: 1) providing information to peers; 2) identifying and using interactive media as the basis for reciprocal, student-to-student exchanges; and 3) arranging interactive activities and facilitating positive social interactions (see Figure 11.1). General and special education teachers, SLPs, instructional assistants, and parents work together to design social supports to meet the needs of individual students and the dictates of educational and social settings and to implement them across the school day. Team members working alone will not be effective because the task is too large for one person, the ideas generated by one team member may be incomplete or off base, and the combined expertise of all team members is needed (Downing, 2005a; Janney & Snell, 2006; Snell & Janney, 2005).

Social supports and facilitation strategies can be identified in the context of regularly scheduled collaborative teaming meetings during which team members develop and review the overall plan of educational and social supports for individual students (Hunt et al., 2003; Hunt et al., 2002). Hunt and her colleagues (2002) investigated the effectiveness of a collaborative teaming process to develop supports for students who used AAC and were members of general education classrooms. The collaborative team included the general education teacher, the inclusion support teacher, the SLP, an instructional assistant, and the child's parents. The major components of the collaborative process were the following: 1) regularly scheduled team meetings; 2) development of supports to increase the focal student's engagement in educational activities, academic progress, communicative competence, and interaction with peers; 3) a built-in accountability system; and 4) flexibility to change ineffectual supports.

Characteristics of effective collaborative teaming were incorporated into the model (Salisbury, Evans, & Palombaro, 1997; Snell & Janney, 2005). Most important, team members shared their expertise, knowledge, and experience to collaboratively create and implement instructional and social supports, curricular adaptations and modifications, and contextual arrangements. In addition, the roles and responsibilities of general and special educators took on the flexibility needed to jointly address the educational and social needs of the students as the team members shared the responsibility for the students' success. The results of the study demonstrated a positive effect on focal student outcomes as well as benefits to members of the educational teams, which included support from other team members and reduced isolation, opportunity to learn from other team members, shared responsibility and increased accountability, and a structure for developing and implementing a comprehensive and cohesive support plan.

CONCLUSION

"One day after school, Sarah was waiting for her dad to pick her up. David came out to the bus pushed by Jerome. Sarah noticed him just as her dad arrived and went over to tell David bye for the day. She took his hand and said, 'Bye, David.' David responded with a big smile, just as her dad walked up. Sarah turned to her dad smiling proudly and said, 'Dad, this is David.' 'I know,' he said, also smiling."

—Morgen Alwell, special education teacher

For David and for Sarah, friendships are essential to their emotional well-being and educational progress. Yet, for many students such as David, positive relationships and friendships with their peers are outside the realm of their educational experience either because they are separated from the social settings and activities of their peer group because of educational placement decisions or architectural and attitudinal barriers or because educational team members are not providing the social supports essential to the development of positive peer relationships. Policy and administrative actions are needed to put an end to the isolation that many students who use AAC experience during their school years by replacing separate educational placements with general education, classroom-based support and eliminating separate buses and bus schedules and architectural barriers that prevent access to educational and social settings and activities. In addition, educational team members must identify membership in peer networks and the development of positive social relationships and friendships with peers as high-priority educational goals. Finally, educational team collaboration is needed to develop and implement cohesive and comprehensive interventions to promote and support social relationships and friendships for students who use AAC across the school years.

REFERENCES

Beck, A.R., Fritz, H., Keller, A., & Dennis, M. (2000). Attitudes of school-aged children toward their peers who use augmentative and alternative communication. *Augmentative and Alternative Communication, 16,* 13–26.

Beck, A.R., & Fritz-Verticchio, H. (2003). The influence of information and role-playing experiences on children's attitudes toward peers who use AAC. *American Journal of Speech-Language Pathology, 12,* 51–60.

Berndt, T.J., & Perry, T.B. (1986). Children's perceptions of friendships as supportive relationships. *Developmental Psychology, 22,* 640–648.

Beukelman, D.R., & Mirenda, P. (2005). *Augmentative and alternative communication: Supporting children and adults with complex communication needs* (3rd ed.). Baltimore: Paul H. Brookes Publishing Co.

Bukowski W.M., Boivin, M., & Hoza, B. (1994) Measuring friendship quality during pre- and early adolescence: The development and psychometric properties of the Friendship Qualities scale. *Journal of Social and Personal Relationships, II,* 471–484.

Bukowski, W.M., Newcomb, A.F., & Hartup, W.W. (1996). Friendship and its significance in childhood and adolescence: Introduction and comment. In W.M. Bukowski, A.F. Newcomb, & W.W. Hartup (Eds.), *The company they keep: Friendship in childhood and adolescence* (pp. 1–15) Cambridge, United Kingdom: Cambridge University Press.

Carter, E., & Hughes, C. (2005). Increasing social interaction among adolescents with intellectual disabilities and their general education peers: Effective interventions. *Research and Practices for Persons with Severe Disabilities, 30* (4), 179–193.

Carter, E.W., & Kennedy, C.H. (2006). Promoting access to the general curriculum using peer support strategies. *Research and Practices for Persons with Severe Disabilities, 31* (4), 284–292.

Carter, M., & Maxwell, K. (1998). Promoting interaction with children using augmentative communication through a peer-directed intervention. *International Journal of Disability, Development and Education, 45* (1), 75–96.

Causton-Theoharis, J., & Malmgren, K. (2005). Increasing peer interactions for students with severe disabilities via paraprofessional training. *Teaching Exceptional Children , 72* (4), 431–444.

Chadsey, J., & Han, G.H. (2005). Friendship-facilitation strategies: What do students in middle school tell us? *Teaching Exceptional Children, 8*(2), 52–57.

Derman-Sparks, L. (1989). *Anti-bias curriculum: Tools for empowering young children.* Washington, DC: National Association for the Education of Young Children.

Downing, J.E. (2005a). Integrating team expertise to support communication. In J.E. Downing (Ed.), *Teaching communication skills to students with severe disabilities* (2nd ed., pp. 201–223). Baltimore: Paul H. Brookes Publishing Co.

Downing, J.E. (2005b). Teaching a wide range of communication skills. In J.E. Downing (Ed.), *Teaching communication skills to students with severe disabilities* (2nd ed., pp. 147–174). Baltimore: Paul H. Brookes Publishing Co.

Falvey, M.A., & Rosenberg, R.L. (1995). Developing and fostering friendships. In M.A. Falvey (Ed.), *Inclusive and heterogeneous schooling: Assessment, curriculum, and instruction* (pp. 267–283). Baltimore: Paul H. Brookes Publishing Co.

Forest, M., & Lusthaus, E. (1989). Promoting educational equality for all students: Circles and maps. In S. Stainback, W. Stainback, & M. Forest (Eds.), *Educating all students in the mainstream of regular education* (pp. 43–57). Baltimore: Paul H. Brookes Publishing Co.

Frederickson, N., & Turner, J. (2003). Utilizing the classroom peer group to address children's social needs: An evaluation of the circle of friends intervention approach. *Journal of Special Education, 36* (4), 234–245.

Fryxell, D., & Kennedy, C.H. (1995). Placement along the continuum of services and its impact on students' social relationships. *Journal of The Association for Persons with Severe Handicaps, 20,* 259–269.

Gershman, E.S., & Hayes, D.S. (1983). Differential stability of reciprocal friendships and unilateral relationships among preschool children. *Merrill-Palmer Quarterly, 29* (2), 169–177.

Giangreco, M.F., Edelman, S.W., Luiselli, T., & MacFarland, S. (1997). Helping or hovering? Effects of instructional assistant proximity on students with disabilities. *Exceptional Children, 64* (7),7–18.

Gibbs, J. (1994). *Tribes: A new way of learning together.* Santa Rosa, CA: Center Source Publications.

Goldstein, H., & Morgan, L. (2002). Social interaction and models of friendship development. In S.F. Warren & M.E. Fey (Series Eds.) & H. Goldstein, L.A. Kaczmarek, & K.M. English (Vol. Eds.), *Communication and language intervention series: Vol. 10. Promoting social communication: Children with developmental disabilities from birth to adolescence* (pp. 5–25). Baltimore: Paul H. Brookes Publishing Co.

Guralnick, M.J. (1980). Social interactions among preschool children. *Exceptional Children, 46* (4), 248–253.

Halvorsen, A.T., & Neary, T. (2001). *Building inclusive schools: Tools and strategies for success.* Boston: Allyn & Bacon.

Haring, T., & Breen, C. (1992). A peer-mediated social network intervention to enhance the social integration of persons with moderate and severe disabilities. *Journal of Applied Behavior Analysis, 25,* 319–333.

Hartup, W.W. (1996). The company they keep: Friendships and their developmental significance. *Child Development, 67,* 1–13.

Howes, C. (1996). The earliest friendships. In W.M. Bukowski, A.F. Newcomb, & W.W. Hartup (Eds.), *The company they keep: Friendship in childhood and adolescence* (pp. 66–86). Cambridge, United Kingdom: Cambridge University Press.

Hughes, C., Copeland, S.R., Guth, C., Rung, L.R., Hwang, B., Kleeb, G., et al. (2001). General education students' perspective on their involvement in a high school peer buddy program. *Education and Training in Mental Retardation and Developmental Disabilities, 36* (4), 343–356.

Hughes, C., Copeland, S.R., Wehmeyer, M., Agran, M., Cai, X., & Hwang, B. (2002). Increasing social interaction between general education high school students and their peers with mental retardation. *Journal of Developmental and Physical Disabilities, 14* (4), 387–402.

Hughes, C., Guth, C., Hall, S., Presley, J., Dye, M., & Byers, C. (1999). They are my best friends: Peer buddies promote inclusion in high school. *Teaching Exceptional Children, 31(5),* 32–37.

Hunt, P., Alwell, M., Farron-Davis, F., & Goetz, L. (1996). Creating socially supportive environments for fully included students who experience multiple disabilities. *Journal of The Association for Persons with Severe Handicaps, 21* (2), 53–71.

Hunt P., Alwell, M., & Goetz, L. (1991). Establishing conversational exchanges with family and friends: Moving from training to meaningful communication. *Journal of Special Education, 25* (3), 305–319.

Hunt, P., Farron-Davis, F., Wrenn, M., Hirose-Hatae, A., & Goetz, L. (1997). Promoting interactive partnerships in inclusive educational settings. *Journal of The Association for Persons with Severe Handicaps, 22* (3), 127–137.

Hunt, P., Hirose-Hatae, A., Goetz, L., Doering, K., & Karasoff, P. (2000). "Community" is what I think everyone is talking about. *Remedial and Special Education, 21* (5), 305–317.

Hunt, P., Soto, G., Maier, J., & Doering, K. (2003). Collaborative teaming to support students at risk and students with severe disabilities in general education classrooms. *Exceptional Children, 69* (3), 315–332.

Hunt, P., Soto, G., Maier, J., Müller, E., & Goetz, L. (2002). Collaborative teaming to support students with AAC needs in general education classrooms. *Augmentative and Alternative Communication, 18,* 20–35.

Janney, R., & Snell, M.E. (2006). *Social relationships and peer support* (2nd ed.). Baltimore: Paul H. Brookes Publishing Co.

Jorgensen, C.M. (2006). Facilitating student relationships: Fostering class membership and social connections. In C.M. Jorgensen, M.C. Schuh, & J. Nisbet (Eds.), *The inclusion facilitator's guide* (pp. 125–137). Baltimore: Paul H. Brookes Publishing Co.

Kennedy, C.H. (2001). Promoting social-communicative interactions in adolescents. In S.F. Warren & M.E. Fey (Series Eds.) & H. Goldstein, L.A. Kaczmarek, & K.M. English (Vol. Eds.), *Communication and language intervention series: Vol. 10. Promoting social communication: Children with developmental disabilities from birth to adolescence* (pp. 307–329). Baltimore: Paul H. Brookes Publishing Co.

Kennedy, C.H., Cushing, L.S., & Itkonen, T. (1997). General education participation improves the social contacts and friendship networks of students with severe disabilities. *Journal of Behavioral Education, 7* (2), 167–189.

Kent-Walsh, J., & McNaughton, D. (2005). Communication partner instruction in AAC: Present practices and future directions. *Augmentative and Alternative Communication, 21* (3), 195–204.

Ladd, G.W. (1990). Having friends, keeping friends, making friends, and being liked by peers in the classroom: Predictors of children's early school adjustment? *Child Development, 61,* 1081–1100.

Ladd, G.W., & Kochenderfer, B.J. (1996). Linkages between friendship and adjustment during early school transitions. In W.M. Bukowski, A.F. Newcomb, & W.W. Hartup (Eds.), *The company they keep: Friendship in childhood and adolescence* (pp. 1–15). Cambridge, United Kingdom: Cambridge University Press.

Light, J.C., Arnold, K.B., & Clark, E.A. (2003). Finding a place in the "social circle of life": The development of sociorelational competence by individuals who use AAC. In D.R. Beukelman & J. Reichle (Series Eds.) & J.C. Light, D.R. Beukelman, & J. Reichle (Vol. Eds.), *Augmentative and alternative communication series: Communicative competence for individuals who use AAC: From research to effective practice* (pp. 361–400). Baltimore: Paul H. Brookes Publishing Co.

Light, J.C., Parsons, A.R., & Drager, K. (2002). "There's more to life than cookies": Developing interactions for social closeness with beginning communicators who use AAC. In D.R. Beukelman & J. Reichle (Series Eds.) & J. Reichle, D.R. Beukelman, & J.C. Light (Vol. Eds.), *Augmentative and alternative communication series: Exemplary practices for beginning communicators: Implications for AAC* (pp. 187–218). Baltimore: Paul H. Brookes Publishing Co.

Lilienfeld, M., & Alant, E. (2005). The social interaction of an adolescent who uses AAC: The evaluation of a peer-training program. *Augmentative and Alternative Communication, 21* (4), 278–294.

McLean, J., & Snyder-McLean, L. (1978). *A transactional approach to early language training.* Columbus, OH: Charles E. Merrill.

Merges, E.M., Durand, V.M., & Youngblade, L.M. (2005). The role of communication partners. In J.E. Downing (Ed.), *Teaching communication skills to students with severe disabilities* (2nd ed., pp. 175–199). Baltimore: Paul H. Brookes Publishing Co.

Meyer, L.H., Park, H.-S., Grenot-Scheyer, M., Schwartz, I.S., & Harry, B. (1998). Participatory research approaches for the study of the social relationships of children and youth. In L.H. Meyer, H.-S. Park, M. Grenot-Scheyer, I.S. Schwartz, & B. Harry (Eds.), *Making friends: The influences of culture and development* (pp. 3–30). Baltimore: Paul H. Brookes Publishing Co.

Millar, S. (2001). Supporting children using AAC in school. In H. Cockerill & L. Carroll-Few (Eds.), *Communicating without speech: Practical augmentative and alternative communication* (pp. 103–123). London: MacKeith Press.

Mirenda, P. (2005). Augmentative and alternative communication techniques. In J.E. Downing (Ed.), *Teaching communication skills to students with severe disabilities* (2nd ed., pp. 89–112). Baltimore: Paul H. Brookes Publishing Co.

Murphy, J., Markovà, I., Moodie, E., Scott, J., & Boa, S. (1995). Augmentative and alternative communication systems used by people with cerebral palsy in Scotland: Demographic survey. *Augmentative and Alternative Communication, 11,* 26–36.

Newcomb, A.F., & Bagwell, C.L. (1996). The developmental significance of children's friendship relations. In W.M. Bukowski, A.F. Newcomb, & W.W. Hartup (Eds.), *The company they keep: Friendship in childhood and adolescence* (pp. 289–321). Cambridge, United Kingdom: Cambridge University Press.

Parker, J.G., & Asher, S.R. (1993). Friendship and friendship quality in middle childhood: Links with peer group acceptance and feelings of loneliness and social dissatisfaction. *Developmental Psychology, 29,* 611–621.

Salisbury, C.L., Evans, I.M., & Palombaro, M.M. (1997). Collaborative problem-solving to promote the inclusion of young children with significant disabilities in primary grades. *Exceptional Children, 63,* 195–209.

Salisbury, C.L., Gallucci, C., Palombaro, M.M., & Peck, C.A. (1995). Strategies that promote social relations among elementary students with and without severe disabilities in inclusive schools. *Exceptional Children, 62,* 125–137.

Sapon-Shevin, M. (1990). Student support through cooperative learning. In W. Stainback & S. Stainback (Eds.), *Support networks for inclusive schooling: Interdependent integrated education* (pp. 65–80). Baltimore: Paul H. Brookes Publishing Co.

Schwartz, I.S., Staub, D., Peck, C.H., & Gallucci, C. (2006). Peer relationships. In M.E. Snell & F. Brown (Eds.), *Instruction of students with severe disabilities* (6th ed., pp. 375–404). Upper Saddle River, NJ: Pearson Education.

Snell, M.E., & Janney, R. (2005). *Teachers' guides to inclusive practices: Collaborative teaming* (2nd ed.). Baltimore: Paul H. Brookes Publishing Co.

Soto, G., Müller, E., Hunt, P., & Goetz, L. (2001). Critical issues in the inclusion of students who use augmentative and alternative communication: An educational team perspective. *Augmentative and Alternative Communication, 17,* 62–72.

Soto, G., & von Tetzchner, S. (2003). Supporting the development of alternative communication through culturally significant activities in shared educational settings. In S. von Tetzchner & N. Grove (Eds.), *Augmentative and alternative communication: Developmental issues* (pp. 287–299). London: Whurr.

Stainback, W., & Stainback, S. (1990). Facilitating peer supports and friendships. In W. Stainback & S. Stainback (Eds.), *Support networks for inclusive schooling: Interdependent integrated education* (pp. 57–64). Baltimore: Paul H. Brookes Publishing Co.

Staub, D., Schwartz, I.S., Gallucci, C., & Peck, C.A. (1994). Four portraits of friendship at an inclusive school. *Journal of The Association of Persons with Severe Handicaps, 19*(4), 314–325.

Turnbull, A., Pereira, L., & Blue-Banning, M. (2000). Teachers as friendship facilitators: Respeto and personalismo. *Teaching Exceptional Children, 32* (5), 66–70.

U.S. Department of Education. (2002). *To assure the free appropriate education of all children with disabilities: Twenty-fourth annual report to Congress on the implementation of the Individuals with Disabilities Education Act.* Washington, DC: Author.

Vandercook, T., & York, J. (1990). A team approach to program development and support. In W. Stainback & S. Stainback, (Eds.), *Support networks for inclusive schooling: Interdependent integrated education* (pp. 95–122). Baltimore: Paul H. Brookes Publishing Co.

von Tetzchner, S., Brekke, K.M., Sjøthun, B., & Grindheim, E. (2005). Constructing preschool communities of learners that afford alternative language development. *Augmentative and Alternative Communication, 21* (2), 82–100.

Warren, S.F., Yoder, P.J., & Leew, S.V. (2002). Promoting social-communicative development in infants and toddlers. In S.F. Warren & M.E. Fey (Series Eds.) & H. Goldstein, L.A. Kaczmarek, & K.M. English (Vol. Eds.), *Communication and language intervention series: Vol. 10. Promoting social communication: Children with developmental disabilities from birth to adolescence* (pp. 121–149). Baltimore: Paul H. Brookes Publishing Co.

12

Integrating Assistive Technology with Augmentative Communication

Yvonne Gillette

———— Keisha is starting first grade and already has technology experience, including a dynamic screen augmentative and alternative communication (AAC) device and a power wheelchair. With powered mobility, she can get from place to place in the school independently, despite her limited hand use. She can send preprogrammed messages to ask and answer questions and sometimes makes comments. She can combine her symbols to generate novel messages from time to time and shows interest in letters and the keyboard. But now the demands of reading, writing, and mathematics across the curriculum will require that she have the tools to participate as independently as possible. She will need these tools to learn as well as to show what she knows. Will she need a teaching assistant to read to her if she cannot hold a book? How will she write her letters, practice spelling, or draw? How can she do her math or use a calculator? These are just some of the questions that began to surface after a successful school year using her AAC device. ————

A considerable body of literature documents the importance of assistive technology (AT) to the academic success and educational inclusion of students with significant disabilities in general and those with augmentative communication needs in particular (Beukelman & Mirenda, 2005b; Edyburn, Higgins, & Boone, 2005; Sturm et al., 2006; see also http://www.cast.org). AAC systems, as delivered by device manufacturers or created by practitioners, are often designed to meet mainly message-sending and/or receiving needs of students. When educational teams and their students who use AAC grapple with the multiple demands of meaningful participation in the classroom as well as access to the general curriculum, the capacities of students' current AAC system must often be enhanced. In the context of this chapter, these enhancements to an AAC system will be considered AT. For these students, the educational team is challenged by the need to *integrate* an often complex array of technologies for learning, mobility, and participation (e.g., Erickson & Koppenhaver, 1998; Erickson, Koppenhaver, Yoder, & Nance, 1997; Koppenhaver, Spadorcia, & Erickson, 1998; Soto, Müller, Hunt, & Goetz, 2001; Sturm, 1998). This chapter discusses current issues and effective practices central to technology integration in the classroom. The chapter begins with a discussion on the concept of technology integration and then moves to the application of technology integration to support the participation of these students in the general curriculum.

TECHNOLOGY INTEGRATION: WHAT DOES IT MEAN?

Edyburn (2001) defined *technology integration* as linking software, media, and other technology tools with instructional objectives to facilitate teaching as well as learning in a process known as *curriculum correspondence*. For students with significant disabilities, additional aspects of technology integration must be considered, namely internal and external technology. *Internal technology integration* refers to the integrated use of all the technological aids each student needs for different functions such as participation, learning, mobility, and communication (Rainey, 2007). The goal of internal technology integration is seamless operation. In an ideal world, a student's access to technology is internally integrated if the technology operates from a single platform with the student as a pilot bringing up environmental controls, such as powerchair controls and tools to listen to books on CD, surf the Internet, draw, write, do math, and e-mail assignments to teachers, as needed. Having access to technology at home, at school, and in the community is essential. Internally integrated technology operates without much setup on the part of the student, teachers, parents, or assistants. *External technology integration* refers to the integration of the student's aids with the learning opportunities available in the student's educational setting (Edyburn, 2001). In the ideal classroom, the student's access to technology is externally integrated if the content within the student's system matches the content provided to the class (i.e., the same textbooks, library time, science experiments, math problems, lunch setting, writing assignments, art projects, and performing arts experiences as other students with similar abilities). In short, internal integration has to do with operating the system, whereas external integration allows the student to gain access to content common to the learning environment he or she shares with the class.

For students who rely on AAC, technology integration may become a complex process as these students may have a personal platform designed to support their communication across multiple environments. When integrating technology with the student's educational needs as defined by his or her individualized education program (IEP), the educational team must consider ways this AAC platform can be designed to meet educational needs. For example, the platform may have screens designed to call the names of others in the classroom, participate in lunch conversations, or ask or respond to questions in class. Teams should also consider AT additions to this platform that may assist the student's performance in educational environments. This might include adding an onscreen keyboard that types directly into a word processor or Internet access to search for information.

Assistive Technology and AAC Integration

The Individuals with Disabilities Education Improvement Act (IDEA) of 2004 (PL 108-446) mandated that the AT needs of all students with disabilities be considered as part of their IEP planning process. According to IDEA 2004, AT includes both devices and services such as evaluation; selection; acquisition; design; customization; maintenance; repair; coordination; intervention; and training for the student, family, and professionals. As such, school personnel are now required to develop policies and procedures for meeting the provision of this law (Blackhurst & Edyburn, 2000).

According to federal law, AT includes both the devices that enhance or change the student's methods of interacting with technology and other learning materials, as well as the services used to select, acquire, implement, and integrate these devices (Edyburn, 2001). Although any generic technology can be considered assistive, specialized AT can provide enhancements to or change methods of teaching and learning to achieve outcomes not possible with generic technology and other learning materials. This can include skills such as writing, communication, reading, studying, math, literacy, recreation, leisure, daily living, art, and transition (Reed & Lahm, 2004). There are a number of tools to assist educational teams as they consider the use of AT during IEP development (see the resources section).

To provide educational opportunities for all students, AT solutions must be integrated with the curriculum and, when possible, with any generic technology available in the student's educational environment, including software and personal computers. Specialized AT is not a "first choice" because generic technology is often less expensive due to its wider use. Sometimes specialized assistive hardware and/or software, however, may be necessary when the student's needs require specialized aids to complete educational tasks more effectively, efficiently, and independently than otherwise possible (Blackhurst, 1997).

When a student uses an AAC device, it needs to be integrated with the rest of the tools and aids the individual uses to participate in the curriculum. In this case, the AAC device is part of the AT system. Yet, AAC differs from educational AT because AAC specifically supports communication as a skill required to succeed in all interactions, settings, and activities, not just educational settings (see Beukelman & Mirenda, 2005a). In some cases, students may have an AAC device already in place, so current school personnel may not have participated in the selection and acquisition of the device. If the school setting is just one of the many places (e.g., home, community) where the student is expected to use the device, it is possible current school personnel may not participate in the selection of the device. Student funding for AAC devices is often supported through public or private health insurance and is covered as a medical necessity. Educational AT can have more specific application to the student's education, and funding for educational AT is supported by an educational entity, such as the student's school district. Although AAC selection involves making the best fit for the student across varied environments, aligning AT, including AAC, with the academic content standards and the student's IEP are specific to the student's educational program.

In the past, the use of a specific AAC platform as a single tool to participate in educational activities was often inhibited due to the use of proprietary software, operating systems, and platform features developed by specific AAC manufacturers. Recent developments, such as using the more generic Microsoft Windows operating system on some AAC devices, provide an opportunity for an integrated platform that runs the communication software but can also run reading and writing programs, educational software, and educational DVDs that the school may already have licensed. When this is the case, the AAC platform may have solved the problem of internal technology integration, leaving only the problem of external technology integration with the curriculum. When incompatibilities between the AAC device and the AT tools exist, however, the educational team must take extra steps to streamline the process of student access to the varied technologies selected to address the student's diverse educational goals. These steps might include 1) providing wireless access to computers through the communication device, 2) finding and funding versions of required software that are compatible with the student's AAC system, 3) simplifying adjustments required to use a device access system with both an AAC device and desktop classroom computers available in varied classrooms throughout the student's day, and 4) ensuring the student has access to technology in his or her home in order to perform homework tasks that might be required of all students (Rainey, 2007).

Model of Technology Integration

Edyburn's (2001) Map of Technology Integration presented a sequence of steps to assist educational teams in the process of integrating technology with the general curriculum (i.e., external integration): selection, acquisition, implementation, and integration.

Selection   The first step, *selection,* involves aligning the student's instructional objectives with necessary technology. The educational team takes an inventory of the student's goals, then selects the technology required to meet them. This process may be as simple as noting the software all students use to meet the same educational objectives or as complex as reviewing web sites and catalogs to find the required technology, then trying various possibilities with the student prior to selection.

_____   Keisha's teacher involved an AT consultant from her school district and also communicated with other teachers and speech-language pathologists (SLPs) who had worked with students with similar profiles. Together, Keisha's educational team created a list of software programs compatible with her communication device that they wanted to try. Some programs provided on-screen options that scanned a keyboard with letters and numbers. Others included programs that allowed the team to import worksheets or reading materials so that Keisha could view them on the screen. Either the district or the software companies provided demonstration programs that Keisha could try. Drawing software also was considered. The AT consultant was essential in this step because the team did not know how to operate the array of programs. _____

Acquisition   The next step, *acquisition* of the selected technologies, may require little more than making sure the technology is available on the days it is needed to the more complex processes of funding and purchasing technology that provides an individualized solution to a particular student's need.

_____   Once Keisha's team narrowed the list, they needed to secure funding and write requisitions. The team also needed to secure time to take part in training and cover the cost of any training the district could not provide. Because Keisha's device was also a computer, they did not need to consider the cost of securing a computer, a workstation, or a switch—all of this was built into her current AAC system. They also did not need to consider the issue of a home system because her system traveled with her to and from school. In the future, however, they might need to consider Internet access because Keisha's family does not have access at home. _____

Implementation   The third step, *implementation,* addresses training needs. The educational team, including the student and family members, should be shown how the technology can support the student's participation in the curriculum across one or more of the four channels of communication and learning—listening, speaking, reading, and writing. Most team members who provide educational services to the student will need to learn to operate and troubleshoot the technology. Systematic instruction should take place for the student and involve team members until they have attained operational competence with the chosen technologies.

_____   Keisha's AT consultant was essential during the process of implementation. She installed the software and contacted the software companies when access or operation of the various components did not appear to be seamless. She provided training for Keisha, the education team at the school, and Keisha's family. She also attached a laminated list of toll-free telephone numbers for the companies that manufactured the various components of Keisha's device so that everyone would have immediate access should a problem arise. _____

Integration   The final step, *integration,* goes beyond the goal of simply enhancing a learning channel, such as speaking or reading, by addressing the details surrounding integration of the technology with actual instructional objectives across the curriculum. This process may go through several iterations as the student's progress is assessed. Continuing iterations may be required to tweak the system, enhance the student's or team's skills, or extend the technology to more curricular opportunities. Extending AT use beyond the initial plan will often continue to require additional technologies, training, and links to the curriculum once the student's previous educational and AT goals have been met.

_____   It was clear to Keisha's team that external integration with the content of the curriculum would be an ongoing process. Some books came on CD; some did not. The team needed to purchase a scanner so that worksheets from workbooks and certain reading materials could be accessible to Keisha. Much of the first-grade curriculum was enhanced by pictures, which were used by all of the students, but Keisha's team knew that the more literate Keisha became, the less she would need to depend on pictures and the more independent she would be within the curriculum. For this reason, everyone supported her efforts to learn about letters, numbers, and print concepts. Time would tell how much curricular customization Keisha would require in the long run because no one yet knew her potential for literacy. _____

There are a number of barriers that may impede the process of integrating AT, such as limited funding, personnel shortages, limited training in AT, and the digital divide—the information imbalance between people with and without access to digital communication and information technology (National Center for Technology Innovation [NCTI], 2006). These barriers frequently result in limited access to technology for students with disabilities, particularly those with multiple disabilities who may require multiple aids to support their listening, speaking, reading, and writing. Although technology developers continue to promote the notion of universal designs that make technology accessible to everyone, including those with disabilities, barriers continue to exist (see http://www.cast.org). Until universal designs are truly universal, AT will continue to be one way to provide the needed link between special education and general education technology and other learning materials.

Technology integration requires the support of the entire educational team—administrators, practitioners, families, and the student. Administrators must agree to provide financial and policy support. Practitioners, such as teachers and SLPs, must continue to use existing technologies and seek opportunities and funding to acquire new technologies and related updates to their technology skills (Smith & Robinson, 2003). Most important, if the plan for AT integration is to succeed, then the student and the family must buy into it and be as integral to it as they can in light of their circumstances and culture (Bailey, Parette, Stoner, Angell, & Carroll, 2006; Huer, Parette, & Saenz, 2001; Parette, Huer, & VanBiervliet, 2005).

THREE KEY CONCEPTS THAT AFFECT TECHNOLOGY INTEGRATION

When practitioners address the complex issues related to AAC/AT[1] integration, it is necessary to consider the intersection between the academic content standards and the technologies students require to communicate and participate in the general curriculum. The following discussion reviews issues that frequently affect the integrated use of AAC/AT, including the operational competence of the student and his or her educational team, the academic content standards, and the IEP. When a student has AAC/AT needs, the IEP provides the plan for the student's operational competence training and for integrating technology with academic content standards.

Operational Competence

_____   Through third grade, Matt participated at school using a modified curriculum of primary concepts and a picture-based dynamic screen system with basic vocabulary. He understood his home, school, and some community environments. Matt's set of symbols consisted of mainly line drawings with a printed message above each symbol. It was difficult to assess his progress because he could not physically access the system. Matt had tried scanning, keyguards, a stylus, and hand braces to help with access. Consequently, operational competence was a big goal. Speed was also a major issue. Matt eventually gained access to items using direct selection with a keyguard on a 12-location dynamic screen, but his accuracy varied due to fatigue and possibly behavioral issues. As Matt entered fourth grade, it appeared that he would still require a modified curriculum and alternative assessment because he did not use a standard symbol system of letters he could spell with, and speed continued to challenge his participation.

_____

Operational competence, as it relates to aided AAC, refers to the individual's ability to effectively control and operate the tools used to communicate (Light, 1989). The technical skills required to use a communication device involve motor, cognitive, linguistic, and perceptual abilities (Rowland & Schweigert, 2003; Treviranus & Roberts, 2003). Successfully using a device is measured in terms of communication accuracy and economy of time and energy (Light, 2003). The student's fluent use of AAC/AT will require *practice*—defined as an investment of time and energy on the part of the student.

---

[1] AAC/AT is used in this chapter as a convention to indicate the intersection between both elements as they contribute to the student's communication and participation in the classroom.

In its definition of AT services, IDEA 2004 specifically addresses AT training as a service required to support the student's education. This training is for the student with the disability, the family, and the professionals who work with the student. Existing literature documents that the success of students with disabilities with AT is directly related to the AT knowledge, skills, and dispositions of the professionals who support the student (Michaels & McDermott, 2003). Including AT training as part of the IEP will ensure that the service is provided. The schools can provide this training in a variety of delivery models, including using an AT specialist or AT vendor, participating in group training sessions, participating in AT conferences, or securing training through web-based workshops. Purchase of AAC/AT must always include follow-up training if the AT tool is to be used effectively. Team members should investigate the availability of training and include any required training as part of the equipment purchase order if it is not included in the purchase price. In addition to training, the team should also investigate the availability of ongoing support, updates, and warranties and/or repair issues because all of these factors can influence the student's operational competence.

Team members who receive technology training and have ongoing support are more likely to use the technology (NCTI, 2006). Team members should not be expected to train themselves, but administrators should hold high expectations for the team members to learn to operate the technology. If team members are competent with the technology, then they can support the student's proficient use of the technology. The goal of the student's operational training and instruction is effective use of the technology to support progress in the academic content standards (Hasselbring & Bottge, 2000; Reichle, Cooley Hidecker, Brady, & Terry, 2003).

It is not enough for the team to understand how to operate the system. Team members must also know how to assess the student's operational competence, provide technological instruction for the student's development of operational competence, and develop plans to move the student forward academically, in part through enhanced operational competence. Students who have operational competence should perform independently on the following tasks:

- Operating the device
- Retrieving new and existing vocabulary
- Integrating AAC/AT use with the classroom activities with increasing independence
- Participating in programming and organizing the device
- Managing, directing, and/or cooperating with activities related to the protection, transport, and repair of the device

Training and practice continue to be important beyond the period of device introduction depending on the rate at which the student develops cognitively, linguistically, and/or motorically. The student's rate of AAC/AT use will affect his or her ability to participate effectively in the classroom, so operational competence should be included in the student's goals. Instructors need to balance the student's access to the general curriculum with opportunities to improve his or her operational competence.

Response rate can be used as a global measure of how well the student's motor, cognitive, linguistic, and perceptual skills are coming together in support of AAC/AT use. Accurate measurement of rate must balance content against speed. Slow rates of responding may indicate that a student is just becoming familiar with the technology or that he or she is creating novel responses to questions or assignments. Both of these scenarios involve motor, cognitive, linguistic, and perceptual abilities. Research on how to maximize these four abilities with AAC/AT is emerging to support educational teams as they attempt to follow evidence-based practices in intervention with AAC/AT (Alper & Raharinirina, 2006; Browder & Cooper-Duffy, 2003; Wilkinson & Hennig, 2007). Despite advances in technology, the use of AAC and AT tools takes extra time (Johnston & Evans, 2005). Effective interventionists can create conditions such as small groups or one-to-one instruction to provide such students with opportunities to communicate without delaying a large group. For example, in a large group, the instructor may ask the focus student a question that requires a single preprogrammed response. In a small group, however, the instructor may ask all students to spend 5 minutes generating written ideas, giving the student with AAC/AT needs time to compose along with his or her group.

Device Customization   Operational competence is also supported by ongoing device customization that will require time and effort. Although some students and families can take responsibility for some of the device customization needed for use across settings and communication partners, a member of the educational team should be identified as primarily responsible for managing the device customization required for curriculum integration. Yet, one team member cannot take on all of the responsibilities related to AAC/AT management and use. Training other members of the team to take on some of the following responsibilities is of paramount importance (Bodine & Melonis, 2005; Rainforth & York-Barr, 1997):

- Updating vocabulary
- Creating displays and overlays
- Protecting and transporting the device and arranging for repairs
- Instructing the student on device operation
- Guiding the content and organization of the device to match the student's need for curricular and social content, his or her organization skills to retrieve messages or combinations of messages, or his or her literacy skills to create information required for the demands of the curriculum

Students with AAC needs must also be included in the processes outlined previously in order to develop self-reliance and communication independence. Students can be involved in choosing their own vocabulary and designing their own displays (Carlson, 1981; Light, Page, Curran, & Pitkin, 2007; Sturm & Clendon, 2004; von Tetzchner & Martinsen, 1996). Students who are given regular instruction on using the device, as well opportunities to use the device throughout their daily curriculum, appear more likely to use the device independently (Reichle et al., 2003).

Due to their complex needs, students who use AAC/AT require flexible schedules of intervention and services delivered by a variety of school staff (Soto et al., 2001; Todis, 2001). Initially, the SLP or AT specialist may need to be heavily involved in implementing the AAC/AT technology including programming the screen; linking the use of this technology to the curriculum; and training the educational team, the family, and the student in initial operational competence. Once the technology is in use, however, more responsibility may fall onto the teacher, family, student, and instructional assistants. The student's operational competence will depend on an effective team that works well together to support the use of the device in the student's daily school routine.

_____   Matt requires considerable support to use his technology due to access problems. His team used the Checklist of Operational Competence (see Figure 12.1) to measure progress in the skills that he needed. They included access goals in his IEP under speech-language pathology and occupational therapy. As noted in the checklist, he had achieved many skills, including turning the device on and off, adjusting the speaker volume, clearing messages, repeating messages, and deleting messages to self-correct. For the next year, the team intends to use more computer technology with Matt and the other children in class. The team hopes to target page navigation, environmental controls, and some computer functions for the coming year, as well as move Matt to competence on the goals he currently requires assistance to complete. The checklist was a useful tool for planning meetings, including the IEP, because the team could place an X next to the targeted goals and then use the "notes" section to record Matt's present level of performance. _____

Check goals	Skill: Operational competencies *The observable behavior*	Notes
	Turn device on and off	*Competence achieved Jan. 15*
	Turn the speaker volume up or down	*Competence achieved Jan. 15*
	Clear the message	*Competence achieved Jan. 15*
	Activate text to repeat what is on the screen	*Competence achieved Jan. 15*
	Delete last letter, word, or message	*Jan. 15, minimal assistance*
X	Navigate to needed page	*Jan. 15, minimal assistance*
	Navigate to needed punctuation, tenses, etc.	
X	Return to "home screen" when finished with page	
X	Navigate through pages (message search)	*Jan. 15, minimal assistance*
	Close "pop-ups"	*N/A*
X	Use "go back" key as needed	*Jan. 15, minimal assistance*
	Activate "speak" operation	*Competence achieved Jan. 15*
	Use word prediction function	
	Scan accurately to message required	
	Navigate to and use any available functions	
	• Print	
	• MP3 functions	
	• Telephone functions	
	• Computer functions	
	• Environmental control functions	
	Individualized functions and features	
X	• Creating and storing messages	*Jan. 15, maximum assistance*
X	• Retrieving stored messages	*Jan. 15, moderate assistance*

Figure 12.1. Sample of a completed Checklist of Operational Competence. (From Perkins, M., Phillips, D., & Henneberry, S. [2007]. *Aligning state standards with IEP goals for AAC users.* Paper presented at the California State University at Northridge Technology and Persons with Disabilities Conference, Los Angeles; adapted by permission.)

Alignment of AAC/AT with Content Standards

_____ Matt's teacher and SLP wanted to align his AAC/AT goal of retrieving messages with an academic content standard. They used a second-grade standard in language arts in the oral communication domain to align with the skill they wanted to achieve—organizing and delivering oral communication and retelling stories, including character, setting, and plot. Matt could achieve this standard using a preprogrammed page of messages and, at the same time, practice his skill in retrieving messages. In addition, he and the SLP could create the screens together in order to begin to address his skill in creating and storing messages.

Reading comprehension is another content standard the team planned to address with technology. Matt had tried books on tape but found following a story or text on a computer that highlighted words as it read to him worked best. It helped him remember, and he began to link the words with meanings he could express, often on the AAC device. In their efforts to help Matt achieve a first-grade reading comprehension standard—retell the central ideas of simple expository or narrative passages—the team planned to provide him with read-aloud software, a headset, and books and texts on CD. Figure 12.2 shows how the team analyzed Matt's AAC/AT needs across the learning channels of speaking, listening, reading, and writing. While this adaptation changed the task to listening comprehension, access to this technology allowed him to participate in a more meaningful way across the curriculum. _____

Each state's academic content standards provide a plan for student learning, a curriculum for all, and a clear target for students to aim toward despite the need for accommodations or modifications (Browder et al., 2007). The Individuals with Disabilities Education Act (IDEA) Amendments of 1997 (PL 105-17) required that all students have access to the general curriculum. Multiple levels of curricular access, however, are required to meet the needs of different students (Wehmeyer, Lance, & Bashinski, 2002). Practitioners who serve students with AAC/AT needs must ensure that these students have goals that align with the academic content standards, that these goals have adequate breadth and depth, that chosen skills have fidelity to the original content, that students have access to the symbolically appropriate AAC/AT they need to achieve these academic goals, and, whenever possible, that students have access to the same AAC/AT during assessment that they use in classroom learning activities (Browder et al., 2007). Browder et al. presented a set of criteria that practitioners can use to determine how well the content of the student's curriculum links to the state's academic standards.

The No Child Left Behind (NCLB) Act of 2001 (PL 107-110) required that all students, including those with disabilities, show annual yearly progress (AYP) in language arts, math, and science, as well as other content required by the state, such as social science or technology. This is in sharp contrast with the previous emphasis on functional curriculum for students with severe disabilities as set out in the Education for All Handicapped Children Act of 1975 (PL 94-142) and IDEA 1990 (PL 101-476). NCLB does not require nor prohibit functional curricular goals; however, academic goals are the only required goals. Professionals serving students in special education should also take note that some states have taken direction from special education practices and applied those practices to general education. For example, Florida and Oregon now include functional domains such as jobs and community skills in the standards for all students. Teaching academic content to students with significant disabilities is a relatively new curricular direction. The rationale is that it is not defensible to systematically omit academic content from the curricular experiences of students with significant disabilities. Notably, it appears the same may soon be said about functional goals for typically developing students (Browder, Spooner, Wakeman, Trela, & Baker, 2006; Wakeman, Browder, Meier, & McColl, 2007).

Language arts is often a primary focus for linking AAC/AT with the academic content standards because the language arts skills of listening, reading, speaking, and writing provide the keys to learning in other academic content areas, such as math and science (Browder et al., 2007; Courtade, Spooner, & Browder, 2007). AAC/AT can provide a means for students with significant disabilities

Period	Class	Activity	AAC/AT tool
1	Opening session	Speaking Listening Reading Writing OC	Dynamic display device with grid software Device, keyguard, hand braces
2	Language arts	Speaking Listening Reading Writing OC	Dynamic display device with grid software Headset Computer with read-aloud software, book on CD
3	Occupational therapy	Speaking Listening Reading Writing OC	Dynamic display device with grid software
4	Science	Speaking Listening Reading Writing OC	Dynamic display device with grid software Headset Read-aloud software, book on CD
5	Lunch	Speaking Listening Reading Writing OC	Dynamic display device with grid software
6	Math	Speaking Listening Reading Writing OC	Dynamic display device with grid software
	Home	Speaking Listening Reading Writing OC	Dynamic display device with grid software Headset Read-aloud software, book on CD

Figure 12.2.   Augmentative and alternative communication (AAC)/assistive technology (AT) integration schedule. (*Source:* Edyburn, 2001.) (*Key:* OC, operational competence.)

to learn academically linked content matched in breadth and depth to their abilities and also provide a way for them to demonstrate their knowledge. The student's ability to use symbols of increasingly abstract representation needs to be considered when customizing curricular content for student access (see Chapter 14 and Beukelman & Mirenda, 2005a).

Practitioners should consider these three levels of symbol use—presymbolic/awareness, concrete symbolic, and abstract symbolic—as they plan access to curricular content. Those who use presymbolic/awareness systems may have some intentionality, such as banging a spoon to be fed, but will need much instruction using photographs or actual objects. Concrete symbol users gain access to a small range of vocabulary and must be taught each symbol to represent a new concept in the unit, such as having a page of locations programmed with a line drawing and a word, to communicate about a specific science experiment or story. Students who use abstract symbols are able to type or select responses that represent a wide range of vocabulary (e.g., a student who can write a paragraph using a keyboard). Although AAC/AT can come into play at all of these levels, the customization of the system should be matched to the student's symbol use based on a functional communication assessment (Browder, Ahlgrim-Delzell, Courtade-Little, & Snell, 2006; Browder et al., 2007).

The specialized needs of a student who relies on AAC will not be unusual when generic technology is used throughout the school's curriculum (Edyburn, 2001; Wehmeyer et al., 2002). In these cases, students with AAC/AT needs will not find themselves alone in using technology approaches. They will be more like everyone else in the classroom. For example, this might apply to a classroom in which students are using laptops and the Internet to find information on a history theme and writing an essay about it. School personnel may also be more open to AT/AAC approaches because they are already familiar with technology principles due to their exposure to generic technology.

Standardized Testing

_____ Matt could not participate in fourth-grade level achievement tests. He had limited reading and keyboard skills, and, in addition, his speed was quite slow. His independent performance in many areas of the curriculum, however, could be measured in alternative ways, primarily by programming his device with a range of vocabulary he could retrieve to answer questions about information in the subject area. Because his AAC/AT technology goals included creating and storing messages, the content in his device will be the source of the questions over which he will be tested. Throughout the year, his practice with retrieving messages and navigating through screens to support oral communication should give him the practice he needs to be successful on the test, but that test will be an alternate form to the ones used by students in fourth grade. Speed will be an issue to be addressed, but teachers should be able to judge an adequate number and range of test items for him in terms of speed as they monitor his progress during the school year. _____

Standards-based testing is another aspect of education in which the use of AAC/AT is critical. NCLB allows states to determine which AT may provide an unfair advantage on the test. In many cases, students who use AT successfully during their school program will be more likely to be approved to use AT in statewide testing than those who do not (Wahl, 2008). For example, the Ohio Administrative Code Rule 3301-13-03 sets out four criteria for allowable accommodations, all of which are designed to ensure that the student using AT does not have an unreasonable advantage during testing (Ohio Department of Education, 2007). One criteria, "the accommodation cannot change or enhance the student's response," is particularly critical in using AAC/AT. The explanation of this accommodation criteria specifically includes problems faced by students who cannot produce written or oral responses without the use of accommodations, such as AT for writing and AAC for responding orally. Note that these accommodations may or may not be allowed during high stakes testing. In the area of reading, for instance, students may be allowed to use read-aloud accommodations for directions, questions, and answer choices but cannot use them for reading passages or selecting on the reading portion of the test because this would measure listening, rather than reading skills. Practitioners who intend to use technology should become familiar with allowable and nonallowable accommodations for statewide testing in their own state, which typically can be found on the state's department of education web site or through the school district's office.

The U.S. Department of Education (2005) provided flexibility for states by allowing for alternate assessment based on modified achievement standards. Three levels of assessment are possible: 1) alternate achievement standards, 2) modified achievement standards, and 3) grade-level achievement standards (see Chapter 1). Browder et al. (2007), through the National Alternate Assessment Center, provided specific criteria to evaluate whether alternate assessments are aligned to the general curriculum. There are other groups and organizations supporting the use of AT in instruction and assessment, such as the State Leaders of Assistive Technology in Education (SLATE) and the Alliance for Assistive Technology Access (see Resources). These groups support the notion that students who require AT for classroom learning also require AT for statewide testing.

Statewide testing only tells part of the story of the student's progress. In addition to statewide testing, alternate or otherwise, schools should provide multiple sources to document student progress during regular classroom assessments to provide supplemental documentation of AYP. These can include portfolios to provide nonstandardized progress reports (e.g., student portfolios). These portfolios can include student work samples to document progress. Other possible data sources are an IEP-linked body of evidence, a performance assessment or direct measure of student skills, a checklist completed by people familiar with the student, or other traditional tests (Browder, Wakeman, & Flowers, 2003; Quenemoen, Rigney, & Thurlow, 2002).

AAC/AT and the IEP

_____ After Matt's team used the Checklist of Operational Competence and the AAC/AT Integration Schedule to gather data for his IEP, they needed to develop IEP goals around the information they gathered. The operational competence goals they had sketched out on the checklist are as follows: 1) using navigation keys such as home, go back, and page; *present level:* minimal assistance; *projected level:* competence; 2) creating and storing messages; *present level:* maximal assistance; *projected level:* moderate assistance; and 3) retrieving stored messages; *present level:* moderate assistance; *projected level:* minimal assistance.

The team determined that Goals 1 and 3 would be addressed in occupational therapy for two 30-minute sessions per week. Goal 2 would be addressed in speech-language pathology service for two 30-minute sessions per week. All skills would also be practiced while Matt worked with academic content, reading, and speaking across the curriculum. His reading comprehension goal would also need to indicate the technology he required to read independently.

A sample literacy goal that applies across the curriculum would be "Using read-aloud computer software installed on his dynamic screen AAC device and a headset, Matt will listen to texts and books on CD and then retell the central idea of the texts and books he reads using dynamic screen-grid software programmed with needed vocabulary on 8 out of 10 trials."

Notice that the SLP would work with the classroom assistant and Matt to create the screens he would need to retrieve vocabulary. In addition, the occupational therapist would spend time with Matt and the assistant to measure the rate of responding with navigation keys and screens he had assisted in creating. Matt would use current access methods for now despite his slow speed, but the occupational therapist could also investigate improved access through other channels, such as eye-gaze technology or improved means of direct select with fingers. The team also determined that although Matt's literacy goal has applications across the curriculum, it would be measured during language arts and science activities, according to the IEP. This was due in part to the fatigue involved with using hands to select from dynamic displays. _____

When a student requires AAC/AT, the IEP should involve strategic planning to provide equipment and services, provide internal integration of required technological components, and delineate external integration with the academic content standards and any functional skills the student may require. The IEP should also include implications for statewide testing. IEP teams should review the present level of performance data to set goals in academic, functional, and AAC/AT skills and document the student's measurable expected level of achievement across these three skill areas. Services and service environments, as well as accommodations, should be itemized with the team considering the student's daily and weekly schedule carefully, determining the time required to achieve each goal, providing the least restrictive environment for the service, noting the accommodations the student will require, and deciding on the extent of involvement for each practitioner providing the program. Once these portions of the IEP are created, statewide testing implications for AAC/AT use should be determined for each of the academic content standards identified in the IEP (Council of Administrators of Special Education [CASE], 2006).

Present Level of Performance   Technology should be a primary theme woven throughout the student's IEP when he or she requires AAC/AT for participation within the typical curriculum or a modified curriculum. Consequently, IEPs can include a statement of the student's present level of academic achievement, functional performance, and AAC/AT operational competence skills. When the student has experience with AAC/AT as a needed skill, care should be taken to point out the contrast between unaided educational performance and any change in performance enhanced by the technology (Bateman & Herr, 2006). This can provide a rationale for continued use of AAC/AT in the classroom and on assessments.

Measurable Annual Goals   Goal statements within the IEP should reference the AAC/AT support the students require to achieve goals. IEPs should also note opportunities within the curriculum to integrate the use of technology, whether the goals are academic or functional (Gillette, 2003; Hitchcock & Stahl, 2003; Purcell & Grant, 2004, 2005). When students require AAC/AT to read in order to gain information, participate in classroom discussions, or complete assignments and activities, their goals should reflect this. Next are some examples of how to embed the use of AAC/AT in goals related to the academic content standards.

- Using a dynamic screen communication device programmed with pictures, the student will participate in weekly classroom discussions about what each student did over the weekend.
- Using a talking word bank preprogrammed with printed words, the student will create a summary of a chapter in the science book as required by the class curriculum.
- After listening to a story through a digital reading program, the student will create an oral book report to be delivered to the class.

Teams that infuse AAC/AT across the student's school program will find that this infusion can have positive effects not only for students who require it but also for other unidentified students who may benefit from the exposure and access that could result.

Operational Competence Goals   Many technological skills are required in order to use a communication device or other technology competently. This technological knowledge may also be considered procedural knowledge or "how to do things" (Basham, 2007; Light, Beukelman, & Reichle, 2003). Opportunities for learning how to use the AAC device or AT should be considered a separate skill as well as one that is integrated within the curriculum. In some states, technology skills are included as one of the content standard areas. When this is the case, the use of AAC/AT technologies may be considered one of the student's technology skills and provide a rationale for practice with these devices as a part of the student's curriculum. When possible, the team should integrate academic content with operational skills across technologies. Practitioners should provide direct instruction as needed to strengthen operational skills (Smith & Robinson, 2003).

Intense, systematic instruction will lead to ease of use not only for the student, but also for practitioners and families, who must be part of the plan and part of the monitoring of the plan. Reichle et al. (2003) listed some of the practices that are necessary in this direct instruction.

- Massing of instructional opportunities
- Tight definition of the behavior that is the target of instruction
- Careful definition of the behavior that will prompt the use of this target
- Definition of the consequences for a correct or incorrect response

Teams should use these practice guidelines to create measurable, operational competence goals. The goals will need to be individualized to the student's technology needs and the student's present and projected level of performance on the goal. Within the IEP, the operational competence goals will often be included as goals of special services, such as communication services provided by the SLP or occupational therapy services, depending on the nature of support the student requires.

Services, Environments, Accommodations, and Statewide Testing   When writing the IEP, the educational team should document the time and personnel allocated to each service, the environment in which the service is to be provided, accommodations, and any AAC/AT that the student will require for learning. AAC/AT should also be provided as an accommodation for testing and statewide assessments, including alternate assessment. These types of decisions should be based on the student's needs, not on issues related to the budget of the school district or the caseloads of the practitioners (Reed & Bowser, 2005). For example, if a student uses an AAC device, then this may include a set amount of service provided by an SLP or AT specialist. It should be noted on the IEP when the family and others on the educational team require training on the operation of the device. Other documentation should include the student's use of AAC/AT in statewide testing. In some cases, education teams of students with significant disabilities may find the need for alternate assessments aligned to the academic content standards. Although states create and validate alternate assessments, districts and individual IEP teams can begin to find ways to document student progress and seek direction from the developing literature (Towles-Reeves & Kleinert, 2006). Technologies will also need to be aligned with the transitional component of the IEP when it is time for transition planning from school to the workplace (Blackhurst, Lahm, Harrison, & Chandler, 1999; Wood, Karvonen, Test, Browder, & Algozzine, 2004).

FIVE PRINCIPLES GUIDING SUCCESSFUL TECHNOLOGY SOLUTIONS

Each student who needs technology for academic and functional success will require a unique solution. A guiding principle for AAC/AT educational integration is "start small and build." Educational teams can easily become overwhelmed with the complexities of AT use. The guiding questions and principles in Table 12.1 are presented to assist teams to develop technology solutions. The five principles, derived from the literature, are expanded in the discussion that follows.

1. **If a student cannot easily gain access to the school's curriculum, then consider AAC/AT solutions.**

AT of all types should be considered at every IEP meeting, including those of students with AAC/AT needs, as mandated under IDEA 1997 and 2004. Specialized or generic technology can support a

Table 12.1.   Guiding questions and principles to assist teams to develop technology solutions

Question	Principle
1. Why use AAC/AT?	If a student cannot easily gain access to the school's curriculum, then consider AAC/AT solutions.
2. What AAC/AT can benefit the student?	Match the student's needs to varied AAC/AT that can promote independent access to the academic content standards and functional skills.
3. How will the team and student learn to use AAC/AT?	Provide training to develop the operational competence of the student and his or her educational team and write it into the individualized education program (IEP).
4. Where will the student use the technology?	Integrate AAC/AT use across the curriculum.
5. When will AAC/AT be used?	Plan AAC/AT use to support curricular units, whether academic or functional.

Key: AAC, augmentative and alternative communication; AT, assistive technology.

variety of academic skills including reading, writing, math, drawing, organization, and research, as well as leisure and social skills (Edyburn, 2000).

2. **Match the student's needs to varied AAC/AT to promote independent access to the academic content standards and functional skills.**

Several tools exist to assist practitioners in finding technology that matches their students' needs (e.g., Reed & Lahm, 2004; Zabala, 2005). For example, a student can read web-based articles using digital reading programs (e.g., Gillette, 2006; Strangman & Dalton, 2005), write and review writing assignments with talking word processors and other computer-based tools (e.g., MacArthur, Ferretti, Okolo, & Cavalier, 2001; Sitko, Laine, & Sitko, 2005; Sturm, Rankin, Beukelman, & Schutz-Meuhling, 1997; Sturm & Rankin-Erikson, 2002), and use a personal digital assistant (PDA) to organize his or her day through the calendar functions and create reminder alarms to stay on schedule (e.g., Gillette & DePompei, 2008). When practitioners are aware of these applications and seek training in their use, all students, including those with AAC needs, will benefit from expanded educational opportunities. In addition, practitioners should note that many dynamic display devices can accept software applications beyond AAC, making the AAC device function not only as a communication tool but also an educational tool.

3. **Provide training to develop the operational competence of the student and his or her educational team to support AAC/AT integration and write it into the IEP.**

Operational competence with any technology takes instruction and practice. As competence grows, the regular use of technology in daily life becomes more likely. It is necessary, then, that IEPs include a plan for training the student and the educational team to operate the device.

As an example of systematic training for the student, the Checklist of Operational Competence (see Figure 12.1) applies to most AAC devices with space to insert other functions as required (Perkins, Phillips, & Henneberry, 2007). This tool is designed to provide practitioners with direction to plan for operational competence training. Practitioners can use the checklist to determine the student's present and projected levels of competence with various device skills, note status on other skills, plan where systematic instruction can take place, determine team member roles in service delivery related to the skill(s), and select specific strategies needed to nurture the growth of the skill.

As a supplement to the checklist, practitioners and their students who struggle with scanning may benefit from an article by Koch (2007). Koch described 13 progressive levels of software use that can provide a guide to teaching scanning. Examples of these levels include cause and effect, errorless choices, match symbol to picture, and answer questions.

4. **Integrate AAC/AT use across the curriculum.**

All students, including students with AAC/AT needs, will find themselves in school contexts that vary widely in the level of generic technology available as well as the technology expertise of the staff. Consequently, the experience and knowledge of the team can affect the external integration of technology with the curriculum as well as the internal integration among the available technologies.

Trends suggest that more learning will depend on technology and, in particular, technologies for learning that are universally designed (Jackson, 2005). Once a tipping point is reached, more practitioners will begin to use technology for learning and find that one of the greatest attributes of technology is the leveling of the playing field—learners of different ability levels will be able to learn together more easily (Gladwell, 2002; Hall, 2002). Between now and then, practitioners can begin to integrate generic and specialized technologies to enhance the four channels of communication—listening, speaking, reading, and writing—during school activities. Communication may no longer be seen as a goal mainly for individuals with disabilities but, instead, a means by which all students engage socially and academically at school, employing whatever technology they require.

Research describes complex and costly interventions that might not easily transfer to the typical classroom (Schlosser et al., 2000; Sonnenmeier, McSheehan, & Jorgenson, 2005). Although these reports describe excellent practices, practitioners in typical settings may find it useful to start small and gradually build technology use across the school life of students with AAC/AT needs. Figure 12.2 is designed to help practitioners visualize that process. The form can easily be adapted to fit a particular school's schedule because it simply includes slots for six class periods, which can be expanded by using more than one form. In the "class" column, the team can enter classes or activities such as opening session, language arts, lunch, and so forth to provide a graphic of the student's day. Next, the "activity" column contains entries to remind the practitioner to consider all four channels of communication (speaking, listening, reading, writing), as well as operational competence, as they integrate ATs to enhance one or more of these channels with the class content (e.g., science, language arts). Finally, in the "AAC/AT tool" column, software and/or hardware technologies can be specifically linked to the channel of communication being enhanced. The chart is not meant to be completely filled out at first, but it should be used as a guide to what is happening now in terms of integrating technology with open slots to show other opportunities available to be completed over time.

5.   **Plan AAC/AT use to support curricular units, whether academic or functional.**

In most cases, students with AAC/AT needs will find themselves at various points across these four dimensions: educational placement, academic participation, social participation, and degree of independence (Beukelman & Mirenda, 2005a). Whatever the student's profile, AAC/AT should be considered and then applied to provide the student with the best curricular option possible within a multilevel curriculum (Wehmeyer et al., 2002). Within all of the curricular areas, instructional unit planning enhanced with technology is becoming a common practice in general and special education. Running parallel to AT developments (e.g., Gardner & Wissick, 2002; Jorgenson, 2005; Schlosser et al., 2000; Smith & Robinson, 2003; Sonnenmeier et al., 2005), the application of generic technology to unit lesson planning is emerging (see, e.g., WebQuest and Kent School District in the resources section). Proper unit planning provides the opportunity for gaining content knowledge as well as developing generic skills such as communicating, writing, reading, and listening. Planning thematic units designed to be accessible for general and special education students will require that all school personnel collaborate to enhance educational outcomes for all students through the use of technology.

Issues for the Present and the Future

Many issues related to AAC/AT integration must be resolved or, at the very least, moved forward if students are to use AAC/AT effectively and efficiently at school for communication and learning. Larger issues often influence the success of AAC/AT integration for students, including 1) creating the conditions for adoption of the device (Todis, 1996); 2) promoting research to support evidence-based practice and policy to support the use of AAC/AT within the school curriculum (Alper & Raharinirina, 2006); 3) collaborating to share effective learning strategies and technology-based learning among the members of the educational team; 4) providing funding that allows for suitable selection and timely acquisition of the technology, both software and hardware; and 5) providing the support required to implement and integrate the technology, such as the costs of training for the team, time for creating links between the technology and the curriculum, and time allocated to operational training for the student.

Although none of these topics can be explored in depth in this chapter, note that all of these issues are interrelated. Devices are often abandoned, and many people assume the reason for the abandonment is because the technology does not really work. Research in the area of AAC device abandonment often settles around a few other issues, such as support and training, attitudes, device characteristics, and fit (e.g., Johnson, Ingelbret, Jones, & Ray, 2006). Although cultural issues may influence the degree of attitudinal support, issues of cost, research, and policy can affect decisions about technology choices and access to training (Wahl, 2008). The interaction among culture, cost, research, and policy can lead to a circle of device success or device abandonment for students, families, and practitioners because they will develop attitudes or offer support based on their personal experience. Consequently, attitudes can be positive when teams experience the rewards of a good match between technology and student. Yet, attitudes will be less than ideal when teams are forced to use a device due to cost rather than fit or if they do not receive the proper training (McSheehan, Sonnemeier, Jorgensen, & Turner, 2006).

Despite these unresolved issues, education teams can often create successful academic and functional outcomes with their students when using AAC/AT. Although everyone involved must contend with issues that interfere with success, finding ways to incorporate AAC/AT into the school curriculum now can help further the causes related to research and policy, which still linger on the horizon.

CONCLUSION

In closing, AAC/AT integration is a big job, but it can have a big payoff—increasing independence for the student in communication and learning opportunities in school and the transition to life beyond school. Each student presents a unique profile influenced not only by cognitive, communication, and motor skills, but also by the attitudes, knowledge, and skills of the student's education team. Teams who advocate for the most seamless internal and external AAC/AT integration possible should find that the efforts made to overcome barriers such as cost and time for one student will pave the way for subsequent students with related needs (NCTI, 2006). Although the communication and learning possibilities are endless, it is necessary to initiate and then gradually build in AAC/AT solutions for each student with AAC/AT needs. Successful solutions can begin to create a culture within schools and communities that can foster greater expectations and more robust outcomes for students who now, through technology, have greater opportunities for success.

RESOURCES

Resources Related to General Education Technology Integration

Discussion and information dissemination platforms that commonly address general education technology integration within the curriculum include the following:

- *eSchools News*—http://www.eschoolnews.com
- *International Society for Technology in Education (ISTE)*—http://www.iste.org
- *WebQuest*—http://www.webquest.org
- *Kent School District*—http://www.kent.k12.wa.us/curriculum/tech/tech_int.html

Resources for AT Consideration During IEP Meetings

- *Hey Can I Try That?*—http://www.wati.org/Curriculum/curriculum.html
- *Assistive Technology Planner, National Assistive Technology Research Institute (NATRI)*— http://www.cec.sped.org/ScriptContent/Orders/ProductDetail.cfm?section=CEC_Store& pc=S5780

Not all students need AT, but for those students who do, AT may change their lives. IEP teams have a major responsibility for ensuring that students with disabilities receive appropriate AT devices and/or services and that AT is used effectively. The Assistive Technology Planner is a practical reference guide for IEP teams as they plan and implement AT as part of a student's IEP. The implementation planning kit contains a user's guide; an implementation planning tool; and individual planners for teachers, administrators, and families.

- *Assistive Technology Quick Wheel*—http://www.cec.sped.org/ScriptContent/Orders/Product Detail.cfm?section=CEC_Store&pc=P5550

- *Assessing Students' Needs for Assistive Technology (ASNAT), Fourth Edition*—http://www.wati.org/Products/products.html

ASNAT is designed to help educational teams assess a student's need for AT. ASNAT provides a wealth of information about AT. The first chapter explains the assessment procedure and forms that the Wisconsin Assistive Technology Initiative has developed to support school teams as they engage in the assessment process. Subsequent chapters provide detailed information on specific categories of AT. The appendix contains resources including print, web, and AT vendors.

REFERENCES

Alper, S., & Raharinirina, S. (2006). Assistive technology for individuals with disabilities: A review and synthesis of the literature. *Journal of Special Education Technology, 21*(2), 47–64.

Bailey, R.L., Parette, H.P., Stoner, J.B., Angell, M.E., & Carroll, K. (2006). Family member's perceptions of augmentative and alternative communication device use. *Language, Speech, and Hearing Services in Schools, 37,* 50–60.

Basham, J.D. (2007). The use of cognitive memory prosthetics for individuals with learning disabilities. *Special Education Technology Practice, 9*(5), 16–21.

Bateman, B.D., & Herr, C.M. (2006). *Writing measurable IEP goals and objectives.* Verona, WI: IEP Resource.

Beukelman, D.R., & Mirenda, P. (2005a). *Augmentative and alternative communication: Supporting children and adults with complex communication needs* (3rd ed.). Baltimore: Paul H. Brookes Publishing Co.

Beukelman, D.R., & Mirenda, P., with Strum, J. (2005b). Literacy development of children who use AAC. In D.R. Beukelman & P. Mirenda, *Augmentative and alternative communication: Supporting children and adults with complex communication needs* (3rd ed., pp. 351–390). Baltimore: Paul H. Brookes Publishing Co.

Blackhurst, A.E. (1997). Perspectives on technology in special education. In A.E. Blackhurst & W.H. Berdine (Eds.), *An introduction to special education* (pp. 199–128). New York: Grune and Stratton.

Blackhurst, A.E., & Edyburn, D. (2000). A brief history of special education technology. *Special Education Technology Practice, 2*(1), 21–35.

Blackhurst, A.E., Lahm, E.A., Harrison, E.M., & Chandler, W.G. (1999). A framework for aligning technology with transition competencies. *Career Development for Exceptional Individuals, 22*(2), 153–183.

Bodine, C., & Melonis, M. (2005). Teaming and assistive technology in educational settings. In D. Edyburn, K. Higgins, & R. Boone (Eds.), *Handbook of special education technology research and practice* (pp. 209–228). Whitefish Bay, WI: Knowledge by Design.

Browder, D.M., Ahlgrim-Delzell, L., Courtade-Little, G., & Snell, M. (2006). General curriculum access. In M. Snell & F. Brown (Eds.), *Instruction for students with severe disabilities* (6th ed., pp. 489–525). Upper Saddle River, NJ: Merrill/Prentice Hall.

Browder, D.M., & Cooper-Duffy, K. (2003). Evidence-based practice for students with severe disabilities and the requirement for accountability in "No Child Left Behind." *The Journal of Special Education, 37*(3), 157–163.

Browder, D.M., Spooner, F., Wakeman, S., Trela, K., & Baker, J.N. (2006). Aligning instruction with academic content standards: Finding the link. *Research and Practice for Persons with Severe Disabilities, 31*(4), 309–321.

Browder, D.M., Wakeman, S.Y., & Flowers, C. (2003). Assessment of progress in the general curriculum for students with disabilities. *Theory Into Practice, 45*(3), 249–259.

Browder, D.M., Wakeman, S.Y., Flowers, C., Rickelman, R.J., Pugalee, D., & Karvonen, M. (2007). Creating access to the general curriculum with links to grade-level content for students with significant cognitive disabilities: An explication of the concept. *Journal of Special Education, 41*(1), 2–16.

Carlson, F. (1981). A format for selecting vocabulary for the nonspeaking child. *Language, Speech, and Hearing Services in Schools, 25,* 11–20.

Council of Administrators of Special Education. (2006). *Response to intervention: An administrator's perspective.* A joint paper by the National Association of State Directors of Special Education and the Council of Administrators of Special Education. Retrieved May 21, 2007, from http://www.casecec.org/rti.htm.

Courtade, G.R., Spooner, F., & Browder, D.M. (2007). Review of studies with students with significant cognitive disabilities which link to science standards. *Research and Practice for Persons with Severe Disabilities, 32*(1), 43–49.

Education for All Handicapped Children Act of 1975, PL 94-142, 20 U.S.C. §§ 1400 *et seq.*

Edyburn, D.L. (2000). Assistive technology and students with mild disabilities. *Focus on Exceptional Children, 32*(6), 1–24.

Edyburn, D.L. (2001). A map of the technology integration process. *Special Education Technology Practice, 4*(1), 28–35.

Edyburn, D.L., Higgins, K., & Boone, R. (2005). *Handbook of special education technology research and practice.* Whitefish Bay, WI: Knowledge by Design.

Erickson, K.A., & Koppenhaver, D.A. (1998). Using the "WriteTalk-nology" with Patrick. *Teaching Exceptional Children, 31*(1), 58–64.

Erickson, K.A., Koppenhaver, D.A., Yoder, D.E., & Nance, J. (1997). Integrated communication and literacy instruction for a child with multiple disabilities. *Focus on Autism and Other Developmental Disabilities, 12,* 142–150.

Gardner, J.E., & Wissick, C.A. (2002). Enhancing thematic units using the world wide web: Tools and strategies for students with mild disabilities. *Journal of Special Education Technology, 17*(1), 27–38.

Gillette, Y. (2003). *Achieving communication independence: A comprehensive guide to assessment and intervention.* Eau Claire, WI: Thinking Publications.

Gillette, Y. (2006). Assistive technology and literacy partnerships. *Topics in Language Disorders, 26*(1), 70–84.

Gillette, Y., & DePompei, R. (2008). Do PDAs enhance the organization and memory skills of students with cognitive disabilities? *Psychology in the Schools, 45*(7), 665–677.

Gladwell, M. (2002). *The tipping point: How little things can make a big difference.* New York: Little, Brown Book Group.

Hall, T. (2002). *Differentiated instruction.* Wakefield, MA: National Center on Accessing the General Curriculum. Retrieved December 30, 2007, from http://www.cast.org/publications/ncac/ncac_diffin struc.html

Hasselbring, T.S., & Bottge, B.A. (2000). Planning and implementing technology programs in inclusive settings. In J.D. Lindsey (Ed.), *Technology and exceptional individuals* (pp. 91–113). Austin, TX: PRO-ED.

Hitchcock, C., & Stahl, S. (2003). Assistive technology, universal design, universal design for learning: Improved learning opportunities. *Journal of Special Education Technology, 18*(4), 45–52.

Huer, M.B., Parette, H.P., & Saenz, T. (2001). Conversations with Mexican Americans regarding children with disabilities and augmentative and alternative communication. *Communication Disorders Quarterly, 22*(4), 197–206.

Individuals with Disabilities Education Act Amendments (IDEA) of 1997, PL 105-17, 20 U.S.C. §§ 1400 *et seq.*

Individuals with Disabilities Education Act (IDEA) of 1990, PL 101-476, 20 U.S.C. §§ 1400 *et seq.*

Individuals with Disabilities Education Improvement Act (IDEA) of 2004, PL 108-446, 20 U.S.C. §§ 1400 *et seq.*

Jackson, R. (2005). *Curriculum access for students with low-incidence disabilities: The promise of universal design for learning.* Wakefield, MA: National Center on Accessing the General Curriculum. Retrieved April 1, 2006, from http://www.cast.org/publications/ncac/ncac_lowinc.html

Johnson, J.M., Inglebret, E., Jones, C., & Ray, J. (2006). Perspectives of speech-language pathologists regarding success versus abandonment of AAC. *Augmentative and Alternative Communication, 22*(2), 85–99.

Johnston, S., & Evans, J. (2005). Considering response efficiency as a strategy to prevent assistive technology abandonment. *Journal of Special Education Technology, 20*(3), 45–50.

Jorgenson, C. (2005). The least dangerous assumption: A challenge to create a new paradigm. *Disability Solutions, 6*(3), 1–15.

Koch, R. (2007). Teaching multiply handicapped switch use to scan: A software guide. *Closing the Gap, 25*(5), 1–9.

Koppenhaver, D.A., Spadorcia, S.A., & Erickson, K.A. (1998). How do we provide inclusive literacy instruction for children with disabilities? In S.B. Neuman & K.A. Roskos (Eds.), *Children achieving: Best practices in early literacy* (pp. 77–96). Newark, DE: International Reading Association.

Light, J. (1989). Toward a definition of communicative competence for individuals using augmentative and alternative communication systems. *Augmentative and Alternative Communication, 5,* 137–144.

Light, J.C. (2003). Shattering the silence: Development of communicative competence by individuals who use AAC. In D.R. Beukelman & J. Reichle (Series Eds.) & J.C. Light, D.R. Beukelman, & J. Reichle (Vol. Eds.), *Augmentative and alternative communication series: Communicative competence for individuals who use AAC: From research to effective practice* (pp. 3–38). Baltimore: Paul H. Brookes Publishing Co.

Light, J.C., Beukelman, D.R., & Reichle, J. (Vol. Eds.). (2003). *Augmentative and alternative communication series: Communicative competence for individuals who use AAC: From research to effective practice.* Baltimore: Paul H. Brookes Publishing Co.

Light, J.C., Page, R., Curran, J., & Pitkin, L. (2007). Children's ideas for the design of AAC assistive technologies for young children with complex communication needs. *Augmentative and Alternative Communication, 23*(4), 274–287.

MacArthur, C.A., Ferretti, R.P., Okolo, C.M.,& Cavalier, A.R. (2001). Technology applications for students with literacy problems: A critical review. *The Elementary School Journal, 101*(3), 273–301.

McSheehan, M., Sonnemeier, R.M., Jorgensen, C.M., & Turner, K. (2006). Beyond communication access: Promoting learning of the general education curriculum by students with significant disabilities. *Topics in Language Disorders, 26*(3), 266–290.

Michaels, C.A., & McDermott, J. (2003). Assistive technology integration in special education teacher preparation: Program coordinators' perceptions of current attainment and importance. *Journal of Special Education Technology, 18*(3), 29–45.

National Center for Technology Innovation. (2006). *Moving toward solutions: Assistive and learning technology for all students.* Washington, DC: U.S. Department of Education, Office of Special Education.

No Child Left Behind Act of 2001, PL 107-110, 115 Stat. 1425, 20 U.S.C. §§ 6301 *et seq.*

Ohio Department of Education, Office of Assessment. (2007). *Ohio statewide testing program rules book.* Columbus, OH: Author.

Parette, H.P., Huer, M.B., & VanBiervliet, A. (2005). Cultural research in special education technology. In D. Edyburn, K. Higgins, & R. Boone (Eds.), *Handbook of special education technology research and practice* (pp. 81–10). Whitefish Bay, WI: Knowledge by Design.

Perkins, M., Phillips, D., & Henneberry, S. (2007). *Aligning state standards with IEP goals for AAC users.* Paper presented at the California State University at Northridge Technology and Persons with Disabilities Conference, Los Angeles.

Purcell, S.L., & Grant, D. (2004). *Using assistive technology to meet literacy standards: Grade 4–6.* Verona, WI: IEP Resources.

Purcell, S.L., & Grant, D. (2005). *Using assistive technology to meet literacy standards: Grade K–3.* Verona, WI: IEP Resources.

Quenemoen, R., Rigney, S., & Thurlow, M. (2002). *Use of alternate assessment results in reporting and accountability systems: Consideration for use based on research and practice* (Synthesis Report 43). Minneapolis: University of Minnesota, National Center on Educational Outcomes. Retrieved January 28, 2008, from http://cehd.umn.edu/NCEO/Online Pubs/Synthesis43.html

Rainey, D. (2007). Technology integration: How to start and when to stop. *Closing the Gap, 26*(1), 1, 10.

Rainforth, B., & York-Barr, J. (1997). *Collaborative teams for students with severe disabilities: Integrating therapy and educational services.* Baltimore: Paul H. Brookes Publishing Co.

Reed, P., & Bowser, G. (2005). Assistive technology and the IEP. Using technology to support struggling readers: A review of the literature. In D. Edyburn, K. Higgins, & R. Boone (Eds.), *Handbook of special education technology research and practice* (pp. 61–80). Whitefish Bay, WI: Knowledge by Design.

Reed, P., & Lahm, A. (2004). *Assessing students' needs for assistive technology: A resource manual for school district teams.* Oshkosh: Wisconsin Assistive Technology Initiative.

Reichle, J., Cooley Hidecker, M.J., Brady, N.C., & Terry, N. (2003). Intervention strategies for communication: Using aided augmentative communication systems. In D.R. Beukelman & J. Reichle (Series Eds.) & J.C. Light, D.R. Beukelman, & J. Reichle (Vol. Eds.), *Augmentative and alternative communication series: Communicative competence for individuals who use AAC: From research to effective practice* (pp. 441–478). Baltimore: Paul H. Brookes Publishing Co.

Rowland, C., & Schweigert, P.D. (2003). Cognitive skills and AAC. In D.R. Beukelman & J. Reichle (Series Eds.) & J.C. Light, D.R. Beukelman, & J. Reichle (Vol. Eds.), *Augmentative and alternative communication series: Communicative competence for individuals who use AAC* (pp. 241–276). Baltimore: Paul H. Brookes Publishing Co.

Schlosser, R., McGhie-Richmond, D., Blackstien-Adler, S., Mirenda, P., Antonius, K., & Janzen, P. (2000). Training a school team to integrate technology meaningfully into the curriculum: Effects on student participation. *Journal of Special Education Technology, 15,* 31–44.

Sitko, M.C., Laine, C.J., & Sitko, C. (2005). Writing tools: Technology and strategies for struggling writers. In D. Edyburn, K. Higgins, & R. Boone (Eds.), *Handbook of special education technology research and practice* (pp. 571–598). Whitefish Bay, WI: Knowledge by Design.

Smith, S.J., & Robinson, S. (2003). Technology integration through collaborative cohorts. *Remedial and Special Education, 24*(3), 154–160.

Sonnenmeier, R.M., McSheehan, M., & Jorgenson, C.M. (2005). A case study of team supports for a student with autism's communication and engagement within the general education curriculum: Preliminary report of the beyond access model. *Augmentative and Alternative Communication, 21*(2), 101–115.

Soto, G., Müller, E., Hunt, P., & Goetz, L. (2001). Critical issues in the inclusion of students who use AAC: An educational team perspective. *Augmentative and Alternative Communication, 17,* 62–72.

Strangman, N., & Dalton, B. (2005). Using technology to support struggling readers: A review of the literature. In D. Edyburn, K. Higgins, & R. Boone (Eds.), *Handbook of special education technology research and practice* (pp. 545–570). Whitefish Bay, WI: Knowledge by Design.

Sturm, J. (1998). Educational inclusion of AAC users. In D.R. Beukelman & P. Mirenda (Eds.), *Augmentative and alternative communication: Management of severe communication disorders in children and adults* (2nd ed., pp. 391–424). Baltimore: Paul H. Brookes Publishing Co.

Sturm, J.M., & Clendon, S.A. (2004). Augmentative and alternative communication, language, and literacy: Fostering the relationship. *Topics in Language Disorders, 24*(1), 76–91.

Sturm, J.M., Rankin, J.L., Beukelman, D.R., & Schutz-Meuhling, L. (1997). How to select appropriate software for computer assisted writing. *Intervention in School and Clinic, 32,* 148–161.

Sturm, J.M., & Rankin-Erikson, J.L. (2002). Effects of hand-drawn and computer-generated concept mapping on the expository writing of middle school students with learning disabilities. *Learning Disabilities, Research, and Practice, 17*(2) 124–139.

Sturm, J., Spadorcia, S., Cunningham, J.W., Cali, K., Staples, A., Erickson, K., et al. (2006). What happens to reading between first and third grade? Implications for students who use AAC. *Augmentative and Alternative Communication, 22*(1), 21–36.

Todis, B. (1996). Tools for the task? Perspectives on assistive technology in educational settings. *Journal of Special Education Technology, 13*(2), 49–61.

Todis, B. (2001). It can't hurt: Implementing AAC technology in the classroom for students with severe and multiple disabilities. In J. Woodward & L. Cuban (Eds.), *Technology, curriculum, and professional development* (pp. 27–46). Thousand Oaks, CA: Corwin Press.

Towles-Reeves, E., & Kleinert, H. (2006) The impact of one state's alternate assessment upon instruction and IEP development. *Aural Special Education Quarterly, 25*(3), 31–39.

Treviranus, J., & Roberts, V. (2003). Supporting competent motor control of AAC systems. In D.R. Beukelman & J. Reichle (Series Eds.) & J.C. Light, D.R. Beukelman, & J. Reichle (Vol. Eds.), *Augmentative and alternative communication series: Communicative competence for individuals who use AAC: From research to effective practice* (pp. 199–240). Baltimore: Paul H. Brookes Publishing Co.

U.S. Department of Education. (2005). *Alternate achievement standards for students with the most significant cognitive disabilities.* Washington, DC: Author. Retrieved January 28, 2008, from http://www.ed.gov/policy/elsec/guid/altguidance.doc

von Tetzchner, S., & Martinsen, H. (1996). Words and strategies: Conversations with young children who use aided language. In S. von Tetzchner (Ed.), *Augmentative and alternative communication: European perspectives* (pp. 65–88). London: Whurr.

Wahl, L. (2008). *No child left behind: Implications for assistive technology.* Retrieved January 20, 2008, from http://www.ataccess.org/resources/nochild.html

Wakeman, S.Y., Browder, D.M., Meier, I., & McColl, A. (2007). The implications of No Child Left Behind for students with developmental disabilities. *Mental Retardation and Developmental Disabilities Research Reviews, 13,* 143–150.

Wehmeyer, M.L., Lance, G.D., & Bashinski, S. (2002). Promoting access to the general curriculum for students with mental retardation: A multilevel model. *Education and Training in Mental Retardation and Developmental Disabilities, 37,* 223–234.

Wilkinson, K.M., & Hennig, S. (2007). The state of research and practice in augmentative and alternative communication for children with developmental/intellectual disabilities. *Mental Retardation and Developmental Disabilities, 13,* 58–69.

Wood, W.M., Karvonen, M., Test, D.W., Browder, D.M., & Algozzine, B. (2004). Promoting student self-determination skills in IEP planning. *Exceptional Children, 36*(3), 8–16.

Zabala, J.S. (2005). *The SETT framework: Critical areas to consider when making informed assistive technology decisions.* Retrieved January 30, 2008, from http://www2.edc.org/NCIP/workshops/sett/SETT_Framework_article.html

III

Supports

13

Supporting Collaborative Teams and Families in AAC

Nancy B. Robinson and Patti L. Solomon-Rice

> The implementation of inclusive education of students with AAC needs requires a collaborative effort by members of educational teams who share a vision of full social and academic participation of students with disabilities within their school communities. (Hunt, Soto, Maier, Müller, & Goetz, 2002, p. 34)

The importance of collaborative teamwork and support for family members to participate in the development of augmentative and alternative communication (AAC) systems for school-age students with AAC needs is extensively described in the literature (Beukelman & Mirenda, 2005; Glennen & DeCoste, 1997; Lloyd, Fuller, & Arvidson, 1997). If students with AAC needs are to fully partici-pate in inclusive general education environments, then the efforts of all members of the educational team need to be coordinated and focused on the provision of necessary educational resources toward that goal. Furthermore, collaborative teamwork and provision of family support are considered to be recommended practice in the development and delivery of AAC services in school settings.

This chapter focuses on the practice of AAC services in school settings within the context of col-laborative teams, which include family members. Several key issues interact to achieve collaborative practice and family support in AAC services. The issues that follow define the scope of this chapter: 1) the rationale, challenges, and strategies for collaborative teaming processes; 2) legal requirements for collaborative practice and family support; 3) family perspectives related to caring for students with complex communication needs; 4) family cultural and linguistic diversity; 5) family perspectives on technology; and 6) strategies to support families as members of the AAC team in the context of family- and student-centered AAC services. Current knowledge, policy, and recommended practices in the provision of AAC services in a collaborative team model are reviewed in relationship to each of the previous issues. Resources for school personnel and family members are provided that offer guidance for collaboration on the AAC team. Collaborative processes for effective AAC teamwork, opportunities and barriers for collaborative teamwork, and strategies to overcome barriers to collab-oration through recommended practice are addressed.

In addition, the families of children with AAC needs encounter a variety of competing demands when raising a child who may have health and physical challenges in addition to complex communication needs. This chapter includes a focus on the stressors that families may encounter and identifies resources to support families to meet their multitude of competing demands in the process of being a full participant with the AAC team. Finally, today's classrooms are rich in cultural and linguistic diversity. The chapter reviews the particular cultural and linguistic diversity issues that are part of the assistive technology (AT)/AAC team process. Strategies to support families of diverse cultural, linguistic, societal, and economic backgrounds are identified, and approaches to include diversity in AAC teams are explored.

DEFINING THE ISSUES

Key issues involved in collaborative AAC services in school settings were listed previously, including collaborative teaming processes, legal requirements, family perspectives, and cultural and linguistic diversity. These issues are further defined to support strategies for successful development of collaborative practice with families and professionals.

Collaborative Teaming

Collaborative teaming requires identifying challenges and developing processes and strategies when implementing AAC services in school settings (Hunt, Doering, Hirose-Hatae, Maier, & Goetz, 2001; Hunt, Soto, Maier, Liboiron, & Bae, 2004; Hunt et al., 2002; Soto, Müller, Hunt, & Goetz, 2001a, 2001b). Challenges facing the practice of collaborative teamwork include uneven levels of AAC experience and limitations of time, technology, funding, and administrative support among school-based programs and professionals (Dowden et al., 2006). Processes for effective collaborative teaming consist of three integral components: 1) regular, positive face-to-face interactions; 2) a structure for addressing issues, performance, and monitoring; and 3) clear individual accountability for agreed-on responsibilities (Salisbury, Evans, & Palombaro, 1997).

Legal Requirements for Team Collaboration and Family Involvement

In addition to the need for collaborative teamwork and support for families in AAC services, legal requirements for team processes and family involvement are also established. The Individuals with Disabilities Education Act (IDEA) of 1990 (PL 101-476), IDEA Amendments of 1997 (PL 105-17), Individuals with Disabilities Education Improvement Act (IDEA) of 2004 (PL 108-446), and Section 504 of the Rehabilitation Act of 1973 (PL 93-112) have specific provisions for team members and family members to jointly develop individualized education programs (IEPs) that include AT and AAC services. The provisions in IDEA 1990, 1997, and 2004 include requirements for a variety of services, including 1) evaluating the needs of a child with disabilities, including a functional evaluation of the child in the child's customary environment; 2) purchasing, leasing, or otherwise providing for the acquisition of AT devices for children with disabilities; 3) selecting, designing, fitting, customizing, adapting, applying, refining, repairing, or replacing AT devices; 4) coordinating and using other therapies, interventions, or services with AT devices, such as those associated with existing education and rehabilitation plans and programs; 5) training or providing technical assistance for a child with a disability or, if appropriate, that child's family; and 6) training or providing technological assistance for professionals, employers, or other individuals who provide services to, employ, or are otherwise substantially involved in the major life functions of children with disabilities (Best, Heller, & Bigge, 2005; Lloyd et al., 1997; National Information Center for Children and Youth with Disabilities [NICHCY], 2007). The need for a collaborative approach to coordinate and maximize AAC resources and services is underscored by the legal policy outlined in IDEA.

Family Roles and Cultural Diversity

Involving family members and addressing the increasing cultural and linguistic diversity in schools and communities are central challenges facing the delivery of AAC services in schools. The roles of family members and students who use AT and AAC are core to all phases of assessment, development, and implementation of AAC services (Beukelman & Mirenda, 2005; Glennen & DeCoste, 1997; Lloyd et al., 1997). Although family participation is identified as a necessary component of effective AAC services, the methods to support family members on collaborative AT and AAC teams are just beginning to be understood and implemented in practice (Bailey, Parette, Stoner, Angell, & Carroll, 2006; Judge, 2002; Parette, Brotherson, & Huer, 2000; Parette & VanBiervliet, 2000).

Recommended professional practices to involve family members in all phases of AAC service delivery are found in the literature. Research by Angelo (2000), Parette and VanBiervliet

(2000), and Parette, Brotherson, and Huer (2000) emphasized the need for professionals to provide family-focused and culturally sensitive interventions in response to the increasing diversity among student populations. Parette and VanBiervliet, in particular, provided seven recommendations for professional practice that are adopted in this chapter as guidelines for AAC teams in school settings.

1. Recognize that families have many demands placed on them coming from both outside and within the family unit.

2. Understand that the presence of a disability in the family affects all family members within the immediate family.

3. Recognize that each child with a disability has unique needs.

4. Identify the child's communication needs in the home, school, and community.

5. Recognize differences and strengths in families.

6. Spend time with each family member before discussing the AAC intervention.

7. Develop competence to provide culturally responsive assessment and intervention services.

THREE LEVELS OF COLLABORATIVE TEAMWORK

Policy, research, and recommended practice regarding AAC service delivery in school settings are focused across three levels: the system, the practitioner, and the family. Required policies, challenges, and research-based strategies to implement collaboration and support for families in AAC services are described at each level.

System Level

Effective collaborative teamwork requires support throughout the service system. Evidence-based research indicates the following needs as critical foundations for successful systems and infrastructure development: 1) administrative support and leadership to develop and sustain collaborative initiatives (Hunt et al., 2001; Hunt et al., 2004; Hunt et al., 2002); 2) time and resources to develop and to sustain collaborative teams (Hunt et al., 2001; Hunt et al., 2004; Hunt et al., 2002); and 3) training and staff development in the provision of AT and AAC services (Hunt et al., 2001; Hunt et al., 2004; Hunt et al., 2002; Soto et al., 2001a, 2001b). Administrative support at the district and local school level are critical for developing and sustaining effective AAC services. As emphasized previously, legal requirements and educational policies established in the United States at the federal and state level provide the foundation for requiring AT (including AAC), including specific provisions of IDEA and the Assistive Technology Act of 1998 (PL 105-394) (National Assistive Technology Technical Assistance Partnership [NATTAP], 1997).

Challenges and Opportunities for System-Level Collaboration in AAC Services   The status of the provision of AAC services in school settings can be best described as uneven (Dowden et al., 2006). Common themes regarding the issues and challenges for implementing comprehensive AAC services in a collaborative team approach are found in the United States and international locales. Sutherland, Gillon, and Yoder (2005) surveyed the status of AAC services throughout New Zealand and identified key systemic variables that affected the provision of AAC services, including: 1) availability of AAC systems, 2) family acceptance of AAC, 3) AAC system abandonment, 4) funding for AAC services, 5) AAC service provision, and 6) administrative processes related to AAC services. The previous issues are further corroborated by previous surveys to assess the needs for AAC services in Nebraska and North Dakota, Australia, Scotland, and South Africa (Alant, 1999; Balandin & Iacono, 1998; Burd, Hammes, Bornhoeft, & Fisher, 1998; King, 1998; Matas, Mathy-Laikko, Beukelman, & Legresley, 1985; McCall & Moodie, 1998; Murphy,

Markova, Moodie, Scott, & Boa, 1995). Each of the previous areas can be discussed as both barriers and opportunities to build AAC services in school systems. The contribution of such survey research in AAC provides a basis for school administrators to examine AAC services at local and regional levels to further determine specific program priorities and initiatives. Taking the view that each of the issues can be framed as an opportunity for program development, school administrators have a basis for district initiatives for building AAC services.

The barriers to implementing collaborative team approaches to AAC services in school settings can be better understood in the context of survey research just discussed. Each of the issues identified by Sutherland et al. (2005) are common across school settings reported by other researchers and have relevance for school-based AAC teams.

AAC System Availability   The limited availability of AAC equipment is a barrier to implementing AAC services (Parette & Dempsey Marr, 1997). Equipment loan systems in school districts, communities, and state programs are often limited to a specific geographical area and inaccessible to a broad population. The perceived barriers to obtaining AAC equipment are often reported by school personnel, thus contributing to unfamiliarity and discomfort with technology in general (Dowden et al., 2006). In addition, school personnel identified a shortage of AAC equipment as a major barrier to services in survey research. This may, in fact, indicate that there is a misperception among professionals that AAC is defined by technology alone. The definition of AAC reaches far beyond high- and low-tech systems and incorporates natural and unaided systems of communication such as sign language (Cress & Marvin, 2003). A lack of understanding of the scope of AAC and potential for application prior to the use of AAC devices certainly leads to gaps in school-based services.

Family Acceptance   Family members' readiness to consider and to implement AAC supports with their children is highly variable, related to familiarity with technology and understanding of alternative methods to supplement communication (Bailey et al., 2006). A family-centered approach is needed when considering using AAC systems (Judge, 2002). In addition, cultural and linguistic differences among families create potential barriers and challenges for the implementation of AAC services in multiple languages (Huer, 2003; McCord & Soto, 2000, 2004; Nigam, 2003). At the school system or district level, provisions to accommodate for translation services and access to training and education for families about the potential application for AAC are needed in multiple languages.

Continuation of AAC Use   Determining appropriate features of AAC systems for individual students and providing the students with a trial period to get familiar with their systems is recommended to support successful and continued use of AAC (Bailey et al., 2006). Decision-making processes for AAC teams that are assessing and selecting appropriate AAC systems are now available to assist in appropriate device selection. For example, the Participation Model developed by Beukelman and Mirenda (1988) and revised through the work of Light, Roberts, Dimarco, and Greiner (1998) and Schlosser et al. (2000) provided a means to guide decision making and intervention through a multiphase assessment process that emphasizes consensus building among team members. Through the application of the Participation Model, AAC teams conduct three phases of assessment that include 1) initial assessment of the individual's current communication needs, characteristics, and communicative environments; 2) detailed assessment of possible future environments and developing a communication system to anticipate future needs; and 3) follow-up assessment to maintain a comprehensive AAC system. A more detailed explanation of the Participation Model can be found in Beukelman and Mirenda (2005).

Although the Participation Model and other multiphase AAC assessment processes include considering multiple environments, individual communication needs, and communication partners, the input of family members and individuals who use AAC is needed to assure that decisions reflect family and individual preferences. Bailey et al. (2006) summarized several key reasons for discontinuation of AAC use that included the pervasive application of professional decision-making approaches rather than consumer/family-centered decision-making processes. The results of family interviews conducted by Bailey et al. indicated a need for increased professional collaboration with families throughout the AAC assessment and system use across settings. School policies and practices also need to include provisions to include perspectives of the family and the student who uses AAC in the decision-making processes. Demonstration and trial use of AAC devices are further recommended to provide an experiential basis for the family, the individual student, and all team members to evaluate necessary features of potential AAC systems.

Service Provision   The issues of AAC service provision in a manner that meets recommended practice for a collaborative approach are complicated by personnel shortages, limitations in AAC, the time-intensive nature of AAC service delivery, AAC expertise, and costs of personnel and AAC services (Dowden et al., 2006; Edgar & Rosa-Lugo, 2007). Within the school-based context for speech-language pathology services, the American Speech-Language-Hearing Association (ASHA; 2002a) advocates for a workload analysis approach to determine caseload size for speech-language pathologists (SLPs). Workload analysis includes considering all activities required for SLPs to adequately serve students in school settings such as assessment, planning, parent communication, and team participation. Based on workload surveys (ASHA, 2006), 50% of SLPs who responded to the survey reported serving children with AAC needs. Of those who reported providing AAC services, the mean number of students served was 5. Although this is a relatively small percentage of an average caseload of 50 students, the time required for provision of AAC services can be expected to exceed the roles and responsibilities for clients with other communication and language needs (Dowden et al., 2006). In addition to the complexity and severity of students' needs, the number of students in special education is rising (ASHA, 2002b). School district policy and practice are faced with multiple challenges when considering personnel needs and workload requirements for speech-language pathology, special education, related services specialists, and general education personnel to adequately serve students with AAC needs.

Funding   The cost for AAC services is an ongoing concern for all school districts and is often considered the most significant barrier to developing AAC systems for students with complex communication needs (Parette & Dempsey Marr, 1997). In addition to the cost of AAC devices, the cost of maintenance, training, and additional AT involved in developing an effective AAC system must be considered. Strategies to reduce costs for expensive technology may include low-tech systems with visual communication methods. Computer technology is also required to create communication boards and picture systems that can be used in addition to expensive speech-generating devices (SGDs; Bailey et al., 2006).

In addition to the costs for technology, personnel positions and considerations for AAC specialists at the school district level add to the cost of providing a system of AAC services. The needs for ongoing training and staff development are further costs that may affect local districts and statewide services.

Evidence-Based Strategies for System-Level Collaboration   Developing systemwide AAC services at the state and district level requires several key components, including the need for administrative leadership, specialized personnel, equipment, and staff training opportunities (Hunt et al., 2001; Hunt et al., 2004; Hunt et al., 2002; Soto et al., 2001a, 2001b). Successful models of collaborative AAC services address several of the previous components. Several state initiatives exist to address the need for developing AAC services due, in part, to the Technology-Related Assistance for Individuals with Disabilities Act of 1988 (PL 100-407) and its amendments in 1994 (PL 103-218) and 1998 (PL 105-394), which gave impetus for state systems to develop AT. A national resource network of AT projects can be accessed through the National Assistive Technology Technical Assistance Project (http://www.resna.org/taproject/index.html). Developing AT systems through school systems is also supported through collaborative partnerships utilizing federal, state,

and local school district partnerships. Wahl (2002) reported increases in the numbers of regional partnerships, with hundreds of school-based programs using AT and AAC services throughout the United States. Sources of funding included federal, state, and private funds, and scope of services included varying levels of assessment, training, consultation, equipment loan, and direct services. Figure 13.1 summarizes guidelines and provides a checklist for developing collaborative initiatives for AAC services.

The following example demonstrates one school-based team facing system-level challenges to develop a collaborative program of AAC services.

_____ Following the completion of a summer course at a local university in AAC, Linda returned to her school district the following semester. As the new specialist in AT, her job role was just becoming defined as the coordinator of AT and AAC assessments for a large rural district with a student body that included many languages and cultural backgrounds, predominantly of Hispanic origin. As a fluent speaker of Spanish, Linda was comfortable that she could provide translation services for assessment purposes and assistance to her colleagues in developing AAC services in both Spanish and English. As the fall semester began, however, Linda realized that her role as the sole professional responsible for all AT and AAC assessments was becoming unmanageable. She was encouraged by three of her colleagues in the district to seek support from her administrator, the special education director, to expand the number of positions dedicated to AT and AAC services. Initially, her requests were denied due to a lack of funding. The director did agree to review the needs and approved two additional positions the following school year.

As the AT specialist in her district, Linda now has two colleagues working with her on the districtwide AT/AAC team, including an SLP and occupational therapist with specialized training in AAC. Through regular meetings and communication with the director, the AT/AAC team has expanded their budget with plans to hold regular staff development workshops in the coming year. Although the needs for additional expertise at the classroom level remain unmet, the team found the support at the district level to discuss and begin to address AT and AAC program needs. _____

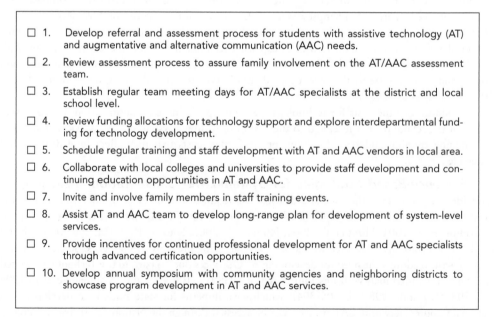

☐ 1.   Develop referral and assessment process for students with assistive technology (AT) and augmentative and alternative communication (AAC) needs.

☐ 2.   Review assessment process to assure family involvement on the AT/AAC assessment team.

☐ 3.   Establish regular team meeting days for AT/AAC specialists at the district and local school level.

☐ 4.   Review funding allocations for technology support and explore interdepartmental funding for technology development.

☐ 5.   Schedule regular training and staff development with AT and AAC vendors in local area.

☐ 6.   Collaborate with local colleges and universities to provide staff development and continuing education opportunities in AT and AAC.

☐ 7.   Invite and involve family members in staff training events.

☐ 8.   Assist AT and AAC team to develop long-range plan for development of system-level services.

☐ 9.   Provide incentives for continued professional development for AT and AAC specialists through advanced certification opportunities.

☐ 10. Develop annual symposium with community agencies and neighboring districts to showcase program development in AT and AAC services.

Figure 13.1.   System-level collaboration checklist. (*Sources:* Hunt, Doering, Hirose-Hatae, Maier, & Goetz, 2001; Hunt, Soto, Maier, Liboiron, & Bae, 2004; Hunt, Soto, Maier, Müller, & Goetz, 2002; Soto, Müller, Hunt, & Goetz, 2001a, 2001b.)

Practitioner Level

The heart of developing effective AAC services for students in school settings lies within the professional team who initiates the development of AT and AAC services for students with complex communication needs. In order to support effective AAC services in school settings, professionals must develop, demonstrate, and embrace skills to facilitate team collaboration (including the special and general education teachers, related services personnel, health professionals, specialized professionals, and instructional assistants as well as families and individuals with AAC needs). Evidence-based practices for effective teaming are identified in the literature and include 1) the development of clear roles and tasks within the team (Hunt et al., 2004; Hunt et al., 2002); 2) a variety of different types of team structures in school settings (Glennen & DeCoste, 1997); 3) clear goals for the team (Beukleman & Mirenda, 2005; Hunt et al., 2004; Hunt et al., 2002); 4) effective interpersonal and communication skills (Thousand & Villa, 1992); and 5) respect for diverse contributions of each member of the AAC team (Beukelman, Burke, Ball, & Horn, 2002; Beukelman, Hanson, Hiatt, Fager, & Bilyeu, 2005; Burke, Beukelman, Ball, & Horn, 2002). Although legal requirements and administrative support provide the necessary conditions to initiate AAC support within schools and districts, the frontline professionals are responsible for service delivery and follow up. The roles among team members include an array of knowledge and skills that must be integrated in AAC service delivery within the context of general education (Hunt et al., 2002; Soto et al., 2001a; Sturm, 1998).

Challenges and Opportunities for Practitioner Collaboration in AAC Services   In spite of personnel shortages and funding limitations, legislation and professional training programs may have an effect in school settings as they create capacity to build and to expand AAC services. For example, Ratcliff, Koul, and Lloyd (in press) surveyed national speech-pathology preprofessional programs regarding the status of teaching in the area of AAC. Of the 168 surveys returned, 52% of respondents reported that an AAC course was required, and 48% reported that it was an elective course in their program. Furthermore, 80% reported that AAC content was infused into other courses. ASHA established new certification requirements for SLPs that include knowledge and skills in the area of AAC (ASHA, 2005). Such increased requirements in AT and AAC at the preprofessional level appear to support the expanded training opportunities in AAC for newly trained professionals in speech-language pathology, special education, and related services.

Many significant challenges and barriers are inherent in the process of developing and maintaining collaborative teamwork in the delivery of AAC services and supports in school settings, including personnel shortages, increasing numbers of referrals for special education services, reported increases in the complexity of student needs in special education, limited time devoted to planning and team development, limited specialized skills in the areas of AT and AAC service provision, family stress, and cultural and linguistic diversity (Dowden et al., 2006; Parette & Dempsey Marr, 1997). Each of these challenges present a set of difficult issues for all professionals in school settings, even those with high levels of expertise in AAC service delivery.

AAC Collaborative Team Models   Recommended practice in the provision of AAC services is based on the following parameters: the need for an array of knowledge and skills, implementation by a collaborative team, a high degree of family involvement, and provision of accommodations for cultural and linguistic diversity among students and their families (Hunt et al., 2002; Judge, 2002; McCord & Soto, 2004; Parette & Dempsey Marr, 1997). A description of approaches to developing collaborative team practice follows with attention to the variety of possible styles of collaboration that may best fit available professional and program resources.

Models of collaborative teamwork are described in traditional and more innovative styles, as follows. Traditionally, team models can be conceptualized as multidisciplinary, interdisciplinary, or transdisciplinary (Glennen & DeCoste, 1997). Briefly, each of these models revolves around professional membership, and family involvement is included as an added component in later phases of team operation. The multidisciplinary model is characterized by team members working in separate settings or separate rooms and coming together to summarize and to integrate their findings. Family members may or may not be present in summary meetings. The interdisciplinary model typically involves more communication among team members throughout the assessment and intervention phases, often with periodic meetings and family consultation. As in the multidisciplinary model, the interdisciplinary team may or may not involve family members until a later stage in the reporting process. The transdisciplinary model, considered the most difficult to achieve, requires that all team members are present during the assessment and planning phases, including family members. This model approaches a collaborative process with family and all team members more than either the multi- or interdisciplinary approach.

The collaborative team model, as described by Glennen and DeCoste (1997), moves beyond all of the traditional approaches with a high priority placed on involving the family and individual from the very outset of the assessment and intervention planning process. Family and individual preferences and needs related to developing AAC systems are considered in the first phase of the collaborative team approach, rather than being conceptualized as a point of "reporting back" following the completion of the assessment by professional members. Parity and equity among all team members, including family members and individuals with AAC needs, are central values and principles of the collaborative team model.

In actual practice, elements of traditional team styles and collaborative practice may be observed. McCormick (2003) described aspects of collaborative practice that include consultation among team members, collaborative consultation, and coteaching. Often, local school and district resources determine what is possible for team members, given time and personnel limitations. In terms of resource demands, the consultation approach requires regular contact among professionals and may vary in the degree of formal time commitments. The collaborative consultation model requires more extensive commitment among team members related to sharing of expertise and planning required for individual students. Often, the collaborative consultation model involves demonstration and peer mentoring (e.g., the SLP implementing vocabulary use for an individual student using an AAC device in regular classroom activities). The most demanding collaborative approach can be found in the coteaching model, in which two professionals with differing but complementary expertise share in AAC service delivery (e.g., the classroom teacher and adapted physical education teacher implementing language arts within a game involving movement).

As discussed in the preceding section, the implementation of collaborative teamwork is affected by the team model (multi-, inter-, and transdisciplinary) in addition to levels of collaboration (collaborative consultation, consultation, or coteaching). Determining the team model and level of collaborative practice may be related to personnel and program resources. For example, team members may work in different settings and be employed by different agencies throughout the community. Elements of collaborative practice as outlined by Hunt et al. (2002) serve as guidelines for achieving recommended practice on behalf of students and families. Commitment to regular team members, frequent communication, family involvement, provisions for cultural and linguistic diversity, staff development, and shared resources are elements of positive collaboration that are common to all models, regardless of the level of collaboration that is determined to be effective in local school settings.

Evidence-Based Practice: Collaborative AAC Teams   Studies have identified key variables for effective collaborative practice in AAC, including professional expertise in AAC, availability of staff training, interpersonal communication skills, and skills for collaboration (Hunt et al., 2001; Hunt et al., 2004; Hunt et al., 2002; Glennen & DeCoste, 1997; Soto et al., 2001a, 2001b; Thousand & Villa, 1992). Hunt et al. (2002) further delineated components of collaborative practice in AAC service delivery that included 1) allocating time and resources for teamwork, 2) identifying innovative communication methods for teamwork, 3) committing to collaboration in the educational process, 4) giving consistent attention to the process of team development and evaluation, and 5) providing knowledge/skill in regard to family needs and supporting family partnerships.

Committing the time to develop team processes that are identified in the research is key to understanding and developing collaborative initiatives in school settings (Thousand & Villa, 1992). The initial stages of goal development often start smoothly and often move into a conflict stage before the team has learned to work through difficult communication and priorities of all members. Stages of team development are often referred to as *forming, storming, norming, and performing*, and the development of interpersonal communication skills is critical to the progress of the team to achieve collaborative work (Thousand & Villa, 1992). In addition to establishing goals, periodic evaluation to determine team effectiveness is an essential component to continued performance (Sadao & Robinson, 2007).

Of the many approaches available for team development, two are particularly relevant to the provision of AAC service. First, Salisbury et al. (1997) developed a collaborative problem-solving process (CPS) to facilitate effective collaborative teaming. The CPS process utilizes a 5-step set of strategies to achieve a positive collaborative outcome. Step 1 identifies the issue. Step 2 generates all possible solutions. Step 3 screens solutions for feasibility. Step 4 chooses the solution to implement, and Step 5 evaluates the solution.

Second, Hunt et al. (2001, 2002, 2004) effectively implemented components of CPS to increase the academic achievement and social participation of students with AAC needs who were members of inclusive classroom settings. Their Unified Plans of Support (UPS) consisted of academic adaptations and communication and social supports developed by a team that included the general education and inclusion support teachers, an instructional assistant, an SLP, and a parent. The main elements of the UPS process are 1) regularly scheduled meetings, 2) development of supports to increase the focus student's academic and social participation in general education instructional activities, 3) a built-in accountability system, and 4) flexibility to change ineffectual supports. Monthly meetings allow for ongoing evaluation and revision of the student's UPS that are implemented though the cooperative efforts of all team members. From the family support perspective, UPS allows the parent an opportunity to provide input to other members of the educational team and hear reports concerning his or her child's progress at regular intervals.

Implementation of the UPS model is highly regarded by parents and professionals (Hunt et al., 2003). Parents highlight the importance of their role in bringing information about their child to the team and the ability to implement the support plan at home. Team members further emphasize the importance of regularly scheduled team meetings on a monthly basis, the shared ownership for developing and implementing support plans, the ability to model implementation of support plans across team members, and the opportunity to be equal team members. The UPS model has been validated in elementary (Hunt et al., 2002) and preschool settings (Hunt et al., 2004).

Skill Development for Practitioners in Collaborative AAC Services

In addition to team development processes, Soto et al. (2001a, 2001b) identified critical professional skills required for effective teamwork in school settings. Soto and colleagues (2001b) conducted focus groups to investigate the professional skills regarded by educational team members as necessary to support students who use AAC in general education classrooms. Necessary skills identified by the focus groups were divided into five themes: 1) collaborative teaming, 2) providing access to the curriculum, 3) cultivating social supports, 4) maintaining AAC system operation, and 5) creating classroom structures that support the learning of heterogeneous groups of students. Furthermore, specific skills were identified as essential by the participants and related to each theme by the researchers (see Table 13.1).

The skills identified by focus group members provide sound guidelines for facilitating family- and student-centered AAC and AT services in K–12 school settings. In addition to identifying professional skills needed to facilitate family- and student-centered AAC and AT services in school settings, it is also useful to identify indicators of success that support family- and student-centered AAC and AT services as a piece of recommended practice guidelines. The focus groups in the previously mentioned Soto and colleagues (2001b) study also identified indicators of success that

Table 13.1.   Themes and skills for effective collaboration

Themes	Skills
Collaborative teaming	Work collaboratively on a multidisciplinary team
	Understand the roles and responsibilities of all members and be willing to be flexible around role boundaries
	Treat one another with respect regardless of professional title or position
	Communicate effectively
	Maintain an action-oriented approach
Access to curriculum	Use the student's augmentative and alternative communication (AAC) system as a means to gain access to the core curriculum
	Have a working knowledge of core curriculum and the ability to contribute to curriculum adaptations and modifications
	Be able to assess the student's learning style to develop appropriate instructional strategies
Cultivating social supports	Facilitate social interactions
	Highlight the uniqueness and attractiveness of the focus student
	Provide support unobtrusively to foster independence and autonomy
AAC system maintenance and operation	Know how to operate, maintain, and integrate all elements of the AAC system
	Know how to obtain technical help and locate resources
	Facilitate student use across classroom activities
	Make vocabulary recommendations
	Familiarize peers with how AAC systems work
Building a supportive classroom community	Use cooperative learning strategies
	Share information with colleagues
	Embrace the student as a rightful member of the classroom

Source: Soto, Müller, Hunt, & Goetz (2001a, 2001b).

supported family- and student-centered AAC and AT services in inclusive classrooms. Collaborative teaming was identified as one of the most important indicators of a successful inclusion program (Soto et al., 2001a). Regular team meetings were identified as needed to develop action-based strategies for mutually defined goals. Accountability, strong leadership, and interpersonal skills were descriptors used to define a functional team. These successful traits for collaborative teaming identified by focus group members provide additional recommended practice guidelines for facilitating family- and student-centered AAC and AT services in K–12 school settings.

Beukelman et al. (2002, 2005) and Burke et al. (2002) completed a series of studies to investigate the influence of learning styles on the performance of AAC team members and found that self-efficacy was related to performance in delivery of AAC services. The importance of self-efficacy as it relates to learning and professional motivation in the collaborative team approach to AAC services is important to meet the work style and learning needs for all team members. Figure 13.2 summarizes key points for team development initiatives to consider when developing collaborative endeavors in AAC.

Table 13.2 provides a summary of resources for school-based teams for the purpose of supporting the development and delivery of collaborative team practices in AAC service delivery. As with all web-based resources, the currency of web sites is transient and requires frequent updating. Resources in Table 13.2 are highlighted related to collaboration at the three levels discussed—school system, practitioner, and family levels.

_____   In a large urban school district, funding for positions and program development in the area of AT and AAC was severely limited. Three specialists, two SLPs, and one special educator with specialized training in AT and AAC were responsible for conducting all AAC assessments and IEP development for students from kindergarten through high school who use AAC.

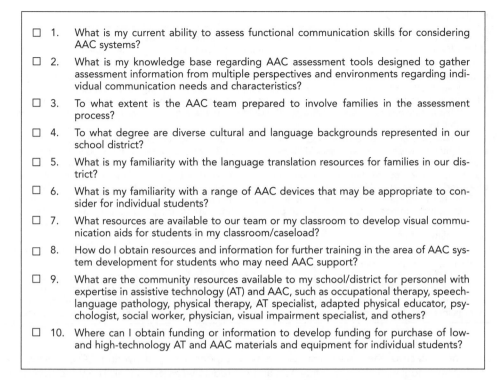

☐ 1. What is my current ability to assess functional communication skills for considering AAC systems?

☐ 2. What is my knowledge base regarding AAC assessment tools designed to gather assessment information from multiple perspectives and environments regarding individual communication needs and characteristics?

☐ 3. To what extent is the AAC team prepared to involve families in the assessment process?

☐ 4. To what degree are diverse cultural and language backgrounds represented in our school district?

☐ 5. What is my familiarity with the language translation resources for families in our district?

☐ 6. What is my familiarity with a range of AAC devices that may be appropriate to consider for individual students?

☐ 7. What resources are available to our team or my classroom to develop visual communication aids for students in my classroom/caseload?

☐ 8. How do I obtain resources and information for further training in the area of AAC system development for students who may need AAC support?

☐ 9. What are the community resources available to my school/district for personnel with expertise in assistive technology (AT) and AAC, such as occupational therapy, speech-language pathology, physical therapy, AT specialist, adapted physical educator, psychologist, social worker, physician, visual impairment specialist, and others?

☐ 10. Where can I obtain funding or information to develop funding for purchase of low- and high-technology AT and AAC materials and equipment for individual students?

Figure 13.2.   Augmentative and alternative communication (AAC) self-efficacy assessment questions. (*Sources:* Parette & Dempsey Marr, 1997; Wilcox, Weintraub, & Aier, 2003.)

Table 13.2.   Resources for collaborative augmentative and alternative communication (AAC) services in school settings

Administrative and system-level collaboration

The National Center for Cultural Competence (NCCC)— The NCCC, located at Georgetown University in Washington, D.C., states that its mission "is to increase the capacity of health and mental health programs to design, implement, and evaluate culturally and linguistically competent service delivery systems." Several tools have relevance for school-based services in AAC, particularly the *Cultural and Linguistic Competence Policy Assessment* (CLCPA) and *A Guide for Advancing Family-Centered and Culturally and Linguistically Competent Care.* Links to both documents are found on NCCC's web site at http://www11.georgetown.edu/research/gucchd/nccc/

Collaborative team development

TOTS-n-TECH (TNT) Efficacy Scale— The TNT web site provides an efficacy scale that can be used to measure providers' and families' perceptions of assistive technology (AT) use with young children (http://asu.edu/clas/tnt/AssisTechConfScale.pdf).

Families, Cultures and AAC Project (VanBiervliet & Parette, 2002)—The Families, Cultures and AAC Project was developed to provide school practitioners and families with accurate, culturally sensitive information about AAC technologies and decision-making strategies. The project resulted in the development of an interactive bilingual CD-ROM for professionals and family members to develop effective AAC competencies. The program includes video clips, educational games, and links to web sites. In addition, it includes bilingual translation in English and Spanish and contains built-in features to make information and activities accessible for people with disabilities. Further information about the CD-ROM and the project can be obtained by contacting the primary author, Alan VanBiervliet, Ph.D., at the University of Arkansas for Medical Sciences, College of Nursing, Nursing Science Department, Little Rock, Arkansas.

Collaboration with families

The Family Center on Technology and Disability (FCTD)—The FCTD is a network of more than 1,900 organizations that include parent support and advocacy groups, disability-specific associations, state and local government agencies, foundations for disability research, national advocacy organizations, and university-based programs (http://www.fctd.info/). Available resources include numerous links to

(continued)

Table 13.2. *(continued)*

information regarding implementing AT, including AAC, in school settings. Family guides are available at http://www.fctd.info/resources/fig/ and contain information in both English and Spanish for families to gain an understanding of the potential applications of AT and AAC in school settings.

Assistive Technology JFK Partners Simple Guides—This web site provides a series of quick guides regarding the application of AT for children with developmental delays, including topics on communication, adaptive skills and cognition, fine motor skills, gross motor skills, self-help, and sensory development (http://jfkpartners.org/PUBLICATIONS.asp). The guides provide a general overview of AT in each developmental area.

YAACK—YAACK provides extensive AAC advocacy, information, and resources for families and professionals (http://www.aac.unl.edu.yaack/d3.html). Ms. Ruth Ballinger developed this web site as part of the requirements for completing her M.Ed. degree in special education at the University of Hawaii. She features resources for families and professionals who work with young children in the development of AT and AAC systems. Ms. Ballinger stated, "The purpose is to provide information and guidance to families, teachers, speech-language pathologists, and anyone else who is involved with a child with special communication needs. It is intended to be easy to understand and practical and cover a wide range of topics dealing with AAC and AAC-related issues of children at various ages and stages of communication ability, with different strengths, disabilities, and learning characteristics."

Message and Context Selection Worksheets (Starble, Hutchins, Favro, Prelock, & Bitner, 2005)—Materials used to facilitate family participation and input include message and context selection worksheets adapted from the Barkley Memorial AAC Centers (available on the University of Nebraska web site at http://aac.unl.edu). The message selection worksheet is designed for parents to determine specific types of messages that were desired but lacking on the child's AAC device. The context selection worksheet is intended for parents to rate priorities for AAC device use in community and home contexts.

Furthermore, each of the AT/AAC specialists was responsible for delivering AAC services in a consultative model with classroom teachers and related services personnel. The three specialists had worked at the district level for many years and had become increasingly distressed at their workload and increasing numbers of students referred for AAC assessment and services. Due to the overall economy of the city schools, the likelihood of additional positions at the district level was limited. The development of a collaborative team model with other professionals within the community appeared to be the only solution.

Through a problem-solving process, the three AT/AAC specialists listed all professionals within the district and urban area with expertise in AAC. In addition, parent advocacy groups were identified with AAC resources and a small loan bank of AAC equipment. Through brainstorming and discussion, a list of 10 additional professionals within the local district and community was developed. As several of the professionals, such as occupational and physical therapists, were employed by the local children's services agency and developmental disabilities programs, an interagency task force was scheduled to address the issues for development of collaborative AAC services. Representation of the parent advocacy group was also included on the task force.

After several weekly meetings, the group obtained support from a professional facilitator employed by the health department to assist the group in defining the needs for AAC services and goals. An initial goal included developing an interagency agreement between the school district, children's services agency, developmental disabilities program, and parent organization to hold regular meetings and AAC training events for professionals and parents in the local area. Funds were obtained through staff development allocations, pooled across agencies. Although the school district AT/AAC team found that AAC service delivery remained uneven, the community team and increased collaboration around AAC services for school-age students encouraged them. ⎯⎯⎯⎯⎯

Family Level

Family inclusion in the collaborative teaming process is perhaps the most crucial element of successful student AAC and AT use over time. Collaboration between practitioners and family members requires that practitioners establish and consistently practice sensitivity toward family needs and diversity in the following areas:

1. Sensitivity to family needs regarding family perspectives, needs, and competing demands related to caring for a student with complex communication needs (Ferguson, 2002; Goldbart & Marshall, 2004; Jones, Angelo, & Kokoska, 1998; Kerr & McIntosh, 2000; McCubbin, Thompson, Thompson, & McCubbin, 1993; Patterson, 1993; Woolfson, 2004)

2. Cultural competence to respond to family diversity issues, such as cultural and linguistic diversity, and varying family structures (Bevan-Brown, 2001; Goode, 2005; Hourcade, Parette, & Huer, 1997; Huer & Saenz, 2002; Kemp & Parette, 2000; Matuszny, Banda, & Coleman, 2007; Parette, VanBiervliet, & Hourcade, 2000; VanBiervliet & Parette, 2002)

3. Time to identify and develop family readiness for AT and AAC (Angelo, 2000; Angelo, Jones, & Kokoska, 1995; Angelo, Kokoska, & Jones, 1996; Parette & Angelo, 1996; Parette & Dempsey Marr, 1997)

4. Professional support for family participation on AAC teams (Hunt et al., 2001; Hunt et al., 2004; Hunt et al., 2002; Salisbury et al., 1997)

5. Implementation of family- and student-centered AT and AAC services in K–12 school settings (Soto et al., 2001a, 2001b)

6. Strategies to build ongoing partnerships with families across school to home settings (Bailey et al., 2006)

7. Training opportunities for families and school personnel related to AAC and the importance of including families in vendor/device training sessions (Parette, VanBiervliet, & Hourcade, 2000).

Family Perspectives, Needs, and Competing Demands Creating linkages between families and schools begins with a clear understanding of parental reactions toward having a child with a disability. Ferguson (2002) identified a dramatic evolution in researcher and practitioner attitudes and supports for students with disabilities and their families beginning in the early 1990s as researchers and practitioners began focusing on how families have adapted and coped with their children with disabilities across the life span. Research models of stress and coping (adaptation) and models of family life course development have influenced attitudes through use of the classic ABCX model developed by Hill (1958). In the ABCX model, the outcome of a family crisis (*X*) is based on the interactions of three factors: *A*, an initial stressor event, combined with *B*, a family's resources for dealing with crisis, and *C*, the family's perception of the stressor event (Hill, 1958; McCubbin et al., 1993; Patterson, 1993). Figure 13.3 provides a schematic of the ABCX model.

Further understanding of the responses of individual families to the stress related to raising a child with a disability is provided through identifying internal and external resources available to families. Internal resources such as belief systems and external resources such as family support and parent-to-parent programs are found to mediate stress and assist in family coping. Woolfson (2004) suggested that parenting beliefs about children with disabilities could also have strong implications for family interactions and the behavior of students with disabilities in school. Kerr and McIntosh (2000) interviewed the parents of children born with limb deficiencies and concluded that parents of children with special needs are uniquely qualified to help each other. Ferguson (2002) identified key points from research on family adaptation to raising a child with a disability, including 1)

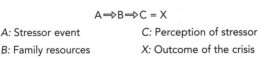

Figure 13.3. The ABCX model. (*Sources:* Hill, 1958; McCubbin, Thompson, Thompson, & McCubbin, 1993.)

patterns of overall adjustment and well-being are similar across groups of families with and without children with disabilities, although there are some differences over the family life course; 2) significant numbers of parents of children with disabilities report numerous benefits and positive outcomes including coping skills (adaptability), family harmony (cohesiveness), spiritual growth or shared values, shared parenting roles, and communication; and 3) having a child with a disability is stressful, although some families are more resilient than others in adapting to stress. Ferguson concluded from research that the factors such as level of disability (severe versus mild) or family structure (single parent versus a two-parent household) may not be as critical as other factors such as the presence/absence of self-injurious behaviors, challenging behaviors, and family income.

Positive outcomes and the negative factors contribute to family adaptation to children with disabilities. Understanding family responses to stress and internal and external resources available to families is linked to developing family support programs in an effort to mediate stress. For example, family support programs offered at schools contribute to how well a family copes with the financial stresses that can be associated with students having AAC needs. It is important for practitioners to recognize family resilience to adapt positively to the stress of having a student with AAC needs. When life cycle issues create increased family stress, external resources from the school can support the family. School supports, when provided at the appropriate time, can facilitate family coping and adaptation to increased stress (Ferguson, 2002).

Although many families successfully cope and adapt to their children with AAC needs, it is important for school practitioners to remain cognizant that families may need support due to increased stress related to having a child with AAC needs. Research findings emphasized the diverse roles of parents as caregivers, advocates, and communication partners for their children. For example, Jones et al. (1998) found in survey research of 59 parents of children ages 3–12 years who used AT and AAC services that both mothers and fathers experienced stress and used external resources differently. Fathers reported they were significantly stressed by their children's moodiness, whereas mothers were significantly stressed by their own depression and relationship with their spouse. Furthermore, mothers reported that they were more likely to rely on their own parents and other professionals for support with their children, whereas fathers relied on their spouses and the parents of their spouses for support. In an ethnographic study by Goldbart and Marshall (2004), parents of children ages 3–11 years with AAC needs reported that they felt "burdened" by their child's AAC needs and found that their capacity to engage in AAC support fluctuated over time. Goldbart and Marshall concluded that school professionals need to be aware of the diversity of families and their varied abilities and resources to support their children in AAC services.

In conclusion, it is incumbent on professionals to put forth the effort needed to understand family perspectives, needs, and competing demands related to caring for students with complex communication needs. Collaborative teaming can be achieved through sensitivity, respectfulness, and acknowledging the family and the expertise that they can provide to practitioners.

Family Cultural and Linguistic Diversity Issues   Professional sensitivity, respect, and acknowledgment for families extend beyond disability to encompass issues of family cultural and linguistic diversity (Parette, VanBiervliet, & Hourcade, 2000). Professionals must take into account and understand how a family's cultural, ethnic, and/or socioeconomic background may affect decision making about using AT with school-age children. Goode (2005) reviewed a number of studies addressing AT and diversity issues and found differences in reaction to AAC and AT across cultures. For example, many Native American and Asian families are reported to value and expect a certain degree of family dependence across family members (Hourcade et al., 1997). In these cultures, the use of AAC and AT to increase independence may not be considered important. AAC devices and AT that draw attention to a child's disability in public places may not be acceptable to families (Parette, VanBiervliet, & Hourcade, 2000). Families from low socioeconomic backgrounds often have pressing concerns about basic needs such as health care, food, work, and transportation. These fundamental needs make it difficult for families from low socioeconomic backgrounds to participate in evaluations and training sessions (Kemp & Parette, 2000). School practitioners must be aware of, sensitive to, and nonjudgmental of cultural, ethnic, and socioeconomic differences.

Decision making regarding AAC systems for school-age children with cultural and linguistic differences must be culturally sensitive to be effective. Parette, Brotherson, and Huer (2000) encouraged the school practitioner to ask a variety of questions when designing a culturally sensitive AT assessment that address the areas of assessment design, professional collaboration, cultural issues, values, family factors, acculturation, ethnicity, social influences, past experiences, and developmental expectations. Furthermore, Hourcade et al. (1997) alerted the school practitioner to be culturally sensitive in the AT/AAC assessment process. Guidelines from the work of these researchers are adapted and summarized in Figure 13.4 and may be useful for administrators and school personnel to consider in developing culturally responsive services in the area of AAC.

Huer and Saenz (2002) reported that there is a scarcity of evidence-based research in the area of AAC services that is relevant to culturally diverse populations and, more specifically, little evidence to support current clinical and educational practices. In order to open a dialogue with researchers who are interested in pursuing culturally sensitive AAC research, Huer and Saenz described a formula, initially introduced by Bevan-Brown (2001), for obtaining accurate research data when working with ethnically diverse groups. Bevan-Brown's six *R*'s formula states that the *right*

Self-assessment

1. How aware am I of my own cultural background, experiences, values, and beliefs?
2. How do my experiences, values, and beliefs affect my interactions with people from various cultures?
3. What is my comfort and experience level with the cultural communities that I serve through the provision of assistive technology (AT)/AAC?
4. Am I flexible when meeting with family members?
5. Do I provide necessary assistance to the family members to ensure their participation in the AT/AAC process?

Cultural knowledge

1. Do I understand the family's attitude regarding disabilities?
2. Do I know who the key decision maker of the family is?
3. Do I understand the family's expectations of me as a professional?
4. Do I understand the importance of extended family?
5. Am I aware of the family's approach to discipline?
6. Do I understand the responsibilities of other siblings in the family setting?

Culturally responsive AT/AAC services

1. Am I aware of what the family expects of me in the AT assessment process?
2. Have I determined whether the family is willing to receive formal AT/AAC services?
3. Does the family accept the idea of AT as a tool to help their child?
4. Does the family's religious affiliation influence their willingness to participate or how they perceive the AT process?
5. Is it possible to meet with the family members in their home prior to the AT assessment?
6. Do I provide information and printed materials related to the AT/AAC assessment process in language spoken by the family?
7. Have I determined whether a community liaison would be the most appropriate contact through which to provide information to or receive information from the family?
8. Have I always made translators available to maintain communication with family members?

Figure 13.4. Discussion guide: Culturally responsive services in augmentative and alternative communication (AAC). (*Sources:* Hourcade, Parette, & Huer, 1997; Parette, 1998.)

person must ask the *right questions* of the *right people* in the *right way* at the *right place* and *right time*. This formula can also be applied to practitioners working with students who use AAC and AT to increase cultural sensitivity when interviewing families. Ideally, people from the family's cultural background should conduct interviews with the family. The right questions to be asked must take into account cultural beliefs about disabilities, cultural values and experiences regarding amounts of independence desired by families, and language familiarity and the amount of information conveyed when translating information. Professional efforts toward mindfulness of family culture during family interviews will greatly facilitate family–professional collaboration and the successful implementation of AAC systems into school and home practices.

In order to build collaborative relationships and partnerships with parents from culturally diverse backgrounds, practitioners must meet two main goals: 1) prevent and break down barriers that may discourage families from becoming involved in using their child's AAC systems, and 2) encourage culturally diverse parents to participate by meeting their need for support and comfortable involvement in their child's successful AAC use at home and in the classroom. Matuszny et al. (2007) described a progressive plan to develop such collaborative relationships that includes parents in the collaborative relationship over time. The progressive plan is best implemented in four phases (see Figure 13.5), which correspond to parts of the school year and include activities intended to establish and enhance parent–professional collaborative relationships. Use of a four-phase plan can help eliminate and prevent barriers to the involvement of culturally diverse families in the special education process. Although the process can be time consuming to implement, the benefits for establishing culturally responsive collaboration with families can be seen to outweigh the efforts involved.

Family Readiness for AAC   Once collaborative and culturally responsive relationships exist between school professionals and families, family readiness for AAC is greatly enhanced, including ability to accept and implement technology in daily settings for communication and learning. Parent and family involvement in AAC intervention programs is desirable, if not essential, for

---

Phase 1: Initiation
Schedule an informal event for school staff and parents to become acquainted prior to the school year.

Phase 2: Building the foundation
Develop a survey for parents to complete regarding preferences and needs for their child.

In the first weeks of school, invite families to the classroom to share basic information regarding family background and culture.

Provide basic information on the classroom or school rules, behavior procedures, and classroom setup as related to the student.

Phase 3: Maintenance and support
Provide continued opportunities for the family to visit the classroom to maintain, support, and continue strengthening the relationship.

Provide information as the parents need it while maintaining informational equity with the family regarding the child's needs and progress.

Use interpreters as needed and share both positive and negative events.

Phase 4: Wrap up and reflection
Repeat the plan with scheduled parent events and visits each year until the student graduates.

Meet with parents to discuss their experiences working with the augmentative and alternative communication (AAC) team.

Complete a collaboration review and reflection worksheet to assist parents to identify what worked, what did not work, and what must be added during subsequent years.

Figure 13.5.   Building collaborative parent–professional relationships. (*Source:* Matuszny, Banda, & Coleman, 2007.)

Table 13.3. Parent perceptions about augmentative and alternative communication (AAC) and assistive technology (AT) needs for their children

Children ages 3–12	Children ages 13–21
1. Learn about AAC devices	1. Learn about AAC devices
2. Plan for future	2. Plan for future
3. Integrate AAC and AT into community settings	3. Integrate AAC and AT into community settings
4. Gain access to computer use	4. Gain access to computer use
5. Find professional support	5. Provide social interactions for their children and other students who use AAC and peers without disabilities
6. Locate volunteers to work with their children	6. Learn programming
7. Obtain funding	7. Learn how to maintain AAC and AT technology
8. Obtain advocacy	

Sources: Angelo & Jones (1991); Angelo, Jones, & Kokoska (1995).

enhancing family readiness and encouraging families to accept and implement technology at home (Angelo et al., 1995). Based on survey research completed in two separate studies with parents of children ages 3–12 years and ages 13–21 years, Angelo and Jones (1991) and Angelo et al. (1996) found both similarities and differences regarding parents' perspectives. Parents of both groups reported their need to learn about AAC devices and plan for the future of their children, to integrate AT and AAC in community settings, and to gain access to computer use. Parents of younger children expressed needs that focused on finding professional support, volunteers to work with their children, funding, and advocacy. Parents of older children emphasized the need for social interaction between other students who use AAC and peers without disabilities and programming and maintaining technology. The importance of professional understanding related to parents' perceptions and use of AAC at differing points in the child's age is critical to respond more precisely to parents' needs and to maintain optimal parent–professional collaboration. Table 13.3 summarizes parent perceptions regarding AAC and AT needs.

A review of the literature by Parette and Angelo (1996) further supported the need for considering family issues prior to the prescription of AAC for children with disabilities. The literature review suggested that failure to consider family issues may contribute to increased family stress and failure of children and families to use AAC devices. Because the family is a system, the events or interventions with one family member is likely to affect the others (Bronfenbrenner, 1979, 1986; Dunst, Trivette, & Deal, 1988, 1994). Thus, from a family perspective, family members can positively or negatively influence the course of AAC intervention, and family acceptance of AAC devices is an important variable in predicting positive outcomes. Noncompliance with AAC intervention often signals a failure to understand family dynamics as well as the needs, preferences, and priorities of family members. The importance of family in all aspects of intervention must be recognized and supported in service delivery approaches. Collaborative teaming creates family readiness for AT and AAC if family values, routines, needs, and resources are collectively considered during the AAC assessment process. When team collaboration with family members is implemented, service plans will be more effective, and device abandonment will occur less frequently.

Supporting Family Participation in Collaborative AAC Services   Collaborative teaming is an ongoing process. Although families may initially accept and participate in the AT and AAC service delivery plan, effective strategies must be implemented to support continued family participation on AAC teams. As mentioned previously, the UPS process provides an example of how to successfully support family participation on AAC teams (Hunt et al., 2001; Hunt et al., 2004; Hunt et al., 2002):

- Schedule monthly meetings at times convenient for parent attendance
- Collaboratively develop supports to increase students' academic and social participation in educational instruction activities
- Maintain an accountability system
- Maintain flexibility to change ineffectual student supports

Team members can incorporate family perspectives in decision making to build on strengths and eliminate weaknesses in the collaborative teaming process. Bailey et al. (2006) examined families' perceptions of the management and use of AAC devices at home and in junior and high school settings for youth with moderate to severe disabilities. In six case studies with families of students who use AAC, family members reported they were involved from the start of the assessment process and therefore felt like part of the team. All participants reported that school professionals had offered information and training, yet some families reported a preference for more extensive information. Areas identified as needing improvement included 1) increased involvement of manufacturers' representatives as integral partners in technology support, 2) continued availability of technical support once the children became more proficient with the device, 3) continued demonstration of professional knowledge about AAC devices as was portrayed in initial team meetings, and 4) more time for training and collaboration between families and professionals. Reported parental expectations included increased independence, communicative competence, and communicative opportunities. Many families expressed gratitude about the support received by the AAC team and recognized the necessity of time for collaboration with professionals.

Much of the stress reported by families was related to the amount of time required to program AAC devices, as several participants reported that the large amount of time they spent programming was due to a lack of training or proficiency with the AAC device. All participants reported benefits of AAC devices for children to include 1) increased number of communication partners, 2) improved degree of independence, and 3) expanded integration of the device in home and community settings. Barriers included technical limitations of the AAC device, such as portability and dependability, inadequate training, and ineffective teaming.

The most effective way to reduce these barriers is to foster open and ongoing communication with families. The previous family perceptions provide important information to school practitioners about how to improve collaborative teaming processes to more fully integrate use of AAC devices from school to home settings. Family perceptions about how to improve partnerships with families across the school to home setting include the following (Bailey et al., 2006):

- Manufacturers' representatives should be integral partners in technology support
- Technical support should remain available once children become proficient with the device
- Professionals should demonstrate knowledge about AAC devices
- More time is needed for training and collaboration between families and professionals in the area of device use and device integration between school and home

Training Opportunities for Families   Families repeatedly report that they desire additional training opportunities to address the use of AAC in school and home settings (Bailey et al., 2006). As stated previously, legal requirements for family information and training have been established within the IEP process. Team members and family members are required to jointly plan the student's IEP, which includes AT and AAC services. Because families are key members of the team, family input is required in the IEP, and requests for family information and training for AT and AAC are to be listed in the IEP as "AT services" (Best et al., 2005; Family Center on Technology Disability [FCTD], 2005). Figure 13.6 provides a checklist for families to use during IEP team meetings to ensure that the team has considered their child's AT needs from the family's perspective and has

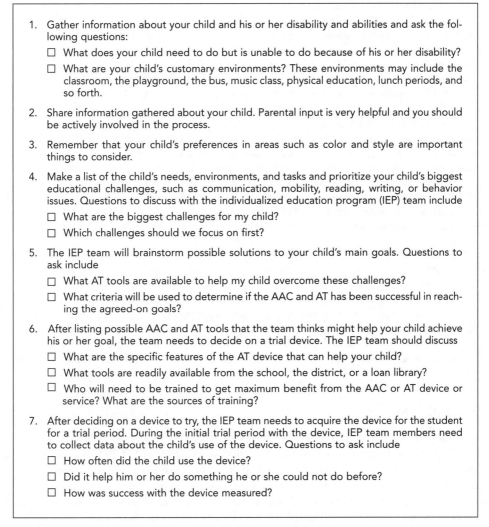

1. Gather information about your child and his or her disability and abilities and ask the following questions:
   ☐ What does your child need to do but is unable to do because of his or her disability?
   ☐ What are your child's customary environments? These environments may include the classroom, the playground, the bus, music class, physical education, lunch periods, and so forth.

2. Share information gathered about your child. Parental input is very helpful and you should be actively involved in the process.

3. Remember that your child's preferences in areas such as color and style are important things to consider.

4. Make a list of the child's needs, environments, and tasks and prioritize your child's biggest educational challenges, such as communication, mobility, reading, writing, or behavior issues. Questions to discuss with the individualized education program (IEP) team include
   ☐ What are the biggest challenges for my child?
   ☐ Which challenges should we focus on first?

5. The IEP team will brainstorm possible solutions to your child's main goals. Questions to ask include
   ☐ What AT tools are available to help my child overcome these challenges?
   ☐ What criteria will be used to determine if the AAC and AT has been successful in reaching the agreed-on goals?

6. After listing possible AAC and AT tools that the team thinks might help your child achieve his or her goal, the team needs to decide on a trial device. The IEP team should discuss
   ☐ What are the specific features of the AT device that can help your child?
   ☐ What tools are readily available from the school, the district, or a loan library?
   ☐ Who will need to be trained to get maximum benefit from the AAC or AT device or service? What are the sources of training?

7. After deciding on a device to try, the IEP team needs to acquire the device for the student for a trial period. During the initial trial period with the device, IEP team members need to collect data about the child's use of the device. Questions to ask include
   ☐ How often did the child use the device?
   ☐ Did it help him or her do something he or she could not do before?
   ☐ How was success with the device measured?

Figure 13.6. Family checklist: Considerations for child's augmentative and alternative communication (AAC) and assistive technology (AT) needs during the individualized education program (IEP) meeting. (*Source:* Family Center on Technology and Disability, 2005.)

included family requests for information and training regarding their child's AT and AAC. Item six on the checklist specifically addresses who will need to be trained to get maximum benefit from AAC and AT services.

Providing appropriate information, training, and related supports is integral to family acceptance of AAC and subsequent use of AAC in the home setting (Parette, VanBiervliet, & Hourcade, 2000). Parette and colleagues reported that families identified needs for AAC information regarding the range of devices available, features of devices, maintenance requirements, cost, funding, teaming issues, and training. Of particular importance to many families was the need for training and information that is accessible and user friendly. Rather than receiving information via lectures, workshops, and handouts, families preferred to receive information and training from family members who already have experience with a particular type of AAC and AT. Finally, families often requested ongoing supports such as demonstrations or technical assistance while they are attempting to implement the training and information received.

The Rosario family is a Latino family from Guatemala newly immigrated to the United States. Eduardo is 8 years old and demonstrates complex communication needs as a result of multiple physical, health, and intellectual disabilities. His speech is unintelligible, and he uses multimodality means to communicate including vocalizing, pointing, gesturing, head shaking, and signing. He signs 20 words idiosyncratically. Family members include Mr. Rosario, a physician who is not licensed to practice medicine in the United States; Mrs. Rosario, a homemaker; and four siblings who demonstrate typical development. Mr. Rosario has had difficulty finding adequate income for his family of five children. Spanish is written and spoken in the home.

The school AAC team meets to collaboratively begin the assessment process. Prior to meeting with the Rosario family, the team brainstorms about how to fully include Mr. and Mrs. Rosario in the assessment process. The team determines that a translator is needed, information must be provided in written form and orally in Spanish, and referrals are needed for agencies to provide information about financial support for insurance, groceries, rent assistance, immigration support, and other areas. The team further determines that following input from the Rosarios about their needs, wants, and priorities for Eduardo's communication, a simple bilingual picture-based communication system can be developed prior to obtaining higher technology devices.

The school AAC team addresses the concerns about the initial visit with the family by contacting a community center to provide the school with a cultural education team knowledgeable in Guatemalan culture; linking the Rosario family to other families who are Spanish speaking for peer support; establishing translation services for the initial parent meeting at school; providing an initial home visit with the teachers and parents to identify priorities for communication; and translating the assessment tools, results, and plans for intervention. As a result of the team collaboration efforts, the Rosario family feels as if they are equal members of the assessment process and are comfortable providing the professional team with information about Eduardo's and the family's needs.

CONCLUSION

The implications for applying collaborative team practice and support for families and individuals with AAC needs are broad and challenging. Several areas were reviewed and discussed in this chapter, including practical clinical and educational applications, considerations for participation in the general curriculum, social interaction for those with AAC needs, involvement and integration of all team members, ethical considerations for professional practice in team settings, family involvement, and cultural adaptations to include people of diverse backgrounds and preferences in the collaborative model.

Applied practice in clinical and educational settings requires considering the realities of professional service delivery. The time constraints and personnel limitations continue to confront all school professionals as significant challenges for practice. In the AAC field, in particular, the time-intensive effort to design appropriate AAC systems is recognized. Creative applications for involving instructional assistants, volunteers, student interns, family members, and all members of the team are needed to achieve optimal support for the students with AAC needs.

Inclusion in the general education curriculum for students with AAC needs requires extensive partnership between special and general educators. Toward that end, goals to support collaborative teaching and learning at all levels are needed. Student–student collaboration can be designed and implemented in cooperative learning models. The support for collaboration centered around the needs of individual students and their need to gain access to the general curriculum requires a common focus from the administration, the classroom team, and family members. Regular communication and teamwork to achieve a coordinated curriculum appears to be a critical area for personnel and material resources.

The application of AAC support outside of the classroom setting may present the most significant challenge for the collaborative team. Social interaction between peers and community members is not a structured learning setting and, thus, outside of the control of educational planning.

Coordination of volunteer efforts such as peer mentors and after-school activities is needed to achieve opportunities for social communication for students with AAC needs. Angelo and Jones (1991) identified family preferences for support to integrate AAC applications in community settings. The focus on application of AAC support outside of classroom settings may emerge as a critical setting to support transition from school to future settings.

Involving and integrating a broad and diverse membership on the AAC collaborative team is needed to provide adequate support for all communication partners and students with AAC needs. The Social Networks approach provides an opportunity to gather perspectives of professional, family, and community membership around the individual with AAC needs (Blackstone & Hunt Berg, 2003). The process of seeking assessment input from key members in an individual's life may serve to integrate significant members on the team and to help the these members gain recognition.

The implementation of AAC services in a collaborative team model implies that training and role sharing will and should occur. The roles of specialized professionals with specific qualifications to conduct assessment and design for AAC systems may often overlap with assessment information from family and community sources. The relationships between professionals, family members, and individuals with AAC needs are part of the collaborative decision-making process and result in effective practice to support communication in multiple environments. Professional responsibility, however, is ethically driven and requires careful analysis and diligence in home, school, and community settings.

In conclusion, processes for effective team development were discussed, and considerations to involve family members of diverse needs and cultural backgrounds were considered. Research informs the practice for collaborative team development and operation in school settings. The research to date outlines many challenges for school-based services given personnel shortages, training needs, and resource limitations. Guidelines for recommended practice provide a beacon to focus our best efforts and to find creative collaborations across classrooms, schools, agencies, communities, and cultures.

REFERENCES

Alant, E. (1999). Students with little or no functional speech in schools for students with severe mental retardation in South Africa. *Augmentative and Alternative Communication, 15,* 83–94.

American Speech-Language-Hearing Association. (2002a). *A workload analysis approach for establishing speech-language caseload standards in the school: Position statement.* Available at http://www.asha.org/policy

American Speech-Language-Hearing Association. (2002b). *A workload analysis approach for establishing speech-language caseload standards in the school: Technical report.* Available at http://www.asha.org/policy

American Speech-Language-Hearing Association. (2005). *Membership and certification handbook of the American-Speech-Language-Hearing Association for speech-language pathology–Effective January 1, 2005.* Retrieved on March 9, 2008, from http://www.asha.org/about/membership-certification/handbooks/slp/slp_standards.htm#Standard%20III:%20Program%20of%20Study%20%E2%80%93%20Knowledge%20Outcomes

American Speech-Language-Hearing Association. (2006). *2006 Schools Survey report: Caseload characteristics.* Rockville, MD: Author. Retrieved on August 7, 2008, from http://www.asha.org/NR/rdonlyres/22D66325-4CE6-460D-8D61-9E0388219EC3/0/SchoolsSurveyCaseloads.pdf

Angelo, D.H. (2000). Impact of augmentative and alternative communication devices on families. *Augmentative and Alternative Communication, 16,* 37–47.

Angelo, D.H., & Jones, S.D. (1991). *Assistive Device Technology Needs Scale.* Bloomsburg, PA: Bloomsburg University.

Angelo, D.H., Jones, S.D., & Kokoska, S.M. (1995). Family perspectives on augmentative and alternative communication: Families of young children. *Augmentative and Alternative Communication, 11,* 193–202.

Angelo, D.H., Kokoska, S.M., & Jones, S.D. (1996). Family perspectives on augmentative and alternative communication: Families of adolescents and young adults. *Augmentative and Alternative Communication, 12,* 13–22.

Assistive Technology Act of 1998, PL 105-394, 29 U.S.C. §§ 3001 *et seq.*

Bailey, R.L., Parette, H.P., Stoner, J.B., Angell, M.E., & Carroll, K. (2006). Family members' perceptions of augmentative and alternative communication device use. *Language, Speech, and Hearing Services in Schools, 37,* 50–60.

Balandin, S., & Iacono, T. (1998). AAC and Australian speech pathologists: Report on a national survey. *Augmentative and Alternative Communication, 14,* 239–249.

Best, S.J., Heller, K.W., & Bigge, J.L. (2005). *Teaching individuals with physical or multiple disabilities* (5th ed.). Upper Saddle River, NJ: Pearson Merrill Prentice Hall.

Beukelman, D.R., Burke, R., Ball, L., & Horn, C.A. (2002). Augmentative and alternative communication technology learning part 2: Preprofessional students. *Augmentative and Alternative Communication, 18,* 250–254.

Beukelman, D.R., Hanson, E., Hiatt, E., Fager, S., & Bilyeu, D. (2005). AAC technology learning part 3: Regular AAC team members. *Augmentative and Alternative Communication, 21,* 187–194.

Beukelman, D.R., & Mirenda, P. (1988). *Augmentative and alternative communication: Supporting children and adults with complex communication needs.* Baltimore: Paul H. Brookes Publishing Co.

Beukelman, D.R., & Mirenda, P. (2005). *Augmentative and alternative communication: Supporting children and adults with complex communication needs* (3rd ed.). Baltimore: Paul H. Brookes Publishing Co.

Bevan-Brown, J. (2001). Evaluating special education services for learners from ethnically diverse groups: Getting it right. *Journal of The Association for Persons with Severe Handicaps, 26,* 138–147.

Blackstone, S.W., & Hunt Berg, M. (2003). *Social networks.* Monterey, CA: Augmentative Communications.

Bronfenbrenner, U. (1979). *The ecology of human development.* Cambridge, MA: Harvard University Press.

Bronfenbrenner, U. (1986). Ecology of the family as a context for human development research perspectives. *Developmental Psychology, 22,* 723–742.

Burd, L., Hammes, K., Bornhoeft, D., & Fisher, W. (1998). A North Dakota prevalence study of nonverbal school aged children. *Language, Speech, and Hearing Services in Schools, 19,* 371–383.

Burke, R., Beukelman, D., Ball, L., & Horn, C. (2002). Augmentative and alternative communication technology part 1: Augmentative and alternative communication specialists. *Augmentative and Alternative Communication, 18,* 242–249.

Cress, C.J., & Marvin, C.A. (2003). Common questions about AAC services in early intervention. *Augmentative and Alternative Communication, 19,* 254–272.

Dowden, P., Alarcon, N., Vollan, T., Cumley, G.D., Kuehn, C.M., & Amtmann, D. (2006). Survey of SLP caseloads in Washington state schools: Implications and strategies for action. *Language, Speech, and Hearing Services in Schools, 37,* 104–117.

Dunst, C.J., Trivette, C.M., & Deal, A.G. (1988). *Enabling and empowering families: Principles and guidelines for practice.* Brookline, MA: Brookline Books.

Dunst, C.J., Trivette, C.M., & Deal, A.G. (Eds.). (1994). *Supporting and strengthening families: Volume 1: Methods, strategies, and practices.* Brookline, MA: Brookline Books.

Edgar, D.L., & Rosa-Lugo, L.I. (2007). The critical shortage of speech-language pathologists in the public school setting: Features of the work environment that affect recruitment and retention. *Language, Speech, and Hearing Services in the Schools, 38,* 31–46.

Family Center on Technology and Disability (FCTD). (2005, February). *Family information guide to assistive technology.* Retrieved January 21, 2008, from http://www.fctd.info/resources/fig/

Ferguson, P.M. (2002). A place in the family: A historical interpretation of research on parental reactions to having a child with a disability. *Journal of Special Education, 36,* 124–130, 147.

Glennen, S.L., & DeCoste, D.C. (1997). Service delivery in AAC. In S.L. Glennen & D.C. DeCoste (Eds.), *The handbook of augmentative and alternative communication* (pp. 21–34). San Diego: Singular.

Goldbart, J., & Marshall, J. (2004). Pushes and pulls on the parents of children who use AAC. *Augmentative and Alternative Communication, 20,* 194–208.

Goode, J. (2005). *Minibiography: Assistive technology and diversity issues.* NECTEC Clearinghouse on Early Intervention & Early Childhood Special Education. Available at http://www.nectac.org/chouse/

Hill, R. (1958). Generic features of families under stress. *Social Casework, 49,* 139–150.

Hourcade, J.J., Parette, H.P., & Huer, M.B. (1997). Family and culture alert! Considerations in assistive technology assessment. *Teaching Exceptional Children, 30* (1), 40–44.

Huer, M.B. (2003). Individuals from diverse cultural and ethnic backgrounds may perceive graphic symbols differently: Response to Nigam. *Augmentative and Alternative Communication, 19,* 137–140.

Huer, M.B., & Saenz, T. (2002). Thinking about conducting culturally sensitive research in augmentative and alternative communication. *Augmentative and Alternative Communication, 18* (4), 267–273.

Hunt, P., Doering, K., Hirose-Hatae, A., Maier, J., & Goetz, L. (2001). Across-program collaboration to support students with and without disabilities in general education classrooms. *Journal for The Association for Persons with Severe Handicaps, 26,* 240–256.

Hunt, P., Soto, G., Maier, J., & Doering, K. (2003). Collaborative teaming to support students at risk and students with severe disabilities in general education classrooms. *Exceptional Children, 69,* 315–322.

Hunt, P., Soto, G., Maier, J., Liboiron, N., & Bae, S. (2004). Collaborative teaming to support preschoolers with severe disabilities who are placed in general education early childhood programs. *Topics in Early Childhood Special Education, 24* (3), 123–142.

Hunt, P., Soto, G., Maier, J., Müller, E., & Goetz, L. (2002). Collaborative teaming to support students with augmentative and alternative communication needs in general education classrooms. *Augmentative and Alternative Communication, 18,* 20–35.

Individuals with Disabilities Education Act Amendments (IDEA) of 1997, PL 105-17, 20 U.S.C. §§ 1400 *et seq.*

Individuals with Disabilities Education Act (IDEA) of 1990, PL 101-476, 20 U.S.C. §§ 1400 *et seq.*

Individuals with Disabilities Education Improvement Act (IDEA) of 2004, PL 108-446, 20 U.S.C. §§ 1400 *et seq.*

Jones, S.D., Angelo, D.H., & Kokoska, S.M. (1998). Stressors and family supports: Families with children using augmentative and alternative communication technology. *Journal of Children's Communication Development, 20,* 37–44.

Judge, S. (2002). Family-centered assistive technology assessment and intervention practices for early intervention. *Infants and Young Children, 15,* 60–68.

Kemp, C.E., & Parette, H.P. (2000). Barriers to minority family involvement in assistive technology decision-making processes. *Education and Training in Mental Retardation and Developmental Disabilities, 35* (4), 384–392.

Kerr, S.M., & McIntosh, J.B. (2000). Coping when a child has a disability: Exploring the impact of parent-to-parent support. *Child: Care, Health, and Development, 26,* 309–322.

King, J. (1998). Preliminary survey of speech-language pathologists providing AAC services in health care settings in Nebraska. *Augmentative and Alternative Communication, 14,* 222–227.

Light, J., Roberts, B., Dimarco, R., & Greiner, N. (1998). Augmentative and alternative communication to support receptive and expressive communication for people with autism. *Journal of Communication Disorders, 31,* 153–180.

Lloyd, L.L., Fuller, D.R., & Arvidson, H.H. (1997). *Augmentative and alternative communication: A handbook of principles and practices.* Boston: Allyn & Bacon.

Matas, J.A., Mathy-Laikko, P., Beukelman, D.R., & Legresley, K. (1985). Identifying the nonspeaking population: A demographic study. *Augmentative and Alternative Communication, 1,* 17–31.

Matuszny, R.M., Banda, D.R., & Coleman, T.J. (2007). A progressive plan for building collaborative relationships with parents from diverse backgrounds. *Teaching Exceptional Children, 39*(4), 24–31.

McCall, F., & Moodie, E. (1998). Training staff to support AAC users in Scotland: Current status and needs. *Augmentative and Alternative Communication, 14,* 228–238.

McCord, S., & Soto, G., (2000). Working with low-income Latino families: Issues and strategies. *Perspectives on Augmentative and Alternative Communication,* 10–12.

McCord, S., & Soto, G. (2004). Perceptions of AAC: An ethnographic investigation of Mexican-American families. *Augmentative and Alternative Communication, 20,* 209–227.

McCormick, L.P. (2003). Policies and practices. In L.P. McCormick, D. Frome Loeb, & R.L. Schiefelbusch (Eds.), *Supporting children with communication difficulties in inclusive settings: School-based language intervention* (2nd ed., pp. 155–187). Boston: Allyn & Bacon.

McCubbin, H., Thompson, E., Thompson, A., & McCubbin, M. (1993). Family schema, paradigms, and paradigm shifts: Components and processes of appraisal in family adaptation to crises. In A. Turnbull, J. Patterson, S. Behr, D. Murphy, J. Marquis, & M. Blue-Bannings (Eds.), *Cognitive coping, families, and disability* (pp. 239–255). Baltimore: Paul H. Brookes Publishing Co.

Murphy, J., Markova, I., Moodie, E., Scott, J., & Boa, S. (1995). Augmentative and alternative communication systems used by people with cerebral palsy in Scotland: A demographic survey. *Augmentative and Alternative Communication, 11,* 26–36.

National Assistive Technology Technical Assistance Partnership (NATTAP). (1997, August). *Collaborative activities of the Tech Act Projects.* Retrieved July 5, 2007, from http://www.resna.org/taproject/library/bulletins/aug97.html

National Information Center for Children with Disabilities (NICHCY). (2007). *NICHCY connections to resources on IDEA 2004.* Retrieved on July 11, 2007, from http://www.nichcy.org/resources/IDEA2004resources.asp

Nigam, R. (2003). Do individuals from diverse cultural and ethnic backgrounds perceive graphic symbols differently? *Augmentative and Alternative Communication, 19,* 135–136.

Parette, H.P. (1998). Cultural issues and family-centered assistive technology decision-making. In S.L. Judge & H.P. Parette (Eds.), *Assistive technology for young children with disabilities: A guide to family-centered services.* Brookline, MA: Brookline Books.

Parette, H.P., & Angelo, D.H. (1996). Augmentative and alternative communication impact on families: Trends and future directions. *Journal of Special Education, 30,* 77–98.

Parette, H.P., Brotherson, M.J., & Huer, M.B. (2000). Giving families a voice in augmentative and alternative communication decision-making. *Education and Training in Mental Retardation and Developmental Disabilities, 35,* 177–190.

Parette, H.P., & Dempsey Marr, D. (1997). Assisting children and families who use augmentative and alternative communication (AAC) devices: Best practices for school psychologists. *Psychology in the Schools, 34,* 337–346.

Parette, H.P., & VanBiervliet, A. (2000). *Culture, families, and augmentative and alternative communication (AAC) impact: A multimedia instructional program for related services personnel and family members.* Available at http://cstl.semo.edu/parette/homepage/research.htm

Parette, H.P., VanBiervliet, A., & Hourcade, J.J. (2000). *Family-centered decision making in assistive technology.* Retrieved February 9, 2007, from http://jset.unlv.edu/15.1/parette/first.html

Patterson, J. (1993). The role of family meanings in adaptation to chronic illness and disability. In A. Turnbull, J. Patterson, S. Behr, D. Murphy, J. Marquis, & M. Blue-Bannings (Eds.), *Cognitive coping, families, and disability* (pp. 221–238). Baltimore: Paul H. Brookes Publishing Co.

Ratcliff, A., Koul, R., & Lloyd, L. (in press). Preparation in AAC: An update for speech-language pathology training. *American Journal of Speech Language Pathology.*

Rehabilitation Act of 1973, PL 93-112, 29 U.S.C. §§ 701 *et seq.*

Sadao, K., & Robinson, N. (2007). *Handbook on developing and evaluating interagency collaboration in early childhood special education programs.* Sacramento, CA: Sacramento County Office of Education.

Salisbury, C.L., Evans, I.M., & Palombaro, M.M. (1997). Collaborative problem solving to promote the inclusion of young children with significant disabilities in primary grades. *Exceptional Children, 63,* 195–209.

Schlosser, R., McGhie-Richmond, D., Blackstien-Alder, S., Mirenda, P., Antonius, K., & Janzen, P. (2000). Training a school team to integrate technology meaningfully into the curriculum: Effects on student participation. *Journal of Special Education Technology, 15,* 31–44.

Soto, G., Müller, E., Hunt, P., & Goetz, L. (2001a). Critical issues in the inclusion of students who use augmentative and alternative communication: An educational team perspective. *Augmentative and Alternative Communication, 17*(2), 62–72.

Soto, G., Müller, E., Hunt, P., & Goetz, L. (2001b). Professional skills for serving students who use AAC in general education classrooms: A team perspective. *Language, Speech, and Hearing Services in Schools, 32*(1), 51–56.

Starble, A., Hutchins, T., Favro, M.A., Prelock, P., & Bitner, B. (2005). Family-centered intervention and satisfaction with AAC device training. *Communication Disorders Quarterly, 27,* 47–54.

Sturm, J. (1998). Educational inclusion of AAC users. In D. Beukelman & P. Mirenda (Eds.), *Augmentative and alternative communicative: Management of severe communication disorders in children and adults* (pp. 391–424). Baltimore: Paul H. Brookes Publishing Co.

Sutherland, D., Gillon, G., & Yoder, D.E. (2005). AAC use and service provision: A survey of New Zealand speech-language therapists. *Augmentative and Alternative Communication, 21,* 295–307.

Technology-Related Assistance for Individuals with Disabilities Act Amendments of 1994, PL 103-218, 29 U.S.C. §§ 2201 *et seq.*

Technology-Related Assistance for Individuals with Disabilities Act Amendments of 1998, PL 105-394, 29 U.S.C. §§ 2201 *et seq.*

Technology-Related Assistance for Individuals with Disabilities Act of 1988, PL 100-407, 29 U.S.C. §§ 2201 *et seq.*

Thousand, J., & Villa, R. (1992). Collaborative teams: A powerful tool in school restructuring. In R. Villa, J. Thousand, W. Stainback, & S. Stainback (Eds.), *Restructuring for caring and effective education: An administrative guide to creating heterogeneous schools* (pp. 73–108). Baltimore: Paul H. Brookes Publishing Co.

VanBiervliet, A., & Parette, H.P. (2002). Development and evaluation of the families, cultures and augmentative and alternative communication (AAC) multimedia program. *Disability and Rehabilitation, 24,* 131–143.

Wahl, L. (2002). *Alliance for Technology access report on the need for assistive technology expertise in education and the creation of new models.* Retrieved February 13, 2008, from http://www.ataccess.org/resources/atk12/Training_Report.pdf

Wilcox, M.J., Weintraub, H.L., & Aier, D., (2003). *Confidence in use of assistive technology by early interventionists.* Paper presented to the annual meeting of Center for Exceptional Children, Division for Early Childhood, Washington, DC. Retrieved July 25, 2008, from http://www.asu.edu/clas/tnt/home_files/r_presentations.htm

Woolfson, L. (2004). Family well-being and disabled children: A psychosocial model of disability-related child behavior proble   ms. *British Journal of Health Psychology, 9,* 1–13.

14

Consideration of Cognitive, Attentional, and Motivational Demands in the Construction and Use of Aided AAC Systems

Krista M. Wilkinson and Shannon C. Hennig

The success of aided augmentative and alternative communication (AAC) for a number of communication goals across a variety of populations of children with communication support needs is now documented by an extensive empirical literature base. Some of the evidence-based benefits of aided AAC include (but are not limited to) enhancing early communication in individuals with severe disabilities (Cosbey & Johnston, 2006; Romski & Sevcik, 1996), providing a bridge to more advanced linguistic functioning (Adamson, Romski, Deffebach, & Sevcik, 1992; Binger & Light, 2007; Romski & Sevcik, 1996; Sturm & Clendon, 2004; Wilkinson, Romski, & Sevcik, 1994), introducing early literacy experiences (Fallon, Light, McNaughton, Drager, & Hammer, 2004), and offering an alternative to challenging behavior (e.g., Bopp, Brown, & Mirenda, 2004; Durand, 1993; Hetzroni & Roth, 2003; see Mirenda, 1997, or Reichle & Wacker, 1993, for reviews).

Given the well-established evidence supporting the efficacy of aided intervention for children with disabilities, the next step is to determine how best to adapt these aided AAC interventions to diverse skills and challenges; preferences; and individual, family, and community considerations brought by each individual with complex communication needs. This approach is consistent with recommendations within traditional speech-based communication and language interventions. In aided AAC, one of the important considerations is the physical structure of the aided display. Unlike spoken communication, aided AAC requires an external physical display or device. Careful construction of this physical aid is critical to maximizing its utility for each individual who will be using it. This chapter discusses strategies for constructing and subsequently using aided AAC systems within the context of school-based communication.

A number of child-based factors influencing communication outcomes in AAC have been delineated in the literature. For instance, level of receptive language appears to be critical in predicting whether children will show fairly rapid and extensive aided communication development (e.g., Romski & Sevcik, 1993, 1996), and preserved visual acuity can influence the learning that occurs (cf. Utley, 2002). Because these child-based factors in learning are covered elsewhere in this book (see Chapters 2 and 3), the discussion is focused on external structural supports of aided AAC systems. The discussion is restricted to visual modes of aided communication. Although the issues of auditory symbols and unaided visual symbols (i.e., signed languages) are equally important, these issues are also equally complex and, in some cases, different from those of visual symbols. Such complex issues are far beyond the scope of a single chapter.

Our discussion is grounded in a basic principle of language intervention in general. As Paul put it, "The goal of our intervention is not only to teach language behaviors but also to make the child a better communicator" (2007, p. 65). With regard to aided AAC, this means not only teaching children to point to symbols but also structuring the aid so children can communicate about topics of interest to them, using the words and voices they would choose for the functions they seek (not the topics, words, or functions the educators, parents, or practitioners might want to hear). We also want to put into place the supports for long-term goals, such as narrative, literacy, or argumentation skills, that will help children advance beyond their current level of functioning. This sounds fairly obvious, but in practice, many systems designed for children do not adhere to this principle; rather, they often reflect adult perspectives, vocabulary words, and reasoning (cf. Light, Drager, & Nemser, 2004).

This chapter begins with a discussion of some of the literature concerning memory and attention that might be relevant to constructing and using aided displays. Then, the chapter examines the unique demands placed by visual-graphic modes of communication and outlines how different kinds of symbols, layouts, and access methods challenge or enhance learners' cognitive, attentional, and memory resources. On the assumption that systematically well-constructed aids lower cognitive demands and enhance users' attention, which, in turn, contribute to better functional communication outcomes, practical suggestions for aid construction are offered. Finally, the cognitive and attentional aspects of naturalistic aided interventions are considered.

ASPECTS OF MEMORY AND ATTENTION RELATED TO AIDED AAC

Among the most unique characteristics of aided AAC is its reliance on a physical visual aid to store and present symbols. This feature presents specific challenges to memory and attention, relative to spoken modes. Perhaps most critical is that even on dynamic displays, aided visual symbols are static or fixed in place during the time they are being displayed; that is, the symbols within a presented array remain in sight even when not being produced by the user or a partner (until the display is removed, the page is turned, or the device turned off). In this way, aided symbols differ from speech, in which the signal is physically present only at the time that it is actually being spoken (cf. Sevcik, Romski, & Wilkinson, 1991). When the vocabulary is more extensive than can be presented in a single array, however, then at least some of the symbols must necessarily be stored "out of sight" on fixed or dynamic display pages that must be actually or virtually located and retrieved for use when necessary.

These characteristics of aided symbols present some challenges that relate to principles of memory and attention from the area of cognitive science. We therefore turn to a general introduction of some basic principles of memory and attention, identifying how they may relate to the task of aided communication. General discussions of many of the attention and memory concepts described in this section can be found in textbooks of cognitive psychology (e.g., Anderson, 2005; Benjafield, 2007).

Recognition versus Recall Memory for Symbol Identification and Retrieval

Because aided symbols are fixed on the display, they offer the user an explicit cue for use. Wilkinson and McIlvane (2002) noted that the presence of a cue allows users of aided AAC to rely on *recognition* memory as compared with *recall* memory. Recall is required when asked the question, "What is the capital of Florida?" and is most typically the type of memory involved when generating spontaneous, nonread spoken language (i.e., when the word, phrase, or sentence to be generated has not been presented immediately prior to production). Recognition memory is tapped when the question, "Is Tallahassee or Atlanta the capital of Florida?" (both cities are capital cities; an alternate could be two cities in Florida). When an individual who relies on AAC is presented with an array of symbols from which to select, the task is often one of recognition (i.e., finding the symbol that matches a referent or concept). An example of these differences is illustrated in Figure 14.1.

Research in cognitive psychology has documented that respondents tend to perform more accurately under recognition tasks than recall tasks (Hamilton & Ghatala, 1994). This has been

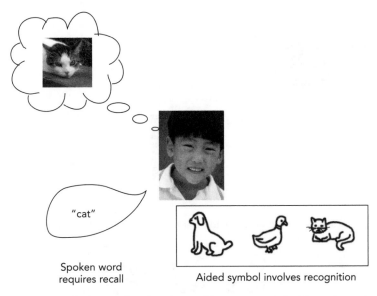

Spoken word
requires recall   Aided symbol involves recognition

Figure 14.1. Illustration of recall and recognition memory recruited by spoken and aided modes (respectively).

observed across individuals of different ages (e.g., Levin, Yussen, De Rose, & Pressley, 1977) and for individuals with some specific forms of amnesia (Kopelman et al., 2007; Volpe, Holtzman, & Hirst, 1986). Furthermore, Craik and McDowd (1998) reported that engaging in a recall task interfered more with other (secondary) task performance than did a recognition task, suggesting that recall involves greater processing demands. The static nature of aided symbols may, therefore, offer a support for lexical retrieval (via recognition) over dynamic and fleeting oral symbols.

Sustained, Selective, and Divided Attention

Although there are potential advantages to exploiting recognition memory through the concrete visual stimuli in aided displays, there are also some trade-offs in terms of attention demands. Many of the trade-offs reflect the fact that the physical display requires a user to scan through the items, at least until the geography of the entire display is committed to memory. An example of the three different forms of attention that will be discussed and how they are influenced by aided communication is presented in Figure 14.2.

Perhaps, most obviously, the scanning capacity of the user is extremely important. If the user has the capacity to scan up to 12 items, then a display of 18 items will exceed his or her capability to scan through the display during the communication event. At least some of the symbols may end up not being used, not for lack of interest on the part of the user but for lack of sufficient attentional resources. *Sustained attention* is the ability to maintain attention across time or effort during any task.

In addition to the demands on the user to sustain attention to scan through a symbol array, the physical display also requires the user to maintain attention to the target item (i.e., whichever symbol he or she starts looking for) while searching through a number of distracting and potentially appealing alternatives. This might be considered a *selective attention* task, which is the ability to focus on a relevant target (in this case, the desired symbol) and exclude attention to irrelevant distracters (Benjafield, 2007). In AAC, a user who begins a search for CAT on a page containing several animals must retain this goal in mind while potentially seeing (and inhibiting response to) DOG, DUCK, and so forth. The ability of a child to maintain selective attention to a stimulus likely

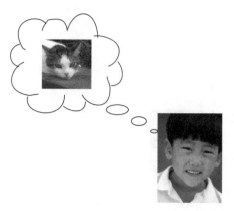

Sustained attention: ability to persist from dog, through duck, to "cat"

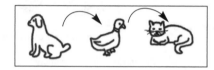

Selective attention: ability to inhibit response to other appealing symbols

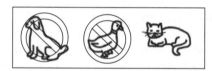

Divided attention: ability to attend to visual display, partner, and/or referent

Figure 14.2.   Illustration of sustained, selective, and divided memory demands of aided augmentative and alternative communication (AAC).

will influence how he or she interacts with a display and warrants consideration when building or using aided AAC.

Finally, in many cases, aided AAC requires the user to divide his or her attention between various ongoing events or activities. The term *divided attention* refers to the ability to attend to multiple tasks or stimuli, perhaps truly simultaneously or perhaps by rapidly switching attention between the two tasks (Benjafield, 2007). In aided communication, users must divide their attention between the display, which they must look at in order to produce a message, and their partner, to whom the message is directed. In many communication events, there are additional stimuli that the user may also have to attend to. At school, for instance, a user of AAC in a geography lesson may have to divide attention between the teacher, his or her aided display, and the map about which they are communicating. Unlike speech, the aided AAC mode requires the user to specifically look away from the other partner and/or referent (the map) while communicating.

Semantic and Episodic Memory

A distinction that has been made for many years in cognitive psychology may be important in the area of aided communication, particularly because of the introduction of using naturalistic visual scenes as methods for presenting aided symbol displays (Drager, Light, Speltz, Fallon, & Jeffries, 2003; Light, Drager, McCarthy, et al., 2004). In the past, symbol displays were either created by hand or with the assistance of technology such as symbol software programs. Because of this, a custom of organizing symbols into Cartesian grids emerged. The advent of early software options allowed people with limited graphic skills to create communication displays for students who use AAC; however, most software programs continued to present individual symbols in fixed rows and columns. Display variations were limited to border color, symbol size, background color, and spacing between symbols.

Researchers and practitioners have begun to use more contextually based, holistic scenes rather than a grid-based presentation of symbols. Visual scenes can take the form of photographs or line drawings with varying degrees of visual complexity, detail, and color. In describing the rationale for using such visual scenes with young learners, Drager and her colleagues (Drager et al., 2003; Light, Drager, McCarthy, et al., 2004) noted that young oral language learners most typically learn to communicate symbolically within a rich, contextually supported environment. Thus, discussions about cereal and milk most typically occur in the morning in the kitchen. Often, these objects are embedded into an activity such as retrieving the milk from the refrigerator or watching someone pouring a drink at the table. The child's experience of the words *cereal* and *milk* occurs in the presence of all of these other contextual cues. Drager and her colleagues argued that we should be presenting visual symbols in a similarly supportive context (e.g., presenting the symbol for MILK within a picture of a kitchen, perhaps in the context of an adult pouring a glass of milk or opening the refrigerator door). Pages designed to promote social communication within an interactive context might include people and objects in the midst of an activity (e.g., playing Peekaboo, jumping into a pool filled with friends and pool toys, cheering at a soccer game) in contrast to a more static portrait of people smiling at the camera or showing objects in an empty room.

Using visual scenes may recruit an important memory function involving the distinction between semantic and episodic memory (e.g., Benjafield, 2007, from Tulving, 1972; see Figure 14.3). *Semantic memory* refers to general knowledge or facts that we know (e.g., the capital of Florida) but have little or no personal detail associated with them—we may not have ever actually visited the capital of Florida, we likely do not remember when or where we learned it, and so forth. Most of our word knowledge, such as symbol meaning, relies on this abstracted semantic memory. *Episodic memory* refers to memories that are directly sited within personal experience and are memories of events that (most typically) involve ourselves. An episodic memory might be remembering that we have visited Tallahassee, how we got there, who we visited, and our emotional state while there.

Presenting symbols within a visual scene may exploit episodic memory as a means to cue or support the learning of the more abstracted word meaning that ultimately becomes integrated as semantic memory. It seems reasonable to suggest that the scene provides the learner with support of

"This is called a ball."   "I remember when
                                   I got this bike."

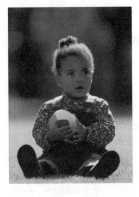   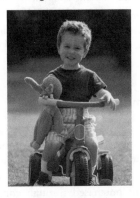

Semantic memory   Episodic memory

Figure 14.3.   Illustration of semantic versus episodic memory types.

personal experience ("I typically find milk in the kitchen") to help him or her learn the individual symbol meaning and location on the device or display (MILK, which is located on the "kitchen" page). Presenting symbols on individual spaces on a grid may not be as likely to bring in this episodic component. Thus, in this presentation, the learning of the symbol meaning (the semantic memory component) occurs without this additional cue.

AAC technologies increasingly have the capacity to accommodate scene-based displays. Yet, despite their advantages, natural or complex visual scenes place unique demands on human visual and cognitive processing and solicit different patterns of attention from viewers (cf. Wilkinson & Jagaroo, 2004). For instance, although visual scenes might provide the episodic cue to support semantic learning, it is also important to consider that they are visually more complex. For clients who are overwhelmed by the visual information in a scene, this type of presentation might reduce attention to the individual symbols by making them too difficult to find (stressing sustained and selective attention). Thus, it is important to be aware of the different supports and challenges offered by either grid or scene-based displays. It seems likely that, as with other things, it will be necessary to further develop assessment tools to determine which type of display may be best for which individuals, under a number of different circumstances.

Summary

Clearly, there are some ways in which aided modes of communication recruit potentially different forms of attention and cognition than oral-aural communication. None of these unique demands are reasons to question the use of aided AAC, given its many benefits. Nonetheless, when practitioners are aware of the unique demands and supports of aided systems, they will be best positioned to construct the most effective display for each individual.

COGNITIVE AND ATTENTIONAL DEMANDS RELATED TO SPECIFIC CLINICAL DECISIONS

In aided AAC, the physical nature of visual symbols and the way they are organized within and across pages often must be determined by practitioners, families, clients, and other stakeholders. It is incumbent on such stakeholders to select symbols and aids that support the learning of the individual child in question. Specific structural aspects of aided displays can affect how readily users find and/or attend to symbols on a display, thus potentially enhancing functional outcomes.

There are many possible avenues concerning structuring aids and interventions to minimize cognitive and attentional demands and thus free up resources for the task of communicating. For the purposes of the rest of this chapter, we have chosen just a few that are fairly fundamental issues within aided AAC. These include selecting the stimuli to be used, organizing the symbols on a grid-based display, and navigating among pages in a display. We will discuss both the typical decisions that need to be made by practitioners as well as how different decisions influence memory or attentional resources.

Selecting Stimulus Type

One of the first decisions facing a practitioner concerns what symbols would be best for a client. Two-dimensional symbols (e.g., photographs, line drawings, written words) are often a natural starting point when considering aided AAC. They are flat, thus appropriate for low-technology (paper-based) books as well as dynamic high-technology displays. They are readily created by hand or purchased through commercially available packages. Two-dimensional symbols, however, are not always the best choice. For example, special considerations emerge when working with children with low vision or severe intellectual disabilities. This section discusses the challenges and supports offered by each symbol type and considers how these factors might influence clinical decisions.

Two-Dimensional Visual Stimuli   The issue of iconicity often arises when considering visual stimuli. *Iconicity* refers to how easily the meaning of each symbol can be guessed, and it was originally believed that the symbols whose meanings were easily guessed facilitated learning and use by reducing the effort required to learn the symbol meaning. Under this logic, increasing iconicity decreased the cognitive or memory load by making the symbol meaning highly apparent. As Stephenson and Linfoot noted, however, the iconicity of any stimulus is "a characteristic determined by the observer, rather than intrinsic to the picture" (1996, p. 246). What this means is that symbols that are iconic to most adults in one community may not be iconic to adults in another community, to children, or to individuals with disabilities. This is a critically important point to keep in mind in any discussion of iconicity.

Early studies sought to examine the relative iconicity of different types of symbols, both across and within symbol sets, on the assumption that a fairly universal "hierarchy" of guessability could be determined. Indeed, studies with a variety of individuals with and without disabilities have suggested that, in general, cut-out photographs are among the most readily guessed visual stimuli, followed by non–cut-out photographs, line drawings, encoded symbols (e.g., Blissymbolics), and finally, nonguessable symbols (e.g., written words; Bloomburg, Karlan, & Lloyd, 1990; Hurlbut, Iwata, & Green, 1982; Mizuko & Reichle, 1989).

Some approaches to iconicity have begun to acknowledge that this seeming hierarchy may be more of a continuum and varies from person to person. Franklin, Mirenda, and Phillips (1996) suggested that individual symbols perceived as highly iconic for preschoolers without disabilities may be fully opaque (nonguessable) for individuals with intellectual limitations. It has also become clear that iconicity is also potentially sensitive to sociocultural experience (Huer, 2003; Nigam, 2003). Differences in experiences with symbols as representations (e.g., early experiences with picture books) may influence the relative ease with which any individual can perceive a relationship between symbols and referents (e.g., Stephenson & Linfoot, 1996). Consequently, hierarchies established within certain social, geographic, linguistic, cultural, or other communities may not be universal.

Using a continuum rather than a hierarchy is important for a number of reasons. First, individual, familial, and cultural variability is accommodated nicely within a continuum because it does not imply a standard or norm from which one might diverge. Second, a continuum allows for more flexible goal selection. A hierarchy implies that symbols that occupy the top of the hierarchy are in some way superior to those at the bottom. A continuum, in contrast, supports the choice of one type of symbol under some circumstances but another type under different circumstances. That is, a continuum allows for movement in either direction, toward either more or less iconic, depending on the communication goal.

Figure 14.4 is a simple illustration of some of the uses (and limitations) of iconicity as a factor in selecting symbols. We might opt to use highly iconic symbols because they reduce the

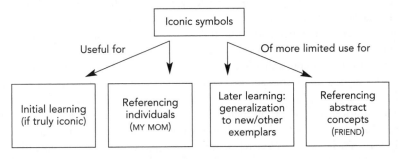

Figure 14.4.   Chart of the uses and limitations of iconicity.

cognitive/memory load on the user, thus making it easier to learn. Indeed, such choices are quite appropriate when the goal is to establish symbol meaning and use rapidly (Bloomburg et al., 1990; Hurlbut et al., 1982; Mizuko & Reichle, 1989). There are other circumstances as well in which it is both desirable and logical for a symbol to be highly specific to its referent. For example, a current photograph of a child's mother may be a more appropriate symbol for MY MOM than a general line drawing of a woman holding a baby.

There is also a trade-off of iconicity with other communication functions. Iconic symbols by their nature resemble specific examples of their referents. Thus, a highly iconic symbol for DOG might be a photograph of a specific dog, such as a large, floppy-eared golden retriever. In potentially enhancing the ability to learn, however, we may sacrifice the ease with which the label is applied to other exemplars of the category that are not quite so physically similar to the picture (e.g., a small, pointy-eared, black-and-white Pekinese). Although learning iconic symbols teaches the child to rely on physical similarity, generalizing to other exemplars requires exactly the opposite—the child must override physical similarities as soon as he or she seeks to extend word meaning past the initial exemplar.

In a similar fashion, the direct ties between iconic symbols and their referents make them difficult to use for abstract concepts. Consider the notion of a friend. I may have a friend named Claire. If I wanted to refer to this individual, then I could refer to her either as "my friend" or "Claire." Referring to her by name is a very concrete means of representing this individual. The notion of a friend, however, is more abstract because a friend cannot be defined through reference to a single individual—even if Claire happens to be my one and only friend. For these concepts, iconic symbols are poor because they cannot capture the functional or abstract aspects; that is, the picture of Claire on my aided display would have the same limitations as her actual name has in spoken language. If we seek to maximize generality of use either across exemplars or in an abstracted fashion, then the highly iconic symbols would be less desirable.

This illustrates the point that iconic symbols could be the most efficient choice in situations in which the most critical short-term goal is rapid acquisition of symbol meaning. They are also valuable components of communication when there is indeed a specific referent (e.g., a photograph of the child's actual mother). In other cases, however, broad usage of symbol meanings, across numerous exemplars, contexts, and/or communication partners may take precedence. This latter situation is particularly true as children enter into school, meet a variety of peers and teachers, and experience the diverse activities across the school day. In this case, the extra time or effort it may take to learn somewhat more opaque symbol meanings may be a worthwhile trade-off. Furthermore, as children's peers begin to enter into literacy-based academic work in the second and third grade, it may be appropriate to provide the user of AAC with literacy-based symbols (even if they function as sight words rather than generative reading) that are compatible with the symbols used by their peers.

Three-Dimensional or Tactile Stimuli   Tactile stimuli or three-dimensional stimuli can also function as aided symbols. Three-dimensional stimuli can be either miniature objects (e.g., scale versions of fast food containers, dollhouse-size furniture) or parts of objects (e.g., the flusher from a toilet, a tab from a soda can). Other tactile symbols include textures, such as sheep's wool or sandpaper, that index specific referents. These kinds of stimuli can be useful with children with significant limitations of cognitive and communication skills (e.g., Kravitz, Littman, & Cassidy, 1996; Rowland & Schweigert, 1989), assuming that three-dimensional stimuli are potentially more physically similar to their referents than flat, two-dimensional graphic stimuli. In other cases, particularly with the tactile stimuli, they are used with children who have visual impairments, allowing for alternative access.

Although intuitively it might seem that miniature objects would generally be superior to real-size object parts or tactile textures, this is not necessarily always the case. Although they do indeed look visually very much like their referents, miniature objects have several potential problems. The first two problems are practical in nature. First, for students with visual impairments, we may question the iconicity of a miniature tactile symbol (small toilet) because that miniature feels to the fingers very different from its real-size counterpart. Second, miniature objects may be less desirable to use for school-age children, particularly older ones, because they or others around them (e.g., peers) may feel that the dollhouse-sized items make the user appear juvenile.

A third problem surrounds using a miniature object as a representation of another object. Studying young children's understanding of scale models, DeLoache (1995; see also 2005) found that most 2½-year-old children had surprising difficulty understanding that miniatures or scale models could be representations (e.g., symbols) for larger objects. In the study, children observed a small Snoopy doll hidden in a miniature version of a large room and then entered the actual larger room to search for Snoopy. The majority of children younger than age 3 did not recognize that they should look for Snoopy in the same place in the larger room as he was hidden in the smaller one. No amount of verbal instruction helped, including the direct command, "Look for Snoopy in the same place in the big room as he was hidden in the little room." Interestingly, when Snoopy's location was pointed out in a photograph of the larger room, the children were easily able to locate him, demonstrating that the problem with the scale object was not due to task or memory demands. By age 3, all children could do the task readily.

DeLoache (2005) argued that the problem is one of "dual representation"—the young child cannot represent the miniature item both as an object and as a representation of something else (i.e., a symbol). Because the photograph is not an interesting object in and of itself, it served more readily as a symbol. But the scale model was too compelling as an object to also be able to serve in its second role as a symbol. Although she has not spoken directly about miniature objects in aided communication, DeLoache (2005) made reference to other functional educational implications of her work. She noted that educational materials that could be manipulated (e.g., rods or objects that represent numerics) and are designed to foster abstract conceptualization of numerosity and mathematics may not in fact do that if the child does not appreciate the representational nature of the objects. There is some limited evidence in the field of AAC that suggests that miniature objects may be more difficult for users with intellectual disabilities to select during matching tasks than some two-dimensional symbols (Mirenda & Locke, 1989). For such individuals, using part of an object (e.g., a flushing handle from an actual toilet) or a relatively iconic two-dimensional symbol (e.g., a clear photograph) might be more useful to the user than a miniature object (e.g., a dollhouse-sized toilet).

Summary and Practical Implications   The type of symbol that is most appropriate for any given individual clearly depends on a number of factors. Although iconic symbols may reduce both memory and attentional demands by making symbol meaning readily transparent, they have some limitations. Two-dimensional iconic symbols may be limited in the ways illustrated in Figure 14.4. Three-dimensional symbols that are highly iconic to adults (miniature objects) may actually introduce some cognitive demands of representation that render them less useful as symbols for some children. In both cases, the additional up-front attention or memory demands of having to learn a symbol–referent relation may be a worthwhile investment to use those items as symbols for a variety of different (generalized) referents.

Organizing Symbols on Grid-Based Displays

Symbols on an AAC device need to be organized because the vocabulary of a student who uses aided AAC is housed on a visual display that is physically external to the communicator (unlike an internalized oral vocabulary). Many children who use AAC cannot arrange their displays independently. The question is how to determine the most effective and efficient layout for any individual child. Looking to the lexical organization of speakers without disabilities is risky, not only because it is difficult to determine the semantic organization of speakers (because the vocabulary is internalized) but also because the lexical organization patterns of individuals without disabilities using speech might not necessarily be representative of the patterns of children (or adults) with communication impairments who use aided communication (cf. Fallon, Light, & Achenbach, 2003; Hux, Rankin, Beukelman, & Hahn, 1993; Wilkinson & Rosenquist, 2006).

We have already discussed some potential benefits and drawbacks of visual scene displays compared with grids. This section focuses exclusively on grid-based displays because they are more commonly used, particularly with school-age individuals.

One method to organize pages on grid-based displays is by semantic/word-class categories. It is tempting to place all the foods together, all the actions together, and so forth. There are cognitive and motor costs, however, for organizing symbols by semantic categories. Although there are exceptions, speakers most typically construct utterances by combining a variety of concepts from different categories. This pattern appears as soon as speaking children begin to combine words; early semantic relations typically include words from two different semantic or word-class categories (e.g., "Mommy go," "bye-bye car"). In aided AAC, an organization based on semantic category within a dynamic display device forces communicators to navigate between multiple pages in order to approximate the utterances produced effortlessly by their speaking peers.

It stands to reason that if page layouts are transparent in their organization to students who use AAC, it might facilitate symbol usage and thus other important functional communication outcomes. Assuming that we must exercise caution when looking at the literature on speech development and that simple semantically based organizations are cumbersome from the standpoint of communication, we must seek other methods for developing the most efficient organization strategies. Some research has examined experimental means for examining lexical organization as it relates to AAC. Two relevant studies are described that offer some strategies for examining lexical organization.

Fallon et al. (2003) asked young, typically developing children to create related displays when given a set of symbols, one by one. The results revealed how children generated relationships between symbols. Although children varied widely from one another, as well as from their own prior arrangements in the previous session, the results revealed some interesting and clinically relevant information. Children typically grouped symbols together in pairs, rather than larger symbol sets. Thus, the symbols DADDY and BOOK were placed together and separate from any others. Children also typically arranged these pairs based on thematic or event relationships between the symbols. Thus, the rationale for DADDY BOOK was, "Daddy goes next to book so he [Daddy] can read a book" (p. 79).

The idea of adding symbols one by one with the end user's input might have clinical value when programming dynamic display devices or creating communication boards. With regard to dynamic display devices, the users could coprogram the device with a teacher, peer, or family member, assisting with various decisions including selecting symbols, background color, spoken message phrasing, and locating and spacing the symbols on a given page or within the overall navigation of the device itself. With regard to communication books, the user could select symbols and place each cut-out symbol, one by one, on his or her board.

Involving the user in construction has several potential advantages. Because the user is involved in construction, it is conceivable that the process itself might have a positive effect on his or her motivation to use and locate a specific symbol. Also, vocabulary and messages are more likely to match the personality of the student who uses AAC. In addition, adding symbols one by one with the end user actively participating and observing leads to discussion regarding the rationale underlying the numerous decisions made in programming each button. This might help ensure that the programmer's logic regarding the organization of the device is not radically different from the end user's logic.

A second method that might be helpful for matching display organization to the user is offered by Wilkinson and Rosenquist (2006). These authors developed and tested a method by which users' appreciation of category relations among symbols could be assessed, which is appropriate for use with individuals with significant intellectual disabilities. The experimental protocol functioned to teach participants to select "as many" available choices from an array of three choices as they felt matched to a target sample. Thus, for instance, participants might view a picture of a golden retriever sample and then be asked to select among choices that included up to three other dogs (Doberman, Chihuahua, terrier). The procedure required participants to indicate when their selections were complete by choosing a "done" key on the computer display on which the choices were being made. Thus, participants learned two things: 1) to select between one and three related items when presented with a sample and 2) to indicate when they felt that they had selected all possible correct available choices. Participants were school-age children with intellectual and receptive vocabulary limitations. Most of the participants learned the task readily with little or no training, and a subgroup of participants who also underwent additional study demonstrated generalization to novel stimuli (birds and trees, after training on dogs and cars) and to different presentation types (auditory-visual matching, after training on visual-visual matching).

This study, although experimental in nature, offers a potential method for examining lexical organization in children, even those with significant intellectual and language limitations. The method could be used to examine whether an individual child understands relationships between items that the practitioner seeks to place on a single page. Imagine, for instance, that the practitioner would like to create a zoo theme page related to a class trip. Does the child understand right away that two physically distinct animals, such as an elephant and a zebra, could be related by virtue of both being zoo animals? Although the applied research has not yet been conducted, conceivably, the child could be presented with a phrase such as "zoo animals" and then be offered an array that contained one or more examples of such animals. The selections by the child would reveal which relations were already existing in the child's lexical structure and which might need to be taught (if we were to put them on a display).

The approach could also be adapted for older children whose goals may include more advanced academic categories, such as geography, natural history, science, and so forth. We might use Wilkinson and Rosenquist's (2006) method to assess existing knowledge about geographic regions (Is New York part of New England?). Or, adapting Fallon et al.'s (2004) approach, a student might demonstrate his or her understanding of curriculum concepts by programming key new vocabulary into his or her dynamic display device. In lieu of a worksheet, the student's homework might be to group states by geographic region. Not only would the student have demonstrated his or her understanding of which states were considered New England versus Southwest but, unlike a worksheet, the student would now have access to this vocabulary on his or her device for future use.

We will be able to match the display organization more closely to the child's own personal preferences as we learn how to assess lexical organization on an individual basis. This should reduce the attentional and memory demands in a number of ways. A child whose array is organized consistently with his or her own internal understanding should logically have a lower demand on selective and sustained attentional resources. If the array is organized to facilitate the child finding the symbol as readily as possible, then the effort of scanning through multiple distracters will be eliminated. Furthermore, such an array will also reduce memory demands because the geography of the array would likely be more readily learned and remembered. With these attentional and memory resources freed up, the child might be able to share attention when necessary (i.e., to dedicate resources to important communication tasks).

Navigation Between Display Pages

It becomes necessary to organize symbols into multiple pages as the size of the vocabulary of a student who uses aided AAC grows beyond the physical dimensions of the paper or screen. One way to do this is to create physical paper pages or overlays in actual books in which navigating consists of physically moving or turning pages. Electronic forms of this involve communication devices containing static or fixed display pages in which physical overlays are placed on the device by the user or support person. For the child with limited motor difficulties and/or attention limitations, however, turning physical pages or waiting for others to shuffle through multiple options may be challenging and frustrating.

In dynamic display devices, pages are typically presented electronically by a computer (either a dedicated communication aid or a multiuse computer), and the task of moving from display page to display page is instantaneous when the navigational link between the pages is activated. As Wilkinson and McIlvane discussed,

> Dynamic displays offer a rapid and independent means of accessing vocabulary, eliminating essential but time-consuming tasks of retaining all overlay pages in one place, locating the appropriate new overlays when a switch is needed, and removing and replacing the current overlay page. (2002, p. 282)

These advantages are substantial for individuals with limited motor skills. Dynamic displays, however, require the individual to understand the "virtual" relationship between different symbol displays. Unlike fixed displays, there is no physical entity that the user can manipulate that indicates that they have switched pages. Thus, there are no motoric or tactile cues, nor are there sounds that indicate the same thing, such as the turning of a page. Furthermore, pages are organized in a similar fashion to a web site, with pages of vocabulary linked in a potentially unlimited variety of ways. To take a very basic example, imagine there is a simple device with three pages arranged thematically—a snack page, a leisure page, and a study page. To gain access to each page, the user must have some linkage symbol that indicates to the computer that it should replace the current display page with the next. We might choose to have two such links on each page (the snack page would contain one link to leisure, another to studying, and so forth). Or, we might choose just to have one link on each page so that the user would simply travel through the links until he or she reached the desired display (thus, the link on the snack page leads to the leisure page, the link on leisure page leads to the study page, and the link on study page leads to the snack page). Or, we might have a central menu page where the links on each theme page connect to; thus, the choice of the theme page occurs only from the central menu page.

Using the links in dynamic displays is actually fairly difficult conceptually. First, there are obvious memory demands involved in remembering the pathways from one page to another. Moreover, the user must understand that the link symbol serves the navigation function, rather than a referential one. In other words, the link symbol must not only represent the page it is linked to but also the concept that it "links" to a page and is not just another communication symbol. How does one best represent this notion of linking? One might select one symbol from the destination page and use it as a "proxy;" thus, a banana might represent the destination of fruits or snacks. The obvious drawback to this method is that a child might have to select one symbol (a picture of a banana) as a navigation link, when in reality the child's intent was to discuss another symbol from that page, such as APPLE. Another drawback to this method is that most pages will consist of diverse words (a theme page, such as zoo, for instance) that are not readily captured by any single member of the page.

Alternative methods have therefore been sought. Some methods within the capacity of technology use shape, relative size, or background color to differentiate linking symbols from communication symbols. Frequently used symbols may be coded by location as well (e.g., link back to the main menu consistently placed in top right corner of each page). In recommendations available on the AAC-RERC web site, Light (n.d.) recommended using screen shots on part or all of the destination pages as the linking symbol. The thumbnail screen shot conveys that it is a linking button and solves the dilemma of how to represent which page the symbol links to. This is particularly useful if the page to be navigated to is thematic in nature, as it is not necessary to select a single symbol. Thus, for a zoo-related page, the user is not forced to choose some individual element, such as ELEPHANT or SOFT-SERVE ICE CREAM, both of which might appear on that page. Pages with many symbols will be difficult to shrink, however, without sacrificing the very visibility that is necessary for it to serve as a thumbnail. Some pages may also better lend themselves to such thumbnails (e.g., a visual scene versus a grid).

Other options include presenting several members in the category (e.g., TIGER, GIRAFFE, MONKEY), a related item (e.g., the zoo logo), or an auditory cue (e.g., the device reads the written symbol aloud when the child interacts with the symbol in some way). If a child is literate or can discriminate sight words, then one can use written labels. Perhaps, in the future, technology will permit navigation between virtual pages to make use of motion cues so that movement to the school page could be accomplished by a school bus appearing to drive down a virtual road (e.g., Jagaroo & Wilkinson, 2008).

Navigation in either type of display requires certain memory skills on the part of the user. The student who uses AAC must remember that the symbols, even those hidden from view, exist within the aided system. Users also must remember either the actual page or the pathway to reach a given symbol in order to navigate to it successfully. For instance, if all pages appear as links on every page display, then the user must simply find the desired next page. When the vocabulary is housed on more than just a few pages, however, this becomes impossible. If there are 10 different display pages and only 20 spots on the display, then half of the vocabulary spots would be taken by these links or navigation symbols. In that event, some organization through a centralized menu page becomes more appealing.

The trade-off in this case, however, is that as soon as we insert intervening pages, we introduce the potential for interference. How many times have we lost our own train of thought during a sentence simply because we heard someone else talking or our eye landed on some unrelated written word that threw us off? In a similar fashion, a child navigating through a display with a certain symbol page in mind might be distracted by the intervening symbols. Although this would never be a reason to not use such a device with any given child, we would want to keep this in mind when choosing or structuring dynamic displays that have this potential, particularly for children with difficulty sustaining attention.

The nearly infinite linking possibilities provided by dynamic display devices create memory challenges for programmers as well. As the number of pages within a device increases, it becomes increasingly difficult to remember the pages and how they link together. Students who use AAC and are developing the ability to organize the pages on their devices often are faced with the task of matching numerous file names to the visual memory of the pages they use on a daily basis. Using thumbnails could be one potential tool to address this challenge. Visual solutions may also need to be incorporated into dynamic display devices to present the internal structure of how the files link to each other in a user-friendly manner. The graphic, branching outlines created with mind-mapping software (e.g., Freemind, Inspiration) might be one source of inspiration to tackle this challenge.

Practitioners may also need to support a student who is capable of using the vocabulary in his or her device, but only if assistance is provided to cope with the navigational demands of the device. The student may require a partner to prompt him or her through the navigational steps (e.g., "First click FUN THINGS, then find BOOKS. Okay, which book do you want to read?") in order to locate a page he or she can independently use for communication. At other times, the situation may demand that a support person quickly navigate to the specific page for the student who uses AAC. For example, if the teacher asks a question that is likely to be answered quickly by a speaking peer, then a support person can intervene to enable the student who uses AAC to find the page with the vocabulary that is needed to answer the question.

In situations with semipredictable vocabulary demands, a series of pages might be programmed so that a selection on one page speaks a message before automatically linking to the next page. This eliminates the need to understand, locate, and activate a linking symbol and allows a user to participate in specific conversational scripts. For example, a telephone script could be segmented into a series of pages. The first page might have a single symbol with the message, HI, THIS IS MARK. When Mark activates this message, the device first speaks the message, then automatically links to a second page with photos of 10 friends. Mark might then select John's photograph to ask, "IS JOHN THERE?", at which point the device automatically links to a topic board with the vocabulary needed to converse with John. Thus, if this student has difficulty with navigation in general or only during demanding and time-sensitive communication situations such as making a telephone call, then he could still successfully meet the communication demands of the situation.

Physical Structure of the Symbol and Aid

We finish with a discussion of some final physical characteristics that may be important in influencing an individual's response to a communication display, irrespective of (or in addition to) the other factors that we have discussed so far. Although there is still more to learn, there are clear indications that the structure of the communication display may influence communication and language outcomes. Sutton and her colleagues (Sutton, Gallagher, Morford, & Shahnaz, 2000; Sutton & Morford, 1998) have examined aspects of morphosyntactic output in children and adults with no communication disorders and whose syntactic skills are known to be intact in spoken modes. When these individuals were asked to create messages with aided symbols, those messages did not always adhere to the syntactic constraints of their spoken language. Because the participants had known capabilities in their spoken language, the alterations to output likely reflect constraints of the aided system (a more detailed examination of issues of morphosyntax in aided AAC is available in Sutton, Soto, & Blockberger, 2002).

The key point for the purpose of this chapter is that the series of studies by Sutton and Morford (1998) and Sutton et al. (2000) offered direct evidence that a nuanced understanding of aided communication requires an understanding of the unique supports and demands of the system being used. At a more basic level of visual perception and attention, Wilkinson and Jagaroo (2004) argued that physical/perceptual aspects of the visual display may influence broader communication goals by making the display more or less easily perceived by a viewer. An analogy for that general approach comes from a common experience among many of us who attempt to cook on a stovetop. At some point we have turned on the wrong burner on the stove, despite years of motor practice at using the dials and a well-established cognitive understanding of the relationships between the dial and the burners. The result is frustration once the inconvenient error is finally realized, and there is a disruption to the timing of the meal. The reason for this error may be that the stovetop design is not an optimal match to how humans process visual information. Conceivably, if we construct the stovetop to be perfectly consistent with human visual processing, then these errors would disappear and the functional outcome (cooking) is made more seamless. Might the same principles apply for aided AAC? Conceivably, if we can match the physical properties of the visual display to the way users process visual information, then we might minimize cognitive demands and enhance attention to displayed symbols.

In this section, we explore some evidence supporting this argument and offer some recommendations concerning device construction. We also review some of the clinical practices concerning setup that offer opportunities for further research.

Role of Color Internally to the Symbol   Color is one of the most important physical dimensions that may foster or inhibit attention to aided communication (see Wilkinson & Jagaroo, 2004, for detailed description). Color was introduced to commercially available symbol sets long ago, and software allows practitioners to directly alter the color of symbol backgrounds and their borders, as well as the symbols themselves. Recommendations for symbol arrangement often include color-coded backgrounds (e.g., Beukelman & Mirenda, 2005; Goossens', Crain, & Elder, 1994) to highlight relationships between symbols (e.g., as a way to group parts of speech or semantically related symbols). Moreover, although the vast majority of communication devices do not incorporate color as a design feature of the device itself, there has been speculation that including color on such devices might enhance their appeal, at least for younger users (Light, Drager, & Nemser, 2004; Light, Page, Curran, & Pitkin, 2007).

There are a few studies within the field that have examined if symbol-internal color does in fact enhance communication outcomes or whether specific strategies for arranging by color are more effective than others. Wilkinson, Carlin, and Jagaroo (2006) examined how rapidly and accurately preschool children without disabilities found symbols in an eight-symbol display. Indeed, children relied on color cues when searching for symbols in an array and were faster and more accurate in finding a target when at least some of the symbols on the array were different colors (as compared with symbols that were all one color). Stephenson (2007) examined whether presence or absence of color in line-drawing symbols influenced matching behavior in individuals with intellectual disabilities. As the author noted, the results are tentative due to high variability. Examination of the data suggests that the role of color may depend on whether it is part of the symbol or the object and whether the picture or the object served as the sample to be targeted. Clearly, further research of this nature is warranted.

Wilkinson, Carlin, and Thistle (2008) followed up on their first study by asking, "How do we arrange symbols on an array if some of them share color?" The study examined whether symbols that share a color (a red strawberry, red cherries) should be placed together, to create a shared location within which to search, or placed separately around the display, to allow each to stand out. The study was conducted with preschool children without disabilities as well as older individuals with Down syndrome. Children of all ages and all developmental levels found a target symbol more rapidly when the symbols that were the same color were clustered together, and younger children and those with Down syndrome who had more limited receptive vocabulary levels also showed better accuracy in the clustered condition as well (older children and those with more advanced vocabularies essentially showed a ceiling effect on accuracy, with more than 95% correct).

These studies would all suggest that symbol-internal color serves to capture attention, allowing the search for individual symbols to move accurately and rapidly and potentially releasing cognitive/attentional resources for other communication functions. Beyond this, there is still much to learn about the role of color, and, of course, its effects are likely to vary by the same child, family, and cultural factors that are important to other outcomes. For instance, the colorful line drawings used as experimental stimuli thus far may be highly attractive to younger school-age children and their peers, and the single-meaning nature of the symbols are appropriate to earlier developmental goals. They may feel juvenile to middle or high school students, however, and the nature of the symbols may not be appropriate to later developmental goals, especially literacy-related academic activities. The role of color as a cue for different goals must be considered when constructing aids for older and/or more developmentally advanced children.

Clinically, the findings that clustering stimuli of the same color influenced the speed of finding a target for older/developmentally advanced students, even though they found the task very easy (as illustrated by ceiling-level accuracy), suggests potential applications for other goals. When planning geography lessons, for instance, it might be useful to cluster regions by color (e.g., New England as red, eastern seaboard as blue), allowing rapid location of the region and then allowing shape and location to indicate individual state identities. This is comparable with the structure of the study in which color served to capture attention to an area of the picture symbol display (red symbols clustered in one place) and form served as the cue to the specific identity of the symbols within (strawberries or cherries). In fact, a brief overview of educational maps demonstrates that clustered color organization is not always represented on commercially available maps. Whether these maps from vendors are best suited to our clinical/academic goals is indeed an empirical question. Similar questions could be asked for a number of other advanced clinical goals, including reading or math.

Role of Color-Coded Backgrounds
Color may play a role not only internally (i.e., the apple symbol itself is colored red) but also on the background of the symbol as an organizing cue. Bailey and Downing (1994) examined color cuing with individuals with multiple disabilities and found that color can be used to attract attention and focus visual attending to an object in adults

with severe intellectual disabilities. A study by Thistle and Wilkinson (2008) examined whether background color cuing facilitates search in preschool children, as well as how the relation of the background color and the symbol color interact. Initial results of this study support the assumption that, indeed, background color cues influence search speed and accuracy.

One way that this can be useful is to highlight elements within social scripts. Within a page of comments, all the positive symbols (COOL, GREAT, AWESOME, FANTASTIC) can be coded one color, and the negative symbols (THAT'S TERRIBLE, OH NO, I'M SO SORRY), a different one. Ideally, of course, the student would carefully select between specific comments. If he or she chooses to focus more on the conversation rather than the specific comment, however, then he or she can still pick any positive comment, and it will likely suit the situation fairly well.

Just as we would use similar colors to group related symbols together, there are situations in which we might use color-coded backgrounds to differentiate between symbols. For example, a feelings page created from one common symbol set often appears to be a sea of floating heads with subtle details differentiating between various emotions such as sad, scared, nervous, and angry. If color backgrounds are added to these same symbols (e.g., red background for angry, blue for sad, black for scared), then they subjectively appear easier to differentiate.

In addition to benefiting the user him- or herself, potential benefit of clustering relates to the partners with whom the user communicates and who are also (ideally) using the aids themselves. Color coding related symbols and using contrasting colors on unrelated symbols may be very useful. Anecdotally, communication partners report that it is easier to find symbols and thus provide augmented input when related symbols are grouped together with color-coded backgrounds. Clearly, all of these clinical practices are ripe areas for research that would provide an evidence base for specific and well justified use of color.

Other Potentially Important Dimensions   Other dimensions of the stimuli that can serve to capture attention also merit consideration. We have already pointed out the argument by Light and her colleagues (Light, Drager, & Nemser, 2004) that aids and displays that are constructed for and/or by adults, which are boxy, colorless computers with symbols organized in a grid layout, may not appeal to children. When children are placed in charge of conceiving an aid for another child, the results are quite different—children add color, multiple functions, and so forth (Light et al., 2007). Would making devices that are more appealing to children enhance the likelihood of use? There is no evidence concerning this question, although DeLoache's (2005) work might have suggested that at least some features that can be manipulated might be distracting to younger children. For older children, overly attractive devices might be distracting in a different way, tempting either the user or his or her friends to play on or with the device at inappropriate times. Most likely, a happy medium between wholly unappealing and overly tempting is necessary.

Some research that has been disseminated through conference presentations and web casts (Light, n.d.) illustrates another occasional gulf between the conceptualizations of adults who make up symbols and young children who are potential users. Light and her colleagues conducted a series of studies looking at children's conceptualizations of symbol meanings from the Mayer-Johnson (1992) Picture Communication Symbol (PCS) set. Many symbol meanings were clear to children (i.e., iconic), but children also raised some questions. For instance, many of the symbols in the PCS dictionary show concepts, such as *want,* through a pair of hands that is reaching for a desired item. Although clear to adults, many children reported being confused or disturbed by the apparently disembodied hands, wondering in some cases why those hands had been "cut off" from the body. When asked themselves to draw the concept of "want," children often drew pictures of two children (fully represented, head to toe) squabbling over some desired item. Children virtually never drew hands or heads without bodies. Again, we do not yet know if changing the symbols might influence children's ability to use those symbols. Now that commercially available symbol sets are beginning to create symbols that incorporate these findings, it will be easier to empirically investigate how children respond to these more detailed, contextual symbols.

We can also consider the actual physical nature of the symbols placed on the displays. If colorful line drawings may be rejected as too juvenile by some children, then it also seems possible that aids and symbols that have desirable physical characteristics might be embraced. Imagine a user of AAC who is interested in Yu-Gi-Oh cards and their related paraphernalia (Yu-Gi-Oh is an imaginary world popular with elementary school children in which the protagonists battle various evil-doers; an associated television show and highly stylized trading cards are often topics of discussion). As noted in the first section, we clearly would want to include content concerning Yu-Gi-Oh on that child's board (thus providing motivating symbols for conversation). We could also make those symbols stand out (thus facilitating attention) by creating them with the distinctive stylized appearance of the actual trading cards. Similarly, for children of all ages who follow specific baseball teams, creating symbols with team-related colors, stylized fonts, or team-logo backgrounds would both allow for rapid identification of team-related symbols in the display and closer affiliation with other like-minded sports fans, who will have little difficulty recognizing one of their own.

RELATION OF MEMORY AND ATTENTION TO NATURALISTIC INTERVENTION APPROACHES

Thus far, we have discussed structuring the specific physical device in ways that will potentially enhance communication outcomes by reducing attention and memory demands, which will free up cognitive resources for the task of communicating. This final section discusses some final characteristics of intervention approaches as they relate to these same issues. We do not focus on the particular methodologies of these approaches, which are described in detail elsewhere in this volume and others. Rather, we identify the ways in which these approaches exploit the factors of interest in this chapter.

Modeling and Augmented Input

Several naturalistic intervention approaches have been described in the literature, including the System for Augmenting Language (SAL; Romski & Sevcik, 1996) and variants on Aided Language Stimulation (ALS; Goossens', 1989). A number of research studies have clearly demonstrated the effectiveness of such modeling and input-based AAC interventions with children with cerebral palsy (Goossens', 1989), intellectual disabilities (Harris & Reichle, 2004; Romksi & Sevcik, 1996; Secvik, Romski, Watkins, & Deffebach, 1995), and autism (Drager et al., 2006; Peterson, Bondy, Vincent, & Finnegan, 1995). Naturalistic approaches are effective not only for teaching important communication functions and symbol meanings but also for promoting more advanced linguistic outcomes such as early morphosyntax (Binger & Light, 2007; Bruno & Trembath, 2006; Wilkinson et al., 1994; see Sutton et al., 2002, for further discussion of nuances of morphosyntax in AAC).

Why might these be such effective approaches from the perspective of attentional and cognitive resources of the child? One reason that aided language input may be effective is that it helps "normalize" the use of visual symbols. A child who is the only student using aided communication may feel (and appear) different from his or her peers. When others use the aided mode, it becomes more typical. Another major function of input is the use of the visual aid for the purposes of enhancing the user's own expressive use. Essentially, the input functions like "immersion" in a foreign language for nonnative speakers, in which the experience of hearing the new language in use is itself a key element by which the learner hones his or her own expressive skill. We do not expect children without disabilities to learn to speak without being spoken to, and, indeed, targeted oral input is a key component of virtually all oral-aural interventions for children with general language impairments. Similarly, when we choose to implement signed languages for children with hearing loss, it seems fairly obvious that a key intervention component is to sign to the child; otherwise, how would he or she learn it? This same fact often seems to be forgotten when we implement aided interventions, however. Finally, the augmented input can serve to support the user's understanding of the language around him or her by supplementing the auditory information with complementing visual information. In this case, for instance, schedule boards might be used to assist a child in planning for the day (or week or month) and understanding what the adults around him or her have planned to do by ensuring that he or she is not solely reliant on auditory information.

Despite understanding the critical importance of input, practitioners and parents often model very infrequently or show only sporadic generalization or maintenance of learned strategies (e.g., Kent-Walsh & McNaughton, 2005; Smith & Grove, 2003). Nonetheless, it is critical for practitioners to provide aided input to communicators using visual aids to foster their enthusiasm and skill as well. Clinically, there are a variety of strategies to allow a student who uses AAC the opportunity to see his or her aided system modeled successfully by others. One simple strategy is to alternate between the student who uses AAC and a competent role model within a communicative context. At the utterance level, a student and therapist might alternate after each phrase (e.g., Practitioner: "HI, HOW ARE YOU?" Student: "I OKAY, AND YOU?" Practitioner: "I AM GREAT, THANKS.") either using the same device or, if resources allow, both parties can easily observe each other's screens/keyboards. At the conversation level, the role model first uses the AAC system to demonstrate an entire conversation (e.g., ordering a soda and entrée at a restaurant), then the student who uses AAC is given an opportunity to attempt a similar conversation.

Similarly, a role model can demonstrate examples of personal narratives (e.g., "The day I met Michael Jordan" or "My flat tire on Highway 101") or academic explanation (e.g., the key elements of the water cycle) on the AAC device and then provide opportunities for the student who uses AAC to do so from his or her point of view. Modeling provides necessary examples to learn from; however, many students may also require direct instruction and scaffolding (e.g., graphic organizers, story maps, explanations of practice with sequencing words such as *first* and *then*) in order to develop the competence to effectively organize these more complex communication acts.

Structured activities can be incorporated into the school day to ensure that the student who uses AAC has opportunities to observe peers modeling the use of the device. Childhood games such as Simon Says and Mother May I are activities with ample built-in repetition that can be readily adapted so that as children take turns being the game leader, they each use the AAC device. A page with directions such as "stop," "turn left," "turn right," and "go over that" can be incorporated into obstacle courses in physical education classes, car rides, or giving directions to locate hidden objects in the classroom by both the student who uses AAC and his or her peers. During a geography lesson, a similar page could be created with the cardinal directions (e.g., north, south) and used during a collaborative group lesson to practice giving directions and locating places on a map.

Joint book reading is another activity that can readily be adapted to incorporate modeling. As an adult reads with a student, the adult can not only pause to allow the student who uses AAC the opportunity to use his or her device to participate in the book reading activity, but the adult can also pause and complete sentences and "read" words using the device him- or herself. For example, while reading the familiar children's book *We're Going on a Bear Hunt* (Rosen, 1989), a teacher might point to the symbols UNDER, OVER, THROUGH, and OH NO as they occur as he or she reads the book. The first few times the book is read, the teacher might also use the device to say the various elements the characters encounter: GRASS, MUD, RIVER, SNOW, CAVE, and, of course, the BEAR. During subsequent readings, the student might increasingly be expected to use his or her device to communicate these words as they occur while the teacher continues to model the words UNDER and OVER. Later, if the student begins to independently communicate THROUGH and RIVER with his or her device, then the teacher might recast and model a symbol combination by verbally saying, "Yes, they went through the river" while also pointing to the symbols THEY, WENT, THROUGH, and RIVER.

This activity extends beyond providing an opportunity for the student to complete repeated phrases. The teacher is also demonstrating the linguistic and operational skills the student is anticipated to develop and use in future lessons. As the student begins meeting these expectations, the teacher progresses to modeling more complex language constructions. This closely mirrors the language-enriching strategies that support oral language development and is, in fact, quite consistent with theories of language development in the field (e.g., Justice & Ezell, 1999).

Including Students Who Use AAC in Group and Community Events

Using aided AAC is also enhanced when the child's aid supports communication in group or community events. Making sure that aided communication allows a child to participate in group or community events moves the aid from the status of "I have to use this because the teacher tells me to" to "I want to use this because it helps me participate." This is an important shift.

We can imagine a number of activities to evaluate whether the communication aid might better support and indeed be an integral aspect of participation for school-age children. For chronologically or developmentally younger children, participation can be enhanced by programming a line from an interactive song that allows the child to engage in a regular circle-time activity. For example, the child might have a line from the song "The Old Lady Who Swallowed a Fly," pressing the symbol to activate the voice output on his or her cue. During class activities, such as cooking, one child can have the role of managing turns. A static display device can be programmed with classmates' names recorded under each photograph, allowing the designated child to be able to respond when the teacher says "Emma, who should help me next?" In this case, Emma has the power to choose any of her classmates. Perhaps even more important in this example, Emma could successfully participate regardless of her ability to discriminate between the symbols. This is because it does not likely matter, really, who Emma picks (she could simply pick randomly)—what is important is that she, Emma, is the one doing the picking. Thus, even for children who are showing inconsistently "correct" selections, an activity structured like this allows them still to be empowered and participatory. Similarly, another student might have a board with recipe ingredients. When the teacher asks, "What should we mix in next?" with regard to the goals of active engagements and participation, it does not much matter if the student who uses AAC selects the flour symbol with the message, "NEXT 2 CUPS OF FLOUR" or the sugar symbol, "1 TABLESPOON OF SUGAR." Both selections are correct because the recipe will work, and the child participating is just as meaningful as his or her peer who yells out, "Salt."

In more advanced academic settings, the user of aided AAC can continue to serve as "moderator" as well. For instance, some schools have all-school activities such as a geography challenge. Although preprogramming a child's device with the correct answer might provide his or her team with an unfair advantage (and asking the entire set of teams to wait while he or she types might be unrealistic), we could provide the child with a role by programming in the questions to be asked, as well as the words CORRECT and WRONG, and then have the child serve as moderator. Other means of promoting participation for a more advanced communicator can be to have the student use AAC to give a presentation, explain how a book relates to personal experience, or share his or her opinion during class discussions. In dramatic arts, children might use aids to participate in plays. Thus, by programming a device to say a few lines, a child might be able to play "Farmer 1" in the fifth-grade production of "Oklahoma," just like his or her peers. Finally, another motivating activity is being able to engage in side conversation during a lecture. Although peers can whisper, silently mouth words, or pass a note to ask, "What page are we on?", most students who use AAC would either have to point silently to symbols or loudly "blurt" out the question with a synthesized voice.

CONCLUSION

Issues of memory and attention in aided AAC are extensive, interrelated, and complex. We sought to examine some of the nuances of how children perceive a visual communication display, what demands that display makes on their cognitive resources, and how to allow children to communicate the diverse functions available to speakers. A child may be motivated to communicate, but only if the available aid contains appealing topics and words that allow communication for more than simply requesting and rejecting. Moreover, even for the most motivated communicator, we must consider the context of how difficult the communication act itself is. If preparing a message taxes both cognitive and attentional resources, then the child might opt simply not to communicate (at least through aided means) at all. Aided AAC interventions of any sort will be most effective if the communication aid itself is structured to 1) communicate messages of relevance to the user, 2) reduce the cognitive load to the greatest extent possible, and 3) use displays that enhance the child's attention to the symbols of greatest relevance.

REFERENCES

Adamson, L.B., Romski, M.A., Deffebach, K., & Sevcik, R.A. (1992). Symbol vocabulary and the focus of conversations: Augmenting language development for youth with mental retardation. *Journal of Speech and Hearing Research, 35,* 1333–1343.

Anderson, J.R. (2005). *Cognitive psychology and its implications* (6th ed.). New York: Worth Publishers.

Bailey, B.R., & Downing, J. (1994). Using visual accents to enhance attending to communication symbols for student with severe multiple disabilities. *RE:View, 26,* 101–119.

Benjafield, J.G. (2007). *Cognition* (3rd ed.). New York: Oxford University Press.

Beukelman, D.R., & Mirenda, P. (2005). *Augmentative and alternative communication: Supporting children and adults with complex communication needs* (3rd ed.). Baltimore: Paul H. Brookes Publishing Co.

Binger, C., & Light, J. (2007). The effect of aided AAC modeling on the expression of multi-symbol messages by preschoolers who use AAC. *Augmentative and Alternative Communication, 23,* 30–43.

Bloomburg, K., Karlan, G., & Lloyd, L. (1990). The comparative translucency of initial lexical items represented by five graphic symbols and sets. *Journal of Speech and Hearing Research, 33,* 717–725.

Bopp, K.D., Brown, K.E., & Mirenda, P. (2004). Speech-language pathologists' roles in the delivery of positive behavior support for individuals with developmental disabilities. *American Journal of Speech-Language Pathology, 13,* 5–19.

Bruno, J., & Trembath, D. (2006). Use of aided language stimulation to improve syntactic performance during a weeklong intervention program. *Augmentative and Alternative Communication, 22,* 300–313.

Cosbey, J.E., & Johnston, S. (2006). Using a single-switch voice output communication aid to increase social access for children with severe disabilities in inclusive classrooms. *Research and Practices for Persons with Severe Disabilities, 31,* 144–156.

Craik, F.M., & McDowd, J.M. (1998). Age differences in recall and recognition. In M.P. Lawton & T.A. Salthouse (Eds.), *Essential papers on the psychology of aging* (pp. 282–295). New York: New York University Press.

DeLoache, J.S. (1995). Early understanding and use of symbols: The model model. *Current Directions in Psychological Science, 4,* 109–113.

DeLoache, J.S. (2005). Mindful of symbols. *Scientific American, 293,* 72–77.

Drager, K.D.R, Light, J.C., Speltz, J.C., Fallon, K.A., & Jeffries, L.Z. (2003). The performance of typically developing 2½ year olds on dynamic display AAC technologies with different system layouts and language organizations. *Journal of Speech, Language, and Hearing Research, 46,* 298–312.

Drager, K.D.R., Postal, V.J., Carrolus, L., Castellano, M., Gagliano, C., & Glynn, J. (2006). The effect of aided language modeling on symbol comprehension and production in two preschoolers with autism. *American Journal of Speech-Language Pathology, 15,* 112–125.

Durand, V.M. (1993). Functional communication training using assistive devices: Effects on challenging behavior and affect. *Augmentative and Alternative Communication, 9,* 168–176.

Fallon, K., Light, J., & Achenbach, A. (2003). The semantic organization patterns of young children: Implications for augmentative and alternative communication. *Augmentative and Alternative Communication, 19,* 74–85.

Fallon, K.A., Light, J., McNaughton, D., Drager, K., & Hammer, C. (2004). The effects of direct instruction on the single-word reading skills of children who require augmentative and alternative communication. *Journal of Speech, Language, and Hearing Research, 47,* 1424–1239.

Franklin, K., Mirenda, P., & Phillips, G. (1996). Comparisons of five symbol assessment protocols with nondisabled preschoolers and learners with severe intellectual disabilities. *Augmentative and Alternative Communication, 12,* 63–77.

Goossens', C. (1989). Aided communication intervention before assessment: A case study of a child with cerebral palsy. *Augmentative and Alternative Communication, 5,* 14–26.

Goossens', C., Crain. S., & Elder, P. (1994). *Engineering the preschool environment for interactive symbolic communication: 18 months to 5 years developmentally.* Birmingham, AL: Southeast Augmentative Communication.

Hamilton, R., & Ghatala, E. (1994). *Learning and instruction.* New York: McGraw-Hill.

Harris, M.D., & Reichle, J. (2004). The impact of aided language stimulation on symbol comprehension and production in children with moderate cognitive disabilities. *American Journal of Speech-Language Pathology, 13,* 155–167.

Hetzroni, O.E., & Roth, T. (2003). Effects of a positive support approach to enhance communicative behaviors of children with mental retardation who have challenging behaviors. *Education and Training in Mental Retardation and Developmental Disabilities, 38,* 95–105.

Huer, M.B. (2003). Individuals from diverse cultural and ethnic backgrounds may perceive graphic symbols differently: Response to Nigam. *Augmentative and Alternative Communication, 19,* 137–140.

Hurlbut, B.I., Iwata, B.A., & Green, J.D. (1982). Nonvocal language acquisition in adolescents with severe physical disabilities: Blissymbol versus iconic stimulus formats. *Journal of Applied Behavior Analysis, 15,* 241–248.

Hux, K., Rankin, J., Beukelman, D., & Hahn, D. (1993). Alternative procedures for neurologically impaired populations. *Augmentative and Alternative Communication, 9,* 119–125.

Jagaroo, V., & Wilkinson, K.M. (2008). Further considerations of visual cognitive neuroscience for aided AAC: The potential role of motion perception systems in maximizing design display. *Augmentative and Alternative Communication, 24,* 29–42.

Justice, L.M., & Ezell, H.K. (1999). Vygotskian theory and its application to assessment: An overview for speech-language pathologists. *Contemporary Issues in Communication Science and Disorders, 26,* 111–118

Kent-Walsh, J., & McNaughton, D. (2005). Communication partner instruction in AAC: Present practices and future directions. *Augmentative and Alternative Communication, 21,* 195–204.

Kopelman, M.D., Bright, P., Buckman, J., Fradera, A., Yoshimashu, H., Jacobson, C., & Colchester, A. (2007). Recall and recognition memory in amnesia: Patients with hippocampal, medial temporal, temporal lobe, or frontal pathology. *Neuropsychologia, 45,* 1232–1246.

Kravitz, E., Littman, S., & Cassidy, K. (1996). *Meeting the communication needs of adults with severe developmental disabilities.* Symposium presented at the 7th Biennial Conference of the International Society for Augmentative and Alternative Communication, Vancouver, British Columbia.

Levin, J.R., Yussen, S.R., De Rose, T.M., & Pressley, M. (1977). Developmental changes in assessing recall and recognition memory capacity. *Developmental Psychology, 13,* 608–615.

Light, J. (n.d.). *Webcasts: AAC interventions to maximize language development for your children.* Available at the AAC-RERC web site: http://www.aac-rerc.com/pages/news/Light_webcast.htm

Light, J.C., Drager, K.D., McCarthy, J., Mellot, S., Millar, D., Parrish, C., et al. (2004). Performance of typically developing four and five-year old children with AAC systems using different language organization techniques. *Augmentative and Alternative Communication, 20,* 63–88.

Light, J., Drager, K.D.R., & Nemser, J.G. (2004). Enhancing the appeal of AAC technologies for young children: Lessons from the toy manufacturers. *Augmentative and Alternative Communication, 20,* 137–149.

Light, J., Page, R., Curran, J., & Pitkin, L. (2007). Children's ideas for the design of AAC assistive technologies for young children with complex communication needs. *Augmentative and Alternative Communication, 23,* 274–287.

Mayer-Johnson, R. (1992). *The Picture Communication Symbols.* Solana Beach, CA: Mayer-Johnson Co.

Mirenda, P. (1997). Supporting individuals with challenging behavior through functional communication training and AAC: Research review. *Augmentative and Alternative Communication, 13,* 207–225.

Mirenda, P., & Locke, P. (1989). A comparison of symbol transparency in nonspeaking persons with intellectual disabilities. *Journal of Speech and Hearing Disorders, 54,* 131–140.

Mizuko, M., & Reichle, J. (1989). Transparency and recall of symbols among intellectually handicapped adults. *Journal of Speech and Hearing Disorders, 54,* 627–633.

Nigam, R. (2003). Do individuals from diverse cultural and ethnic backgrounds perceive graphic symbols differently? *Augmentative and Alternative Communication, 19,* 135–136.

Paul, R. (2007). *Language disorders from infancy through adolescence* (2nd ed.). St Louis: Mosby.

Peterson, S.L., Bondy, A.S., Vincent, Y., & Finnegan, C. (1995). Effects of altering communicative input for students with autism and no speech: Two case studies. *Augmentative and Alternative Communication, 11,* 93–100.

Reichle, J., & Wacker, D.P. (Eds.). (1993). *Communicative alternatives to challenging behavior: Integrating functional assessment and intervention strategies.* Baltimore: Paul H. Brookes Publishing Co.

Romski, M.A., & Sevcik, R.A. (1993). Language comprehension: Considerations for augmentative and alternative communication. *Augmentative and Alternative Communication, 9,* 281–285.

Romski, M.A., & Sevcik, R.A. (1996). *Breaking the speech barrier: Language development through augmented means.* Baltimore: Paul H. Brookes Publishing Co.

Rosen, M. (1989). *We're going on a bear hunt.* New York: Margaret K. McElderry.

Rowland, C., & Schweigert, P. (1989). Tangible symbols: Symbolic communication for individuals with multisensory impairments. *Augmentative and Alternative Communication, 5,* 226–234.

Sevcik, R.A., Romski, M.A., Watkins, R., & Deffebach, K. (1995). Adult partner-augmented communicative input to youth with mental retardation using the System for Augmenting Language. *Journal of Speech and Hearing Research, 38,* 902–912.

Sevcik, R.A., Romski, M.A., & Wilkinson, K.M. (1991). Roles of graphic symbols in the language acquisition process for persons with severe cognitive disabilities. *Augmentative and Alternative Communication, 7,* 161–170.

Smith, M.M., & Grove, N.C. (2003). Asymmetry in input and output for individuals who use AAC. In D.R. Beukelman & J. Reichle (Series Eds.) & J.C. Light, D.R. Beukelman, & J. Reichle (Vol. Eds.), *Augmentative and alternative communication series: Communicative competence for individuals who use AAC: From research to effective practice* (pp. 163–195). Baltimore: Paul H. Brookes Publishing Co.

Stephenson, J. (2007). The effect of color on the recognition and use of line drawings by children with severe intellectual disabilities. *Augmentative and Alternative Communication, 23,* 44–55.

Stephenson, J., & Linfoot, K. (1996). Pictures as communication symbols for students with severe intellectual disability. *Augmentative and Alternative Communication, 12,* 244–255.

Sturm, J.M., & Clendon, S.A. (2004). Augmentative and alternative communication, language, and literacy. *Topics in Language Disorders, 24,* 76–91.

Sutton, A., Gallagher, T., Morford, J., & Shahnaz, N. (2000). Relative clause sentence production using AAC systems. *Applied Psycholinguistics, 21,* 473–486.

Sutton, A., & Morford, J. (1998). Constituent order in picture pointing sequences production by speaking children using AAC. *Applied Psycholinguistics, 19,* 525–536.

Sutton, A., Soto, G., & Blockberger, S. (2002). Grammatical issues in graphic symbol communication. *Augmentative and Alternative Communication, 18,* 192–204.

Thistle, J., & Wilkinson, K.M. (2008). *The effects of background color on speed of locating a symbol: Implications for AAC display design.* Manuscript under review.

Tulving, E. (1972). Episodic and semantic memory. In E. Tulving & W. Donaldson (Eds.), *Organization of memory* (pp. 382–403). New York: Academic Press.

Utley, B.L. (2002). Visual assessment considerations for the design of AAC systems. In D.R. Beukelman & J. Reichle (Series Eds.) & J. Reichle, D.R. Beukelman, & J.C. Light (Vol. Eds.), *Augmentative and alternative communication series: Exemplary practices for beginning communicators: Implications for AAC* (pp. 353–394). Baltimore: Paul H. Brookes Publishing Co.

Volpe, B., Holtzman, J., & Hirst, W. (1986). Further characterization of patients with amnesia after cardiac arrest: Preserved recognition memory. *Neurology, 36,* 408–411.

Wilkinson, K.M., Carlin, M., & Jagaroo, V. (2006). Preschoolers' speed of locating a target symbol under different color conditions. *Augmentative and Alternative Communication, 22,* 123–133.

Wilkinson, K.M., Carlin, M., & Thistle, J. (2008). The role of color cues in facilitating accurate and rapid location of aided symbols by children with and without Down Syndrome. *American Journal of Speech-Language-Pathology, 17,* 179–193.

Wilkinson, K.M., & Jagaroo, V. (2004). Contributions of principles of visual cognitive science to AAC system display design. *Augmentative and Alternative Communication, 20,* 123–136.

Wilkinson, K.M., & McIlvane W.J. (2002). Considerations in teaching graphic symbols to beginning communicators. In D.R. Beukelman & J. Reichle (Series Eds.) & J. Reichle, D.R. Beukelman, & J.C. Light (Vol. Eds.), *Augmentative and alternative communication series: Exemplary practices for beginning communicators: Implications for AAC* (pp. 273–322). Baltimore: Paul H. Brookes Publishing Co.

Wilkinson, K.M., Romski, M.A., & Sevcik, R.A. (1994). Emergence of visual-graphic symbol combinations in children with mental retardation using an augmented communication system. *Journal of Speech and Hearing Research, 37,* 883–896.

Wilkinson, K.M., & Rosenquist, C. (2006). Demonstration of a method for assessing semantic organization and category membership in individuals with autism spectrum disorders and receptive vocabulary limitations. *Augmentative and Alternative Communication, 22,* 242–257.

Index

Page numbers followed by *f* indicate figures; those followed by *t* indicate tables.